Pediatric Management of Autism

Editors

PAUL H. LIPKIN
JOSHUA B. EWEN

PEDIATRIC CLINICS
OF NORTH AMERICA

www.pediatric.theclinics.com

Consulting Editor
TINA L. CHENG

April 2024 • Volume 71 • Number 2

ELSEVIER

1600 John F. Kennedy Boulevard • Suite 1800 • Philadelphia, Pennsylvania, 19103-2899

http://www.theclinics.com

THE PEDIATRIC CLINICS OF NORTH AMERICA Volume 71, Number 2
April 2024 ISSN 0031-3955, ISBN-13: 978-0-443-18409-3

Editor: Kerry Holland
Developmental Editor: Saswoti Nath

The Pediatric Clinics of North America (ISSN 0031-3955) is published bimonthly by Elsevier Inc., 360 Park Avenue South, New York, NY 10010-1710. Months of issue are February, April, June, August, October, and December. Periodicals postage paid at New York, NY and additional mailing offices. Subscription prices are $290.00 per year (US individuals), $368.00 per year (Canadian individuals), $440.00 per year (international individuals), $100.00 per year (US students and residents), $100.00 per year (Canadian students and residents), and $165.00 per year (international residents and students). For institutional access pricing please contact Customer Service via the contact information below. To receive students/resident rare, orders must be accompanied by name of affiliated institution, date of term, and the signature of program/residency coordinator on institution letterhead. Orders will be billed at individual rate until proof of status is received. Foreign air speed delivery is included in all *Clinics* subscription prices. All prices are subject to change without notice. **POSTMASTER: Send address changes to *The Pediatric Clinics of North America*, Elsevier Health Sciences Division, Subscription Customer Service, 3251 Riverport Lane, Maryland Heights, MO 63043. Customer Service: 1-800-654-2452 (US and Canada). From outside of the US and Canada: 1-314-447-8871. Fax: 1-314-447-8029. For print support, E-mail: JournalsCustomerService-usa@elsevier.com. For online support, E-mail: JournalsOnlineSupport-usa@elsevier.com.**

Reprints. For copies of 100 or more, of articles in this publication, please contact the Commercial Reprints Department, Elsevier Inc., 360 Park Avenue South, New York, NY 10010-1710. Tel.: 212-633-3874; Fax: 212-633-3820; E-mail: reprints@elsevier.com.

The Pediatric Clinics of North America is also published in Spanish by McGraw-Hill Inter-americana Editores S.A., Mexico City, Mexico; in Portuguese by Riechmann and Affonso Editores, Rua Comandante Coelho 1085, CEP 21250, Rio de Janeiro, Brazil; and in Greek by Althayia SA, Athens, Greece.

The Pediatric Clinics of North America is covered in *MEDLINE/PubMed (Index Medicus)*, *Excerpta Medica*, *Current Contents*, *Current Contents/Clinical Medicine*, *Science Citation Index*, *ASCA*, *ISI/BIOMED*, and *BIOSIS*.

PROGRAM OBJECTIVE
The goal of the *Pediatric Clinics of North America* is to keep practicing physicians and residents up to date with current clinical practice in pediatrics by providing timely articles reviewing the state-of-the-art in patient care.

TARGET AUDIENCE
All practicing pediatricians, physicians, and healthcare professionals who provide patient care to pediatric patients.

LEARNING OBJECTIVES
Upon completion of this activity, participants will be able to:
1. Review the variety of screening tools developed and tested to identify early signs of autism.
2. Discuss how pediatricians can support autistic patients and their families during the transition from pediatric care to adult care.
3. Recognize health issues affect autistic people across the life course and public health strategies can help mitigate them.

ACCREDITATIONS
Physician Credit

The Elsevier Office of Continuing Medical Education (EOCME) is accredited by the Accreditation Council for Continuing Medical Education (ACCME) to provide continuing medical education for physicians.

The EOCME designates this journal-based activity for a maximum of 14 *AMA PRA Category 1 Credit*(s)™. Physicians should claim only the credit commensurate with the extent of their participation in the activity.

All other healthcare professionals requesting continuing education credit for this journal-based activity will be issued a certificate of participation.

ABP Maintenance of Certification Credit

Successful completion of this CME activity, which includes participation in the activity and individual assessment of and feedback to the learner, enables the learner to earn up to 14 MOC points in the American Board of Pediatrics' (ABP) Maintenance of Certification (MOC) program. It is the CME activity provider's responsibility to submit learner completion information to ACCME for the purpose of granting ABP MOC credit.

DISCLOSURE OF CONFLICTS OF INTEREST
The EOCME assesses conflict of interest with its instructors, faculty, planners, and other Individuals who are in a position to control the content of CME activities. All relevant conflicts of interest that are identified are thoroughly vetted by EOCME for fair balance, scientific objectivity, and patient care recommendations. EOCME is committed to providing its learners with CME activities that promote improvements or quality in healthcare and not a specific proprietary business or a commercial interest.

The planning committee, staff, authors, and editors listed below have identified no financial relationships or relationships to products or devices they or their spouse/life partner have with commercial interest related to the content of this CME activity:
Jennifer L. Ames, PhD; Somer Bishop, PhD; Jamie K. Capal, MD; Thomas D. Challman, MD; Lisa A. Croen, PhD; Elizabeth A. Cross, PhD; Meghan N. Davignon, MD; Inge-Marie Eigsti, PhD; Jill Escher; Joshua B. Ewen, MD; Whitney Guthrie, PhD; Alycia Halladay, PhD; Elizabeth A. Hayes, MD; Luther Kalb, PhD, MHS; Steven M. Lazar, MD, MEd; Michelle Littlejohn; Carmen Lopez-Arvizu, MD; Amy Lutz, PhD; Rajkumar Mayakrishnan, BSc, MBA; Scott M. Myers, MD; Kate Neamsapaya; Lindsay Olson, PhD; Suzanne Rybczynski, MD, MSHCM; Gloria Satriale, Esq, EdD; Navjot Sidhu, MD; Margaret C. Souders, PhD, CRNP; Audrey Thurm, PhD; Roma A. Vasa, MD; Lee Elizabeth Wachtel, MD; Kate E. Wallis, MD, MPH; Arthur Westover, MD; Zoe Wong

The planning committee, staff, authors, and editors listed below have identified financial relationships or relationships to products or devices they or their spouse/life partner have with commercial interest related to the content of this CME activity:
Amanda E. Bennett, MD, MPH: Researcher: F. Hoffmann-La Roche Ltd, Acadia Pharmaceuticals Inc., Jazz Pharmaceuticals, Inc., Maplight

Shafali Jeste, MD: Advisor: Ionis Pharmaceuticals, Inc.; Consultant: F. Hoffmann-La Roche Ltd

Paul Lipkin, MD: Advisor: Sarepta, Inc, Earlitec

Jay A. Salpekar, MD: Consultant: Cerevel Therapeutics; Researcher: Jazz Pharmaceuticals, Inc.

Lawrence Scahill, MSN, PhD: Consultant: Johnson & Johnson, Impel Pharmaceuticals Inc., Cogstate Ltd.,; Patent Beneficiary: F. Hoffmann-La Roche Ltd, Yamo Pharmaceuticals, AbbVie, Inc.

UNAPPROVED/OFF-LABEL USE DISCLOSURE
The EOCME requires CME faculty to disclose to the participants:
1. When products or procedures being discussed are off-label, unlabelled, experimental, and/or investigational (not US Food and Drug Administration [FDA] approved); and
2. Any limitations on the information presented, such as data that are preliminary or that represent ongoing research, interim analyses, and/or unsupported opinions. Faculty may discuss information about pharmaceutical agents that is outside of FDA-approved labelling. This information is intended solely for CME and is not intended to promote off-label use of these medications. If you have any questions, contact the medical affairs department of the manufacturer for the most recent prescribing information.

TO ENROLL
To enroll in the *Pediatric Clinics of North America* Continuing Medical Education program, call customer service at 1-800-654-2452 or sign up online at http://www.theclinics.com/home/cme. The CME program is available to subscribers for an additional annual fee of USD 313.00.

METHOD OF PARTICIPATION
In order to claim credit, participants must complete the following:
1. Complete enrolment as indicated above.
2. Read the activity.
3. Complete the CME Test and Evaluation. Participants must achieve a score of 70% on the test. All CME Tests and Evaluations must be completed online.

In order to claim MOC points, participants must complete the following:
1. Complete steps listed above for claiming CME credit
2. Provide your specialty board ID#, birth date (MM/DD), and attestation.
3. Online MOC submission is only available for the American Board of pediatrics' (ABP) Maintenance of Certification (MOC) program

CME INQUIRIES/SPECIAL NEEDS
For all CME inquiries or special needs, please contact elsevierCME@elsevier.com

Contributors

CONSULTING EDITOR

TINA L. CHENG, MD, MPH
BK Rachford Professor and Chair of Pediatrics, University of Cincinnati, Director, Cincinnati Children's Research Foundation, Chief Medical Officer, Cincinnati Children's Hospital Medical Center, Cincinnati, Ohio

EDITORS

PAUL H. LIPKIN, MD
Professor of Pediatrics, Kennedy Krieger Institute, The Johns Hopkins University School of Medicine, Baltimore, Maryland

JOSHUA B. EWEN, MD
Division Head of Developmental-Behavioral Pediatrics, Irene Heinz Given and John LaPorte Given Research Professor in Pediatrics, Ann & Robert H. Lurie Children's Hospital of Chicago, Department of Pediatrics at Northwestern University Feinberg School of Medicine, Chicago, Illinois; Adjunct Associate Professor, Department of Neurology, The Johns Hopkins University School of Medicine, Department of Psychological and Brain Sciences (joint appointment), The Johns Hopkins University, Baltimore, Maryland

AUTHORS

JENNIFER L. AMES, PhD
Research Scientist, Division of Research, Kaiser Permanente Northern California, Oakland, California

JULIA ANIXT, MD
Professor of Pediatrics, University of Cincinnati College of Medicine, Director of The Kelly O'Leary Center for Autism Spectrum Disorders, Division of Developmental and Behavioral Pediatrics, Cincinnati Children's Hospital Medical Center, Cincinnati, Ohio

AMANDA E. BENNETT, MD, MPH
Associate Professor, Department of Pediatrics, The University of Pennsylvania Perelman School of Medicine, Autism Integrated Care Program, Division of Developmental and Behavioral Pediatrics, The Children's Hospital of Philadelphia, Philadelphia, Pennsylvania

SOMER BISHOP, PhD
Professor, Department of Psychiatry and Behavioral Sciences, UCSF Weill Institute for Neurosciences, University of California, San Francisco, San Francisco, California

MEGAN E. BONE, MD
Assistant Professor, Department of Neurology, The Johns Hopkins University School of Medicine, Department of Neurodevelopmental Medicine, Kennedy Krieger Institute, Baltimore, Maryland

JAMIE K. CAPAL, MD
Associate Professor of Pediatrics and Neurology, Carolina Institute of Developmental Disabilities, University of North Carolina at Chapel Hill, Chapel Hill, North Carolina

THOMAS D. CHALLMAN, MD
Medical Director, Geisinger Autism and Developmental Medicine Institute, Geisinger Commonwealth School of Medicine, Lewisburg, Pennsylvania

WENDY CORNELL, MEd
ECHO Autism Communities, University of Missouri School of Medicine, Department of Special Education, College of Education and Human Development, Columbia, Missouri

LISA A. CROEN, PhD
Senior Research Scientist, Division of Research, Kaiser Permanente Northern California, Oakland, California

ELIZABETH A. CROSS, PhD
Assistant Professor, Department of Psychiatry and Behavioral Sciences, Clinical Child Psychologist, Center for Autism and Related Disorders, The Johns Hopkins School of Medicine, Baltimore, Maryland

MEGHAN N. DAVIGNON, MD
Kaiser Permanente Roseville Medical Center, Pediatric Subspecialties, Regional Medical Director of Pediatric Developmental Disabilities, Roseville, California

AMIE DUNCAN, PhD
Associate Professor of Pediatrics, University of Cincinnati College of Medicine, Division of Behavioral Medicine and Clinical Psychology, Cincinnati Children's Hospital Medical Center, Cincinnati, Ohio

JENNIFER EHRHARDT, MD, MPH
Associate Professor of Pediatrics, University of Cincinnati College of Medicine, Division of Developmental and Behavioral Pediatrics, Cincinnati Children's Hospital Medical Center, Cincinnati, Ohio

INGE-MARIE EIGSTI, PhD
Director, Connecticut Autism and Language Lab (CALL), Co-Director, Cognitive Neuroscience of Communication T32 Training Program, Director of Research, Institute for the Brain and Cognitive Sciences, Department of Psychological Sciences, Professor of Clinical Psychology, University of Connecticut, Storrs, Connecticut

JILL ESCHER, JD
President, National Council on Severe Autism, San Jose, CA

WHITNEY GUTHRIE, PhD
Assistant Professor, Division of Developmental and Behavioral Pediatrics and Department of Child and Adolescent Psychiatry and Behavioral Sciences, Center for Autism Research and Clinical Futures, The Children's Hospital of Philadelphia, Departments of Psychiatry and Pediatrics, Perelman School of Medicine, University of Pennsylvania, Philadelphia, Pennsylvania

ALYCIA HALLADAY, PhD
Chief Science Officer, Autism Science Foundation, New York, New York

ELIZABETH A. HAYES, MD
Associate Program Director, Ambulatory and Community Pediatrics, Kaiser Permanente Oakland Medical Center, Oakland, California

SHAFALI S. JESTE, MD
Chief, Division of Neurology, Co-Director, Neurological Institute, Las Madrinas Chair, Chief of Neurology, Children's Hospital Los Angeles, Professor of Neurology and Pediatrics, Keck School of Medicine of USC, Los Angeles, California

LUTHER KALB, PhD, MHS
Assistant Professor, Wendy Klag Center for Autism and Developmental Disabilities, Johns Hopkins Bloomberg School of Public Health, Kennedy Krieger Institute, Baltimore, Maryland

STEVEN M. LAZAR, MD, MEd
Assistant Professor, Pediatrics and Pediatric Neurology and Developmental Neuroscience, Meyer Center for Developmental Pediatrics and Autism, Associate Program Director, Neurodevelopmental Disabilities Residency, Baylor College of Medicine, Texas Children's, Hospital, Houston, Texas

CARMEN LOPEZ-ARVIZU, MD
Medical Director, Psychiatric Mental Health Program, Kennedy Krieger Institute, Baltimore, Maryland

AMY LUTZ, PhD
Department of History and Sociology of Science at the University of Pennsylvania, Philadelphia, Pennsylvania

SCOTT M. MYERS, MD
Associate Professor of Pediatrics, Department of Clinical Science, Geisinger Commonwealth School of Medicine, Geisinger Autism and Developmental Medicine Institute, Lewisburg, Pennsylvania

KATE NEAMSAPAYA, BA
Department of International Health, Johns Hopkins Bloomberg School of Public Health, Baltimore, Maryland

MARY L. O'CONNOR LEPPERT, MB, BCh
Associate Professor, Department of Pediatrics, The Johns Hopkins University School of Medicine, Department of Neurodevelopmental Medicine, Kennedy Krieger Institute, Baltimore, Maryland

CHARLES OBERWEISER, CPA, PhD
Assistant Professor, Schlief School of Accountancy, Stephen F. Austin State University, Nacogdoches, Texas

CRYSTALENA OBERWEISER
Human Differently, Nacogdoches, Texas

LINDSAY OLSON, PhD
Postdoctoral Scholar, Department of Psychiatry and Behavioral Sciences, UCSF Weill Institute for Neurosciences, University of California, San Francisco, San Francisco, California

ELLY RANUM, MD
Department of Pediatrics, University of Missouri School of Medicine, Columbia, Missouri

SUZANNE RYBCZYNSKI, MD, MSHCM
Chief Medical Officer, East Tennessee Children's Hospital, Knoxville, Tennessee; Adjunct Assistant Professor, Department of Pediatrics, Johns Hopkins School of Medicine, Kennedy Krieger Institute, Baltimore, Maryland

JAY A. SALPEKAR, MD, FANPA, FAES, DFAACAP
Director, Neuropsychiatry Center, Kennedy Krieger Institute, Associate Professor of Psychiatry and Neurology, The Johns Hopkins University School of Medicine, Baltimore, Maryland

GLORIA M. SATRIALE, JD, EdD
Mission for Educating Citizens with Autism; Preparing Adolescents and Adults for Life, Downingtown, Pennsylvania

LAWRENCE SCAHILL, MSN, PhD
Professor of Pediatrics, Emory University School of Medicine, Director of Clinical Trials, Marcus Autism Center, Atlanta, Georgia

NAVJOT SIDHU, MD
Fellow, Division of Developmental and Behavioral Pediatrics, The Children's Hospital of Philadelphia, Philadelphia, Pennsylvania

KRISTIN SOHL, MD, FAAP
Professor, Department of Pediatrics, ECHO Autism Communities, University of Missouri School of Medicine, Columbia, Missouri

MARGARET C. SOUDERS, PhD, CRNP
Assistant Professor, The University of Pennsylvania School of Nursing, The Children's Hospital of Philadelphia, Philadelphia, Pennsylvania

AUDREY THURM, PhD
Professor, Intramural Research Program, Neurodevelopmental and Behavioral Phenotyping Service, National Institute of Mental Health, Bethesda, Maryland

ROMA A. VASA, MD
Director of Psychiatric Services, Center for Autism Services, Science and Innovation, Kennedy Krieger Institute, Department of Psychiatry and Behavioral Sciences, Johns Hopkins University, Baltimore, Maryland

LEE ELIZABETH WACHTEL, MD
Medical director, Neurobehavioral Unit Kennedy Krieger Institute, Professor, Department of Child and Adolescent Psychiatry, Johns Hopkins University School of Medicine. Baltimore, Maryland

KATE E. WALLIS, MD, MPH
Assistant Professor, Department of Pediatrics, Perelman School of Medicine, University of Pennsylvania, and Attending Physician, Division of Developmental and Behavioral Pediatrics, PolicyLab, Clinical Futures, and Center for Autism Research, Children's Hospital of Philadelphia, Philadelphia, Pennsylvania

ARTHUR WESTOVER, MD
Associate Professor, Department of Psychiatry, UT Southwestern Medical Center, Dallas; Director of Adult Autism Services, Department of Psychiatry, and Medical Director, UT Southwestern Behavioral Health Clinic, Richardson/Plano Campus, Richardson, Texas

ZOE WONG, BS
Clinical Research Assistant, The Children's Hospital of Philadelphia, Center for Autism Research, Sidney Kimmel Medical College, Thomas Jefferson University, Philadelphia, Pennsylvania

Contents

> Autism has been the subject of large-scale public health investment. These investments are increasingly shifting toward mitigating the lifelong disability and impairment associated with autism. Key efforts include bolstering screening schedules, accelerating the path to diagnosis and early entry into evidence-based therapies, and providing preventive management of common co-occurring conditions. Enhancing their implementation will necessitate addressing neurodiversity and health equity. Pediatric primary care teams continue to be important stewards in population-level initiatives to promote autistic health. To thrive in this role, these providers will benefit from specific educational and logistical supports from the health care system.

> Screening for autism is recommended in pediatric primary care. However, the median age of autism spectrum disorder (ASD) diagnosis is substantially higher than the age at which autism can reliably be identified, suggesting room for improvements in autism recognition at young ages, especially for children from minoritized racial and ethnic groups, low-income families, and families who prefer a language other than English. Novel approaches are being developed to utilize new technologies in aiding in autism recognition. However, attention to equity is needed to minimize bias. Additional research on the benefits and potential harms of universal autism screening is needed. The authors provide suggestions for pediatricians who are considering implementing autism-screening programs.

> This article discusses the diagnostic criteria for autism spectrum disorder (ASD), as well as other neurodevelopmental disorders that may be confused with or co-occur with ASD. Practitioners involved in diagnostic assessment of ASD must be well versed in the features that differentiate ASD from other conditions and be familiar with how co-occurring

conditions may manifest in the context of ASD. ASD symptoms present differently across development, underscoring the need for training about typical developmental expectations for youth. Periodic reevaluations throughout development are also important because support needs for individuals with autism change over time.

Steven M. Lazar, Thomas D. Challman, and Scott M. Myers

Autism spectrum disorder (ASD) is clinically and etiologically heterogeneous. A causal genetic variant can be identified in approximately 20% to 25% of affected individuals with current clinical genetic testing, and all patients with an ASD diagnosis should be offered genetic etiologic evaluation. We suggest that exome sequencing with copy number variant coverage should be the first-line etiologic evaluation for ASD. Neuroimaging, neurophysiologic, metabolic, and other biochemical evaluations can provide insight into the pathophysiology of ASD but should be recommended in the appropriate clinical circumstances.

Julia S. Anixt, Jennifer Ehrhardt, and Amie Duncan

Pediatricians have a critically important role in the care of children with autism, including conducting developmental screening to support early diagnosis and intervention, advising families about evidence-based treatments for autism spectrum disorder, and supporting families' emotional health as they care for a child with a developmental disability. The purpose of this article is to provide pediatricians with information about evidence-based autism treatments and how to determine which interventions are appropriate for children across the autism spectrum at different ages and developmental stages.

Megan E. Bone and Mary L. O'Connor Leppert

The diagnosis of autism spectrum disorder (ASD) brings a lifetime of considerations for individuals and their families. The core symptoms of ASD vary in severity and influence behavior and function across all environments. Co-occurring medical, mental health, cognitive, language, learning, and behavioral differences add challenges to those associated with core symptoms. Navigating the preschool, school, and transition ages in the educational setting requires continual reassessment of the strengths, weaknesses, and needs of the student to provide appropriate placement and services.

Jamie K. Capal and Shafali S. Jeste

Epilepsy is one of the most common comorbidities in individuals with autism spectrum disorders (ASDs). Risk factors include the presence of developmental delay/intellectual disability, female sex, age, and an underlying genetic condition. Due to higher prevalence of epilepsy in

ASD, it is important to have a high index of suspicion for seizures and refer to a neurologist if there are concerns. Genetic testing is recommended for all children with ASD but it becomes more high yield in children with epilepsy and ASD.

Sleep problems are common in children with autism spectrum disorder (ASD), with 40% to 80% prevalence. Common disorders include insomnia, parasomnias, and circadian rhythm sleep-wake disorders. These problems have a multifactorial etiology and can both exacerbate and be exacerbated by core ASD symptoms. Sleep problems also impact the health and quality of life of both patients and their caregivers. All children with autism should be regularly screened for sleep problems and evaluated for co-occurring medical contributors. Behavioral interventions with caregiver training remain first-line treatment for sleep disorders in both neurotypical and neurodiverse youth.

Children with autism are at high risk for experiencing a mental health crisis, which occurs when psychiatric and behavioral symptoms become a danger and caregivers do not have the resources to safely manage the event. Our current mental health systems of care are not fully prepared to manage crisis in autistic individuals, due to the shortage of available mental health providers and programs that are tailored for autistic children. However, new strategies to address crisis are gradually emerging. This article provides a framework to define crisis and implement prevention and intervention approaches that could potentially mitigate risk for crisis.

Persons with autism spectrum disorder (ASD) may have other psychiatric conditions that warrant treatment. Symptoms may not be easy to discern from rigidity or irritability that are sometimes considered to be constituent parts of ASD. Pathophysiology that involves hyperexcitable neurons and anomalous connectivity may provide justification for using psychopharmacologic agents, although nonmedical strategies may also be effective. Hyperactivity, irritability, and tantrums with or without aggression may be rational targets for psychopharmacological intervention. The best-studied drug class to date has been the second-generation antipsychotics targeting irritability.

PEDIATRIC CLINICS OF NORTH AMERICA

Foreword

Autism Today

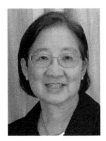

Tina L. Cheng, MD, MPH
Consulting Editor

The history of autism is a fascinating and somewhat controversial story. Ancient human history suggests that the condition existed long before Swiss psychiatrist Eugen Bleuler coined the term "autism" in the early twentieth century. Bleuler contributed to psychiatry in describing "schizophrenia," "schizoid," and "autism" in the early 1900s. The concept of autism was used to describe severe cases of schizophrenia.[1] Bleuler's four A's of fundamental symptoms of schizophrenia included Alogia, Autism, Ambivalence, and Affective blunting with delusion considered an episodic accessory symptom.[2] The Greek word "autós" meaning self was the root for "Autism" describing self-admiration and withdrawal within self.

Research pioneers in the 1940s included Leo Kanner. Working separately, Kanner described severely affected children. Later, Hans Asperger described very able children with autism. Autism had many names in the 1950s and 1960s, including Kanner syndrome, early infantile autism, hyperkinetic disease, childhood disintegrative disorder, and Heller disease (based on the 1908 description by Austrian educator Theodor Heller), also known as dementia infantilis. Some children lived in institutions for "mental defectives."

As science has evolved, so have the terms used. In 2013, the American Psychiatric Association merged four distinct autism diagnoses into one umbrella diagnosis of autism spectrum disorder (ASD). This included autistic disorder, childhood disintegrative disorder, pervasive developmental disorder–not otherwise specified, and Asperger syndrome.

Research on causes and treatments continue to advance while the prevalence of children with autism grows. The Centers for Disease Control and Prevention estimated that in 2000, 1 in 150 children aged 8 years had autism. This has risen rapidly in 2020 to 1 in 36 children aged 8 years (approximately 4% of boys and 1% of girls).[3] While there has been positive advancement in family engagement and greater acceptance of neurodiversity, there is continued work to do. Accelerated research is needed on the complex genetic and environmental factors contributing to autism, while we also address

Pediatr Clin N Am 71 (2024) xv–xvi
https://doi.org/10.1016/j.pcl.2024.01.009
0031-3955/24/© 2024 Published by Elsevier Inc.

pediatric.theclinics.com

the growing need among the children and families in our care. This issue offers the state-of-the-art to guide us.

Tina L. Cheng, MD, MPH
Cincinnati Children's Hospital Medical Center
University of Cincinnati
Cincinnati Children's Research Foundation
3333 Burnet Avenue MLC 3016
Cincinnati, OH 45229-3026, USA

E-mail address:
Tina.cheng@cchmc.org

REFERENCES

1. Evans B. How autism became autism: the radical transformation of a central concept of child development in Britain. Hist Human Sci 2013;26(3):3–31. https://doi.org/10.1177/0952695113484320. PMID: 24014081; PMCID: PMC3757918.
2. Arantes-Gonçalves F, Gama Marques J, Telles-Correia D. Bleuler's psychopathological perspective on schizophrenia delusions: towards new tools in psychotherapy treatment. Front Psychiatry 2018;9:306. https://doi.org/10.3389/fpsyt.2018.00306. PMID: 30065668; PMCID: PMC6056670.
3. Maenner MJ, Warren Z, Williams AR, et al. Prevalence and characteristics of autism spectrum disorder among children aged 8 years—autism and developmental disabilities monitoring network, 11 sites, United States, 2020. MMWR Surveill Summ 2023;72(No. SS-2):1–14.

Preface

Pediatric Management of Autism

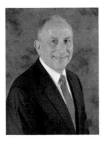 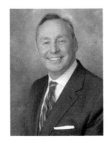

Paul H. Lipkin, MD   Joshua B. Ewen, MD
Editors

Autism is among the most common health conditions in general pediatrics, surpassed only by asthma, bone, joint, or muscle problems, and other neurodevelopmental and behavioral conditions.[1] However, it began its existence as a clinical entity within the medical field of psychiatry. While other early descriptions exist, it was the account of a psychiatrist, Leo Kanner at Johns Hopkins,[2] that ignited awareness and the line of autism research that evolved to what it is today. It was not until later in the twentieth century that the neurologic basis of the condition was better appreciated,[3,4] diversifying the range of clinicians involved in autism. Pediatric interest in the care and management of children with autism accelerated in the 1990s with the rise of neurodevelopmental and developmental-behavioral specialists. Autism's high prevalence in child health was highlighted with the creation of the Autism and Developmental Disabilities Monitoring (ADDM) Network of the Centers for Disease Control and Prevention in 2000,[5] at which time autism was thought to affect one in every 150 children. Current estimates from ADDM now put its prevalence at approximately one in 36 children, affecting all racial, ethnic, and socioeconomic groups, with four boys affected to every girl.[6]

Given autism's high prevalence and workforce limitations among psychiatric, pediatric, and neurologic specialists,[7,8] the general pediatric clinician is now charged with screening for this disorder and assuring each child gets evaluated and diagnosed.[9] They also now assume long-term monitoring and management responsibilities for the child within the primary care pediatric home. With this issue of *Pediatric Clinics of North America*, our aim is to provide the pediatric generalist with actionable steps that they can deliver to the child with autism, supporting their medical, social, and community-participation needs from early childhood through transition to adult care. We have invited a group of pediatric and related experts in the care of children with autism from throughout the United States to write a collection of reviews outlining the many needs of the autistic child as well as providing the pediatric clinician with a toolbox

Pediatr Clin N Am 71 (2024) xvii–xix
https://doi.org/10.1016/j.pcl.2024.01.010

of effective assessment and intervention steps. The articles are ordered across the chronology of childhood, beginning first with fundamental public health and biomedical perspectives on autism, followed by articles dedicated to early childhood (eg, screening, diagnosis), the school-aged years and associated medical conditions (eg, home and school needs, epilepsy, sleep, psychopharmacology), and then the teen years with transition to adult care.

It is typical in works about autism for editors to provide notes about the terms used to label the condition and the individuals affected by it, given the often-heated debates about terminology. Our approach as editors of this issue has been to take a light hand and to let the authors speak for themselves. However, the evolution of the language, the debates that drive this evolution, and the differing prioritizations reflected in those debates should be instructive to the clinician. Namely, while some medical and psychological comorbidities of autism demand intervention because they create distress (eg, anxiety and sleep dysfunction) or safety risks (eg, epilepsy, depression, and harmful behavior), many features of the condition are not inherently distress-inducing or dangerous for the individual and therefore create disability primarily through the interactions between the individual and environment. Developmental diagnoses are, after all, sociologic constructs, and while opposing parties to the language debates of any generation may have differing priorities, each evolutionary leap in language reflects a new facet of understanding and support. For examples, person-first language (eg, "the child with autism") was intended to highlight the individuality of all autistic individuals—that they cannot and should not be reduced simply to their diagnosis. A more recent trend toward identity-first language (eg, "the autistic teenager") reflects, in a sense, a reclamation and demedicalization of the term as well as a growing organization of self-advocates aiming to create a social environment more welcoming to and accommodating of autistic individuals. Very recently, there has been a movement to define the construct of profound autism, reflecting concerns that those with the greatest support needs and least opportunity to communicate their desires may not share the same priorities as self-advocates who do have. The term "Autism Spectrum Condition," common in the United Kingdom, contrasts with the *Diagnostic and Statistical Manual of Mental Disorders* (Fifth Edition) diagnosis[10] of "Autism Spectrum Disorder," by both demedicalizing the terminology and highlighting that the diagnosis may not be lifelong for some. This focus on terminology and the sociology that underlies it emphasizes that the role of the individual pediatric clinician is not only to treat dangerous and distressing medical and psychiatric needs but also to help their patients and families navigate systems and society in order to maximize quality of life, communication, self-actualization, adaptive skills, and desired community participation. And the pediatric community has a role in advocacy toward those goals—an undertaking for which it has proven highly effective time and time again.

We hope that the reader finds this to be a comprehensive and up-to-date guide for everyday use in the clinical office setting, offering a unique perspective and guide on the health care and related care needs of the child for the primary care clinician and others caring for children with autism. We also hope that it offers the reader the latest evidence-based knowledge on these subjects. Research on autism has ballooned over the past two decades, establishing the role of biomedical and psychosocial factors on quality of life and adaptive function. We hope that the pediatric clinician will benefit from this issue as they provide care to children with this common condition.

DISCLOSURE

No disclosures to be made.

Dr P.H. Lipkin is on the Scientific Advisory Board for Sarepta, Inc. He receives research grant funding from the American Foundation for Suicide Prevention and the Patient-Centered Outcomes Research Institute. Dr J.B. Ewen has consulted for Novartis AG and receives research grant funding from the National Institutes of Health.

Paul H. Lipkin, MD
Kennedy Krieger Institute
Johns Hopkins University School of Medicine
707 North Broadway
Baltimore, MD 21205, USA

Joshua B. Ewen, MD
Ann & Robert H. Lurie Children's Hospital
of Chicago
225 East Chicago Avenue, Box 119
Chicago, IL 60611, USA

E-mail addresses:
lipkin@kennedykrieger.org (P.H. Lipkin)
jewen@luriechildrens.org (J.B. Ewen)

REFERENCES

1. US Department of Health and Human Services HRaSA, Maternal and Child Health Bureau. The health and well-being of children: a portrait of states and the nation, 2011–2012. Rockville (MD): US Department of Health and Human Services; 2014.
2. Kanner L. Autistic disturbances of affective conduct. Nervous Child 1943;2: 217–50.
3. DeMyer MK. Research in infantile autism: a strategy and its results. Biol Psychiatry 1975;10(4):433–52.
4. Rutter M. Concepts of autism: a review of research. J Child Psychol Psychiatry 1968;9:1–25.
5. Autism and Developmental Disabilities Monitoring Network Surveillance Year 2000 Principal Investigators, Centers for Disease Control and Prevention. Prevalence of autism spectrum disorders—autism and Developmental Disabilities Monitoring Network, six sites, United States, 2000. MMWR Surveill Summ 2007; 56(1):1–11.
6. Maenner MJ, Warren Z, Williams AR, et al. Prevalence and characteristics of autism spectrum disorder among children aged 8 years—Autism and Developmental Disabilities Monitoring Network, 11 Sites, United States, 2020. MMWR Surveill Summ 2023;72(2):1–14.
7. Bridgemohan C, Bauer NS, Nielsen BA, et al. A workforce survey on developmental-behavioral pediatrics. Pediatrics 2018;141(3):e20172164.
8. Rimsza ME, Ruch-Ross HS, Clemens CJ, et al. Workforce trends and analysis of selected pediatric subspecialties in the United States. Acad Pediatr 2018;18(7): 805–12.
9. Hyman SL, Levy SE, Myers SM, et al. Identification, evaluation, and management of children with autism spectrum disorder. Pediatrics 2020;145(1):e20193447.
10. American Psychiatric Association. Diagnostic and statistical manual of mental disorders, 5th edition: DSM-5. Arlington (VA): American Psychiatric Publishing; 2013.

Health Care for Autistic Children
A Public Health Perspective

Jennifer L. Ames, PhD[a],*, Meghan N. Davignon, MD[b],
Elizabeth A. Hayes, MD[c], Lisa A. Croen, PhD[a]

KEYWORDS

- Autism • Screening • Public health • Co-occurring conditions • Neurodiversity
- Health care • Transition • Medical home

KEY POINTS

- Autism has been the subject of large-scale public health investment, including national surveillance, pediatric screening, and health insurance coverage for autism-related therapies.
- However, health issues affect autistic people across the life-course and public health strategies can help mitigate them, with the pediatric medical home serving as the first-line provider.
- It is important for health care systems to recognize autistic people as a significant clinical population.
- Pediatric primary care teams have a key role in setting the course of positive health trajectories for autistic people and their families.

Autism has been the subject of large-scale public health investment, from the Centers for Disease Control and Prevention's (CDC) establishment of a national surveillance system to efforts to implement universal screening in early childhood and mandate insurance coverage for autism therapies. Today, over 1.5 million autistic children live across the United States[1] and represent a significant segment of the pediatric population. However, this population often experiences greater unmet health care needs and poorer physical, mental, and behavioral health outcomes than their peers with other chronic conditions.[2] Without adequate health care management and transition planning, these health challenges may worsen and bring about more health problems

[a] Division of Research, Kaiser Permanente Northern California, 4480 Hacienda Drive, Building B, Pleasanton, CA 94588, USA; [b] Kaiser Permanente Roseville Medical Center, 1600 Eureka Road, Building C, Department of Pediatric Subspecialties, Roseville, CA 95661, USA; [c] Kaiser Permanente Oakland Medical Center, Department of Pediatrics, 275 West Macarthur Boulevard, Oakland, CA 94611, USA
* Corresponding author.
E-mail address: Jennifer.L.Ames@kp.org

Pediatr Clin N Am 71 (2024) 111–125
https://doi.org/10.1016/j.pcl.2024.01.002
0031-3955/24/© 2024 Elsevier Inc. All rights reserved.

pediatric.theclinics.com

as autistic youth age into adulthood. This article summarizes the key issues facing pediatric primary health care providers (PCPs), such as pediatricians, family medicine physicians, nurse practitioners, and physician assistants. As the first-line providers for autistic children, PCPs set the course for public health within the medical home, including promotion of positive health trajectories for autistic people and their families.

SURVEILLANCE

Autism became a public health priority when the CDC, under the auspices of the Children's Health Act of 2000, established a national autism surveillance system called the Autism and Developmental Disabilities Monitoring (ADDM) Network.[3] Every 2 years the ADDM network conducts active surveillance of 8-year-old children in multiple communities across the United States, identifying children with autism through a comprehensive review of the state's health and education records. The ADDM network has tracked a rapid rise in the prevalence of autism over the last 2 decades, from 1 in 150 children in 2000 to 1 in 36 in 2020. ADDM's spotlight on autism coincided with major clinical changes, including the broadening of diagnostic criteria and growth of universal developmental surveillance, standardized screening, and referral in general pediatrics.[4] Thus, through these concerted shifts in care practices, which have driven better detection of autism and at earlier ages, PCPs have greatly aided epidemiologic surveillance.[4,5]

Nevertheless, evidence suggests the rising prevalence might be influenced by trends, such as higher survival rates in preterm infants, median parental age, and levels of environmental pollutants.[6] While research into autism's etiology shows that rare, highly penetrant genetic variants account for only a small part of the prevalence, most autism cases seem to stem from a complex interplay of early-life genetic and environmental factors. Regardless of what underlies the rising prevalence, we now recognize that children on the autism spectrum represent a significant slice of the pediatric clinical population.[5]

AUTISM SCREENING

An autism diagnosis is a key that unlocks access to developmental and support services. Prompt engagement with these services is associated with better long-term outcomes for children with autism.[7] Thus, universal autism screening is an integral public health strategy for earlier and wider identification of autism and access to services.[8] Instrumental to these efforts is the growth in use of the Modified Checklist for Autism in Toddlers, Revised with Follow-up (M-CHAT-R/F), a short and cost-effective screener that flags children with early signs of autism and other developmental conditions. Since 2006, the American Academy of Pediatrics (AAP) has recommended general developmental surveillance at every preventive visit throughout childhood and standardized developmental screening at specific preventive visits (9, 18, 24, and 30 months), with autism-specific screening, particularly with the M-CHAT-R, at 18 and 24 months.[5,9] Standardized autism screening, either by the pediatric provider or by other staff, has led to dramatic improvements in identifying autism overall and at earlier ages.[4,10] Screening performance of the M-CHAT-R improves even further with use of structured follow-up questions for children with medium likelihood of autism and a second M-CHAT administration at 24 months.[10] Although up to 72% of PCPs use standardized autism screeners today,[4,11] more work is needed, including allowing sufficient time and staffing (**Table 1**), to address the persistently low implementation of screening protocols as recommended.[10]

Table 1
Summary of actions to address the public health of autistic children

Topic	Ideal State	What Needs to Happen to Get There
General approaches		
Neurodiversity-informed care practices/accommodations	• Quiet waiting rooms with dimmer lights • Allow augmentative and alternative communication devices • Social stories in advance of uncomfortable procedures such as immunizations or blood draws • Communication accommodations such as speaking slowly, in concrete terms, waiting for patient to process information, and sitting side by side rather than forcing eye contact	• Training to increase knowledge and comfort working with autistic patients • Investment in clinical support staff: Patient and family navigators, behavioral health specialists, nurses, social workers, medical assistants, etc.
Family-provider relationships	• Caregiver and provider partnership in health care decision-making, transition planning • Primary health care providers (PCP) recommend safe and evidence-based complementary and alternative medicine (CAM) with family • Caregiver-mediated therapies used when appropriate • Caregiver and family health and well-being screened and supported by health care system • Parent support groups	• Further research on long-term outcomes following caregiver-mediated therapies • Continuing clinical education on evidence-based CAM and autism therapies. • Clinical coordination to support the health of the child as well as their family
Specific practices		
Screening	• Universal autism screening (eg, M-CHAT-R) at 18-mo and 24-mo well-child visits	• Adequate time/staffing • Integration into electronic health records • Clinical training and refreshers to support developmental screening best practices • Care coordination to support completion of screening on schedule • Improving availability of downstream services
Assessment/diagnosis	• After positive screen, child promptly seen by specialist team for formal autism assessment • PCP can reliably diagnose overt autism without specialist	• Increase accessibility and availability of specialists, shorten wait times • Care coordination to make sure children with diagnostic referral are not lost to follow-up • Train general PCPs to diagnose autism and speed path to services

(continued on next page)

Table 1
(continued)

Topic	Ideal State	What Needs to Happen to Get There
Referral/treatment	• Child referred to personalized plan of evidence-based services and supports • Initiate therapies as early as possible • Monitor for improvements in relevant child outcomes	• Expand evidence base to understand which therapies work best for which children • Care coordination to assist families with timely initiation and managing multiple therapies for their children
Co-occurring conditions	• Screening for common co-occurring conditions • Anticipatory guidance for health management • Referral to specialists, therapies, and/or medication as appropriate • Ongoing management and continuation of care	• Growing pediatric PCPs' knowledgeability and comfort with treating common mental and physical health issues in autistic patients • Longer appointment lengths to address medical complexity • Tailored anticipatory guidance for autistic patients (eg, diet, physical activity, sleep) • Care coordination to connect patient and families to specialist(s) and manage co-occurring conditions
Transition	• Transition planning starts between ages 12 and 14, transition readiness built gradually • Warm handoff between pediatric and adult provider • Pediatric PCP follows up with adult PCP to confirm successful transition of care	• Departmental written transition policies; resources for families • Provider and clinical team training on transition best practices (Medical school and/or specialized training programs) • Clinic tracking of transition-age patients • Longer appointment lengths or annual transition-oriented visits • Lines of communication created between pediatric and adult care • Care coordination to connect patient and families to adult care and assist with medical documentation for health conservatorships, education, and employment services
Autism care advocacy	• Insurance reimbursement and expanded access to services • Involvement in consensus recommendations developed by the AAP • Connect families to community-supports	• Clinical champions within health care systems and national policy committees

Despite enhanced screening, the median age of diagnosis has plateaued at age 4 in the United States, suggesting that screening is not the only lever for altering developmental trajectories.[12] After screening, a child is typically referred to a specialized team for formal diagnostic assessment. Scaling diagnostic services to the surge in referrals from expanded screening has been difficult, partly due to a shortage of developmental-behavioral pediatricians and lengthy diagnostic assessments.[13] This has led to long wait times for appointments and, without strong follow-up by the health care system, many families, disproportionally from marginalized groups, are at risk of falling out of the process.[14,15] Furthermore, these care specialists are typically located near urban centers and are often completely inaccessible to children living in more rural communities.[15] Thus, the diagnostic bottleneck and limited accessibility of evaluations still hinder earlier diagnosis, squandering time during a critical window when developmental trajectories are most sensitive to intervention.[16] Earlier intervention, especially before the age of 3, has been shown to significantly reduce the social, communication, and behavioral impairments associated with autism and lifelong disability.[7]

The step from diagnosis to support services is yet another critical juncture for families in the complex care path for autistic children. While private health insurers are required to cover health care therapies for autism (another major success for lowering barriers to care for this population), these interventions are not accessible to families until the child receives a diagnosis.[15] Families commonly feel overwhelmed by balancing an intense schedule of multiple interventions, including applied behavioral analysis, occupational therapy, speech therapy, community support services, and/or school services, and often navigate these services with little support for care coordination.[17] Furthermore, the benefits of these services are not distributed equally across the autism spectrum and the intensity, quality, and monitoring of these services are highly variable. This is partly because many services are delivered outside the primary health care system, resulting in less oversight and inconsistent tracking of outcomes meaningful to patients and their families. Thus, the evidence base remains limited in understanding which interventions work best for which children.[18]

Opportunities for Primary Care Providers in Promoting Screening and the Early Autism Care Path

As the first-line clinical professionals in the autism care path, PCPs are important allies in implementing public health strategies, but they have received little support to take on this responsibility.[15] For example, PCPs endorse the need for enhanced training to increase their awareness and confidence in caring for autistic children.[15] Physician and non-physician members of the care team are particularly poised to benefit from specialized training on screening best practices, where confusion remains around how to effectively manage a positive screen, including the administration of follow-up questions and subsequent screens and referrals.[10]

Beyond screening, recent evidence suggests that PCPs can also reliably diagnose autism, especially among young children with overt signs.[19] Expanding diagnostic services to pediatric primary care will alleviate the diagnostic bottleneck, speeding up the path to diagnosis and timely initiation of intervention services within an optimal developmental window. PCPs also have a large influence on referring patients for genetic testing, which can open more avenues of health screening, resources, and therapies, as well as advance scientific discovery.[15]

There is also a need for building the PCP's knowledge in how to triage families to the appropriate care path, whether that is referral to a specialist and/or directly to services within the school or community.[15] Providers who make appropriate referrals to specialists and services are considered more competent and trustworthy by caregivers.[20] However, to be effective in this role, PCPs need a stronger evidence base of what therapies work for which children, especially with respect to long-term outcomes.[18] Despite many therapies for autistic children, there is still a paucity of resources targeting autism's core symptoms and limited understanding of the cost-effectiveness of treatment modalities, especially in combination.

THE IMPORTANCE OF PREVENTIVE CARE FOR CO-OCCURRING CONDITIONS

Pediatric care for autistic children also entails addressing a wide range of co-occurring psychiatric, medical, and behavioral conditions that are more common in autistic children compared to non-autistic children, including attention deficit hyperactivity disorder, depression, anxiety, epilepsy, gastrointestinal issues, sleep disorders, elopement, and suicidality.[21] Many of these conditions emerge during childhood and adolescence and can contribute to poorer quality of life, injury, high health care needs, trauma, and mortality into adulthood.[22,23] Given this complexity, autistic children may require multiple types of specialized pediatric care, necessitating care coordination.[24] While medically complex children like those with cystic fibrosis or type 1 diabetes often receive coordinated, specialist care, workforce challenges in developmental-behavioral pediatrics[13] leave many autistic children mainly reliant on their PCP as their medical home.[25] Thus, PCPs are oftentimes the first-line providers to screen for and treat new symptoms and open the referral path to pediatric specialists when needed. However, many PCPs feel under-equipped to care for autistic children, citing lack of time and limited knowledge about tailoring anticipatory guidance and treatment for this population.[20] For example, when mental health specialists are not readily available within their network, PCPs might hesitate to prescribe psychotropics and other medications for autistic children's psychiatric symptoms.[26] Clinical guidelines on the long-term effects of some of these medications, some of which are prescribed to autistic children off-label, in combination with other medications, and at younger ages than their typical use, are currently lacking.

The Transition to Adulthood Sets a Long-Term Trajectory

Poor health management and diminished well-being can adversely affect the patient's long-term success in other domains including education, independent-living, and employment.[27] Thus, the transition to adulthood is a particularly vulnerable period for autistic adolescents and their families as numerous developmental and societal changes, including loss of educational and developmental support services, coincide.[28] Strain on youth and their families is further compounded by evolving medical needs that often go unmet, including sexual and reproductive health care, when the adolescent's care team shifts from pediatrics to adult medicine.[29,30] Studies suggest that autistic youth receive fewer transition resources than their peers with other special health care needs (SHCN) and often experience steeper declines in utilization of outpatient health services in young adulthood than non-autistic youth with intellectual disabilities.[25,31] This disparity may be attributable to lack of awareness and experience caring for autistic patients among adult care providers, who tend to underestimate the number of autistic patients in their care.[32,33] Increased ED visits, hospitalizations, and inpatient psychiatric visits among autistic young adults compared with non-autistic peers further point to inadequate access to primary and preventive care during the transition years.[34]

Systematic reviews of health care transition interventions demonstrate that structured transition processes for youth with SHCN have positive impacts on treatment adherence, patient experiences, service utilization, and population health.[35] Got Transition—a partnership of the Health Resources & Services Administration's (HRSA) Maternal and Child Health Bureau and the National Alliance to Advance Adolescent Health—has developed a 6-step system of health care transition best practices[36] which has been endorsed by the American Academies of Pediatrics and Family Medicine.[37] Implementing these best practices, which include transition-oriented health care visits starting at age 12, a warm hand-off between pediatric and adult PCPs, and planning discussions with families, will require institutional investment in pediatric infrastructure, such as patient tracking, longer appointment lengths, and clinical support staff. Innovative care models for transitioning autistic youth, from targeted transition protocols and clinics to specialized training and mentoring programs for pediatric providers, are emerging.[35,38,39] These initiatives often start with local clinical champions but require institutional support for scalability and sustainability.

CHALLENGES CASCADE TO THE FAMILY

The child's behavioral and medical challenges and the logistics of autism-related care, including costs, time, and transportation, have implications for the well-being of their families. Caregivers of autistic children report difficulty maintaining social well-being, employment, housing, finances, and physical and mental health.[5,17,40] They also commonly perceive that health care providers have limited autism competency and knowledge, which can further compound their stress and exhaustion.[41] Many also worry about their child's future care but receive little guidance on how to prepare for the transition to adulthood.[42]

Caregiving stress and dissatisfaction with available therapeutic options leads some families to turn to complementary and alternative medicine (CAM). While some CAM can be beneficial, some approaches are expensive, risky, and not evidence-based, which can make CAM a problematic topic and source of tension between PCPs and caregivers.[43] Families may not disclose CAM treatments to their child's provider out of concern for the provider's knowledge or disapproval of these alternatives.[44] These issues can hinder shared decision-making between the PCP and caregiver, have negative consequences for the child, and enable health misinformation, such as anti-vaccine sentiments, to spread.[43] The AAP affirms that the PCP has a bioethical obligation to educate families about the harms and benefits of CAMs, as with all treatments.[45] Their guidelines advise the provider to approach CAM discussions with an open mind, knowledgeability of the CAM evidence base (see National Center for Complementary and Alternative Medicine (www.nccam.nih.gov)), and respect for cultural beliefs or values around health.[46] Nevertheless, these conversations require significant provider time, including literature review, and can be fraught when the evidence base for a CAM's safety and efficacy is limited.[45]

Parent-Mediated Therapies

The caregiver is an autistic child's most important advocate. Partnering with the caregiver in their child's autism care path can bring significant benefits to the whole family and alleviate burdens on the health care system. For example, providing the caregiver with information and resources as they navigate their child's care can empower them in care coordination and decision-making. Parent-mediated early interventions and coaching have also shown promise in improving family interactions and child language skills and reducing the severity of some behaviors.[47] Interventions delivered as group classes additionally help parents find social support and community and mitigate feelings of helplessness and isolation. While these approaches have been received positively by families, they need further study, especially with respect to long-term outcomes and effectiveness in different settings and populations.[48,49]

Parental depression can accompany a child's diagnoses of co-occurring psychiatric conditions and autism-related behaviors.[50] These symptoms not only decrease the parent's quality of life but also may lower engagement and benefits from autism therapies, including parent-mediated approaches.[51] Routine screening for parental mental health is recommended by the AAP and is required in some states, at least for Medicaid patients.[52] However, many pediatric PCPs and health care systems are not well-equipped to incorporate this screening into standard practice, and do not address needs of parents once identified. Nonetheless, this population would benefit from enhanced screening and support to address their stress and mental health.

EMPOWERING PRIMARY HEALTH CARE PROVIDERS TO SUPPORT AUTISTIC HEALTH
Medical School, Residency, and Continuing Education

Providers report limited clinical training in autism as a barrier to knowledgeability and confidence in caring for autistic patients.[26,53] Given the life-course aspects of autistic health and the increased dependence on primary care as the medical home,[54] advancing autism as a core competency in medical training would better prepare clinicians to manage the special health care needs of this growing population.[5] Despite the recognized educational gaps, medical and nursing schools have had limited capacity, with respect to curricula space and availability of knowledgeable academic faculty, to incorporate autism and other condition-specific trainings.[55,56]

Expansion and augmentation of pediatric residency programs have shown promise in promoting autism knowledge and care competency among providers. While the Accreditation Council for Graduate Medical Education (ACGME) currently does not specifically mandate autism training in General Pediatrics, they require a month-long residency rotation in developmental and behavioral pediatrics, which can be spread out longitudinally.[57] The AAP also endorses the "Autism Case Training (ACT): A Developmental-Behavioral Pediatrics Curriculum"; this is a freely-available, 7-module teaching tool which addresses best practices for early autism screening and early interventions, referrals, and autism-specific anticipatory guidance.[57] These programs boost autism competency in residents, but their full implementation is challenging due to tight clinical schedules and limited teaching capacity of developmental-behavioral pediatricians, who are in short supply.[58]

Continuing education (CE) has been a popular and important avenue for making pediatric care teams aware of the benefits of screening, enhance the rigor of their screening practices, and allow them to confidently and efficiently shepherd families toward the appropriate care path.[53,56] Building knowledge about treatment options is a particular priority for CE, as many providers are wary of boosting autism screening when they feel uncertain about the efficacy and availability of treatment options for their patients, especially in a quickly changing evidence landscape.[12] Innovative models such as the ECHO autism training are also low-cost, low-resource tools that build pediatric competencies, especially in community-based clinical settings outside of academic medical centers.[38,59] While these programs are growing more accessible and appear efficacious in the short term, an evaluation of their influence on long-term clinical practices would inform how to best make use of the provider's limited time and energy for CE.[53] To pragmatically fit within provider's schedules, CE should be designed with ease of access (online and/or asynchronous) and low time commitment (intensive or small investments over longer periods).[53]

Lastly, providers will benefit from clinical organizations' continued updates of clinical consensus statements,[5,9] dissemination of resources such as the AAP autism toolkit (https://publications.aap.org/toolkits/pages/Autism-Toolkit), and enhanced coordination between the health care system and school and community-based developmental services. For example, PCPs indicate needing more clinical guidance on services provided through the educational system, respite care for families, and community-based services, including parent support groups.[26,60]

Clinical Support and Structural Changes

As outlined earlier, PCPs play a key role in the care of autistic patients, including autism screening, coordinating the early care path to services internal and external to the health system, screening and preventive care of co-occurring mental and physical health conditions, and the transition to adult care. All these activities are time-intensive and PCPs need clinical support to thrive as the medical home for autistic patients. Multiple logistical constraints, including documentation burdens, scheduling inflexibility, and reimbursement restrictions, can make it challenging for PCPs to identify their autistic patients and follow through with referrals and care coordination. However, PCPs who have been able to implement practice level changes, including developmental screening, care coordination, and extended appointment lengths, have reported greater confidence in addressing autism-specific needs.[26]

Health care systems also need investment in personalized care approaches for autistic patients. Patient and family navigators, behavioral health specialists, nurses, social workers, medical assistants, and other care partners within the primary care clinic can facilitate individualized care plans and enhance screening and care coordination.[26] Alternative models such as complex care clinics implement multidisciplinary care teams, longer appointments, and coordinated care plans to improve quality of care. However, they have been challenging to fairly evaluate due to their high upfront costs, with studies not lasting long enough to capture their long-term benefits.[61] Telemedicine may further reduce costs of these clinics and improve accessibility, especially in rural areas.

NEURODIVERSITY-INFORMED CARE

Health care can also be strengthened with neurodiversity-informed care practices. The neurodiversity movement shifts away from a deficit-based understanding of autism, recognizing instead that ways of thinking, behaving, and communicating are traits spanning a multidimensional spectrum in the population. This approach in health care advances a social rather than medicalized model of disability, in which the emphasis is on altering the environment rather than altering the person to promote health and well-being.[62]

For a PCP, this approach can be woven into care in several ways. For example, the health care environment can be made more autism-friendly with communication strategies, and sensory and environmental accommodations (see **Table 1**),[63] without which health care environments may trigger challenging child behaviors and negatively impact care.[20] Families often prefer providers knowledgeable about autism, not just for specialized treatment but to ensure their child's communication style is accommodated in all care.[63] This approach also encompasses adapting health interventions and health educational resources, including physical activity, diet, and sleep, to the needs of autistic patients.[64] In addition, autism-friendly clinics have implemented patient and family navigation, peer support, and autism training programs for residents and the rest of the care team.[65–67]

HEALTH EQUITY ISSUES

The adoption of universal screening and state insurance mandates for autism care has made significant inroads in addressing racial/ethnic disparities in autism diagnosis.[68] The gap in median age of autism diagnosis among Black and Hispanic children compared to non-Hispanic White counterparts has closed in some parts of the United States.[3] However, socioeconomic disparities in diagnostic screening, utilization of evidence-based treatments, and lifelong health status remain.[69] Black autistic children experience intellectual disability at higher rates than their White counterparts, possibly due to disparities in timely and equitable access to therapies, especially within key developmental windows in early childhood.[14] These issues can be further compounded by clinical biases such as overdiagnosis of behavioral disorders in Black and Hispanic children.[70]

Health disparities may also extend to autistic females and people with gender expansive identities.[30] For example, current diagnostic methods, validated in largely male samples, may lead to delayed diagnosis in girls who will often collect multiple other psychiatric diagnoses (eg, anorexia, anxiety, and depression) in the years leading up to their autism diagnosis.[71] Girls are also more likely than boys to report social "masking" of autism symptoms to fit in at school.[71] At the intersection of autism and gender expansive identities, which are more common among autistic than non-autistic people, there may be increased risk of health care barriers, mental health challenges, and poorer quality of life.[30]

Advocacy for Services and Supports

There are opportunities for PCPs to advocate for better care and supports for this population, both as clinical champions within their health care systems and at the national policy level (see **Table 1**). PCPs are trusted authorities in their communities and can advocate for inclusivity of neurodivergent children in health-promoting, community-based activities.

SUMMARY

While etiologic studies advancing our understanding of the neurobiology of autism remain important, mounting evidence calls for a shift in public health strategies toward mitigating the lifelong disability and impairment associated with autism. These strategies include bolstering screening schedules, accelerating the path to diagnosis and early entry into evidence-based therapies, and preventive management of common co-occurring conditions. A thoughtful approach to their implementation will necessitate addressing neurodiversity and health equity. PCPs and other pediatric providers continue to be key stewards in population-level initiatives to promote autistic health as well as the health of other pediatric populations with complex chronic conditions. However, it is essential for health care systems and medical educators to provide supports for PCPs to promote autistic health via structural changes such as support for universal developmental and autism screening, longer visits for complex patients, care coordination among service providers, as well as training opportunities and resources starting early in medical education and continuing throughout the years of clinical practice.

CLINICS CARE POINTS

- Implementing effective autism screening necessitates integrating universal screening protocols into regular health checks at key developmental stages, supported by adequate staffing, training, and care coordination to ensure timely and comprehensive follow-up services.

- Creating a neurodiversity-informed healthcare environment requires training healthcare professionals in autism-specific accommodations such as sensory friendly waiting areas and communication supports.
- Effective management of co-occurring conditions in autistic children requires tailored anticipatory guidance and longer appointment times for complex cases, complemented by coordinated care connecting patients and families with appropriate pediatric, and as they transition, adult specialists.
- Providers report that limited clinical training in autism during medical school, residency, and continuing education is a barrier to confidently caring for autistic patients.

DISCLOSURE

The Authors have nothing to disclose.

REFERENCES

1. Kogan MD, Vladutiu CJ, Schieve LA, et al. The Prevalence of Parent-Reported Autism Spectrum Disorder Among US Children. Pediatrics 2018;142(6). https://doi.org/10.1542/peds.2017-4161.
2. Karpur A, Lello A, Frazier T, et al. Health Disparities among Children with Autism Spectrum Disorders: Analysis of the National Survey of Children's Health 2016. J Autism Dev Disord 2019;49(4):1652–64.
3. Maenner MJ, Warren Z, Williams AR, et al. Prevalence and Characteristics of Autism Spectrum Disorder Among Children Aged 8 Years - Autism and Developmental Disabilities Monitoring Network, 11 Sites, United States, 2020. MMWR Surveill Summ 2023;72(2):1–14.
4. Lipkin PH, Macias MM, Baer Chen B, et al. Trends in Pediatricians' Developmental Screening: 2002 2016. Pediatrics 2020;145(4). https://doi.org/10.1542/peds.2019-0851.
5. Hyman SL, Levy SE, Myers SM. Executive Summary: Identification, Evaluation, and Management of Children With Autism Spectrum Disorder. Pediatrics 2020; 145(1). https://doi.org/10.1542/peds.2019-3448.
6. Lyall K, Croen L, Daniels J, et al. The Changing Epidemiology of Autism Spectrum Disorders. Annu Rev Public Health 2017;38:81–102.
7. Reichow B, Hume K, Barton EE, et al. Early intensive behavioral intervention (EIBI) for young children with autism spectrum disorders (ASD). Cochrane Database Syst Rev 2018;5(5):Cd009260.
8. Lipkin PH, Macias MM. Promoting Optimal Development: Identifying Infants and Young Children With Developmental Disorders Through Developmental Surveillance and Screening. Pediatrics 2020;145(1). https://doi.org/10.1542/peds.2019-3449. Added reference: Council on Children With Disabilities; Section on Developmental Behavioral Pediatrics; Bright Futures Steering Committee; Medical Home Initiatives for Children With Special Needs Project Advisory Committee. Identifying infants and young children with developmental disorders in the medical home: an algorithm for developmental surveillance and screening [published correction appears in Pediatrics. 2006 Oct;118(4):1808-1809]. Pediatrics. 2006; 118(1):405-1809. doi:10.1542/peds.2006-1231.

9. Johnson CP, Myers SM. American Academy of Pediatrics Council on Children With D. Identification and evaluation of children with autism spectrum disorders. Pediatrics 2007;120(5):1183–215.

10. Wieckowski AT, Williams LN, Rando J, et al. Sensitivity and Specificity of the Modified Checklist for Autism in Toddlers (Original and Revised): A Systematic Review and Meta-analysis. JAMA Pediatr 2023;177(4):373–83.

11. Lipkin PH. Screening Success in the Age of Autism. JAMA Pediatr 2023. https://doi.org/10.1001/jamapediatrics.2022.5972.

12. Klin A, Micheletti M, Klaiman C, et al. Affording autism an early brain development re-definition. Dev Psychopathol 2020;32(4):1175–89.

13. Bridgemohan C, Bauer NS, Nielsen BA, et al. A Workforce Survey on Developmental-Behavioral Pediatrics. Pediatrics 2018;141(3). https://doi.org/10.1542/peds.2017-2164.

14. Constantino JN, Abbacchi AM, Saulnier C, et al. Timing of the Diagnosis of Autism in African American Children. Pediatrics 2020;146(3). https://doi.org/10.1542/peds.2019-3629.

15. Malik-Soni N, Shaker A, Luck H, et al. Tackling healthcare access barriers for individuals with autism from diagnosis to adulthood. Pediatr Res 2022;91(5):1028–35.

16. Dawson G, Jones EJ, Merkle K, et al. Early behavioral intervention is associated with normalized brain activity in young children with autism. J Am Acad Child Adolesc Psychiatry 2012;51(11):1150–9.

17. Moh TA, Magiati I. Factors associated with parental stress and satisfaction during the process of diagnosis of children with Autism Spectrum Disorders. Research in Autism Spectrum Disorders 2012;6(1):293–303.

18. Franz L, Goodwin CD, Rieder A, et al. Early intervention for very young children with or at high likelihood for autism spectrum disorder: An overview of reviews. Dev Med Child Neurol 2022;64(9):1063–76.

19. Penner M, Senman L, Andoni L, et al. Concordance of Diagnosis of Autism Spectrum Disorder Made by Pediatricians vs a Multidisciplinary Specialist Team. JAMA Netw Open 2023;6(1):e2252879.

20. Wilson SA, Peterson CC. Medical care experiences of children with autism and their parents: A scoping review. Child Care Health Dev 2018;44(6):807–17.

21. Rosen TE, Mazefsky CA, Vasa RA, et al. Co-occurring psychiatric conditions in autism spectrum disorder. Int Rev Psychiatry 2018;30(1):40–61.

22. Schendel DE, Overgaard M, Christensen J, et al. Association of Psychiatric and Neurologic Comorbidity With Mortality Among Persons With Autism Spectrum Disorder in a Danish Population. JAMA Pediatr 2016;170(3):243–50.

23. Sikora DM, Vora P, Coury DL, et al. Attention-deficit/hyperactivity disorder symptoms, adaptive functioning, and quality of life in children with autism spectrum disorder. Pediatrics 2012;130(Suppl 2):S91–7.

24. Peacock G, Amendah D, Ouyang L, et al. Autism spectrum disorders and health care expenditures: the effects of co-occurring conditions. J Dev Behav Pediatr 2012;33(1):2–8.

25. Rast JE, Shattuck PT, Roux AM, et al. The Medical Home and Health Care Transition for Youth With Autism. Pediatrics 2018;141(Suppl 4):S328–34.

26. Mazurek MO, Harkins C, Menezes M, et al. Primary Care Providers' Perceived Barriers and Needs for Support in Caring for Children with Autism. J Pediatr 2020;221:240–5.e1.

27. Anderson KA, Sosnowy C, Kuo AA, et al. Transition of Individuals With Autism to Adulthood: A Review of Qualitative Studies. Pediatrics 2018;141(Suppl 4): S318–27.

28. Roux AM, Shattuck PT, Rast JE, et al. National Autism Indicators Report: Transition into Young Adulthood. In: Life Course Outcomes Research Program. Philadelphia, PA: A.J. Drexel Autism Institute, Drexel University; 2015.

29. Lounds J, Seltzer MM, Greenberg JS, et al. Transition and change in adolescents and young adults with autism: longitudinal effects on maternal well-being. Am J Ment Retard 2007;112(6):401–17.

30. Graham Holmes L, Ames JL, Massolo ML, et al. Improving the Sexual and Reproductive Health and Health Care of Autistic People. Pediatrics 2022;149(Suppl 4). https://doi.org/10.1542/peds.2020-049437J.

31. Nathenson RA, Zablotsky B. The Transition to the Adult Health Care System Among Youths With Autism Spectrum Disorder. Psychiatr Serv 2017;68(7):735–8.

32. Nicolaidis C, Raymaker DM, Ashkenazy E, et al. "Respect the way I need to communicate with you": Healthcare experiences of adults on the autism spectrum. Autism 2015;19(7):824–31.

33. Zerbo O, Massolo ML, Qian Y, et al. A Study of Physician Knowledge and Experience with Autism in Adults in a Large Integrated Healthcare System. J Autism Dev Disord 2015;45(12):4002–14.

34. Gilmore D, Krantz M, Weaver L, et al. Healthcare service use patterns among autistic adults: A systematic review with narrative synthesis. Autism 2022;26(2): 317–31.

35. Schmidt A, Ilango SM, McManus MA, et al. Outcomes of pediatric to adult health care transition interventions: An updated systematic review. J Pediatr Nurs 2020; 51:92–107.

36. Got Transition Center for Health Care Transition Improvement. Six Core Elements of Health Care Transition 2.0. The National Alliance to Advance Adolescent Health. Updated March 12, 2019. Available at: https://www.gottransition.org/resourceGet.cfm?id=206.

37. White PH, Cooley WC. Transitions Clinical Report Authoring G, American Academy Of P, American Academy Of Family P, American College Of P. Supporting the Health Care Transition From Adolescence to Adulthood in the Medical Home. Pediatrics 2018. https://doi.org/10.1542/peds.2018-2587.

38. Mazurek MO, Stobbe G, Loftin R, et al. ECHO Autism Transition: Enhancing healthcare for adolescents and young adults with autism spectrum disorder. Autism 2020;24(3):633–44.

39. Fernandes P, Timmerman J, Hotez E, et al. A Residency Program Curriculum to Improve Health Care Transitions for Autistic Individuals. Pediatrics 2022; 149(Suppl 4). https://doi.org/10.1542/peds.2020-049437U.

40. Vasilopoulou E, Nisbet J. The quality of life of parents of children with autism spectrum disorder: A systematic review. Research in Autism Spectrum Disorders 2016;23:36–49.

41. Dovgan K, Mazurek MO. Impact of multiple co-occurring emotional and behavioural conditions on children with autism and their families. J Appl Res Intellect Disabil 2019;32(4):967–80.

42. Ames JL, Mahajan A, Davignon MN, et al. Opportunities for Inclusion and Engagement in the Transition of Autistic Youth from Pediatric to Adult Healthcare: A Qualitative Study. J Autism Dev Disord 2022. https://doi.org/10.1007/s10803-022-05476-4.

43. Levy SE, Frasso R, Colantonio S, et al. Shared Decision Making and Treatment Decisions for Young Children With Autism Spectrum Disorder. Acad Pediatr 2016;16(6):571–8.

44. Smith CA, Parton C, King M, et al. Parents' experiences of information-seeking and decision-making regarding complementary medicine for children with autism spectrum disorder: a qualitative study. BMC Complement Med Ther 2020;20(1):4.

45. Gilmour J, Harrison C, Cohen MH, et al. Pediatric use of complementary and alternative medicine: legal, ethical, and clinical issues in decision-making. Pediatrics 2011;128(Suppl 4):S149–54.

46. American Academy of Pediatrics. Counseling families who choose complementary and alternative medicine for their child with chronic illness or disability. Committee on Children With Disabilities. Pediatrics 2001;107(3):598–601.

47. Nevill RE, Lecavalier L, Stratis EA. Meta-analysis of parent-mediated interventions for young children with autism spectrum disorder. Autism 2018;22(2):84–98.

48. Oono IP, Honey EJ, McConachie H. Parent-mediated early intervention for young children with autism spectrum disorders (ASD). Cochrane Database Syst Rev 2013;(4):CD009774.

49. Shalev RA, Lavine C, Di Martino A. A Systematic Review of the Role of Parent Characteristics in Parent-Mediated Interventions for Children with Autism Spectrum Disorder. J Dev Phys Disabil 2020;32(1):1–21.

50. Zablotsky B, Anderson C, Law P. The association between child autism symptomatology, maternal quality of life, and risk for depression. J Autism Dev Disord 2013;43(8):1946–55.

51. Feinberg E, Augustyn M, Fitzgerald E, et al. Improving maternal mental health after a child's diagnosis of autism spectrum disorder: results from a randomized clinical trial. JAMA Pediatr 2014;168(1):40–6.

52. Hagan JF, Shaw J, Duncan P. Bright futures. Itasca, IL: American Academy of Pediatrics; 2017.

53. Clarke L, Fung LK. The impact of autism-related training programs on physician knowledge, self-efficacy, and practice behavior: A systematic review. Autism 2022;26(7):1626–40.

54. Croen LA, Zerbo O, Qian Y, et al. The health status of adults on the autism spectrum. Autism 2015;19(7):814–23.

55. Gardner MR, Suplee PD, Jerome-D'Emilia B. Survey of Nursing Faculty Preparation for Teaching About Autism Spectrum Disorders. Nurse Educ 2016;41(4): 212–6.

56. Carbone PS. Moving from research to practice in the primary care of children with autism spectrum disorders. Acad Pediatr 2013;13(5):390–9.

57. Major NE. Autism education in residency training programs. AMA J Ethics 2015; 17(4):318–22.

58. Froehlich TE, Spinks-Franklin A, Christakis DA. Ending Developmental-Behavioral Pediatrics Faculty Requirement for Pediatric Residency Programs—Desperate Times Do Not Justify Desperate Actions. JAMA Pediatr 2023;177(10):999–1000.

59. Buranova N, Dampf M, Stevenson B, et al. ECHO Autism: Early Intervention Connecting Community Professionals to Increase Access to Best Practice Autism Intervention. Clin Pediatr (Phila) 2022;61(8):518–22.

60. Zwaigenbaum L, Nicholas DB, Muskat B, et al. Perspectives of Health Care Providers Regarding Emergency Department Care of Children and Youth with Autism Spectrum Disorder. J Autism Dev Disord 2016;46(5):1725–36.

61. Simon TD, Whitlock KB, Haaland W, et al. Effectiveness of a Comprehensive Case Management Service for Children With Medical Complexity. Pediatrics 2017; 140(6). https://doi.org/10.1542/peds.2017-1641.

62. Haegele JA, Hodge S. Disability Discourse: Overview and Critiques of the Medical and Social Models. Quest 2016;68(2):193–206.

63. Morris R, Greenblatt A, Saini M. Healthcare Providers' Experiences with Autism: A Scoping Review. J Autism Dev Disord 2019;49(6):2374–88.

64. Curtin C, Bowling AB, Boutelle KN, et al. Chapter Eight - Lifestyle intervention adaptations to promote healthy eating and physical activity of youth with intellectual and developmental disabilities. In: Riggs NR, Rigles B, editors. International review of research in developmental disabilities. Academic Press; 2021. p. 223–61.

65. O'Hagan B, Krauss SB, Friedman AJ, et al. Identifying Components of Autism Friendly Health Care: An Exploratory Study Using a Modified Delphi Method. J Dev Behav Pediatr 2023;44(1):e12–8.

66. O'Hagan B, Sonikar P, Grace R, et al. Youth and Caregivers' Perspective on Teens Engaged as Mentors (TEAM): An Inclusive Peer Mentoring Program for Autistic Adolescents. J Autism Dev Disord 2022. https://doi.org/10.1007/s10803-022-05543-w.

67. Broder-Fingert S, Qin S, Goupil J, et al. A mixed-methods process evaluation of Family Navigation implementation for autism spectrum disorder. Autism 2019; 23(5):1288–99.

68. Maenner MJ, Shaw KA, Bakian AV, et al. Prevalence and Characteristics of Autism Spectrum Disorder Among Children Aged 8 Years - Autism and Developmental Disabilities Monitoring Network, 11 Sites, United States, 2018. MMWR Surveill Summ 2021;70(11):1–16.

69. Chavez AE, Feldman MS, Carter AS, et al. Delays in autism diagnosis for U.S. Spanish-speaking families: The contribution of appointment availability. Evid Based Pract Child Adolesc Ment Health 2022;7(2):275–93.

70. Mandell DS, Ittenbach RF, Levy SE, et al. Disparities in diagnoses received prior to a diagnosis of autism spectrum disorder. J Autism Dev Disord 2007;37(9): 1795–802.

71. Lai MC, Lombardo MV, Auyeung B, et al. Sex/gender differences and autism: setting the scene for future research. J Am Acad Child Adolesc Psychiatry 2015;54(1):11–24.

Screening for Autism

A Review of the Current State, Ongoing Challenges, and Novel Approaches on the Horizon

Kate E. Wallis, MD, MPH[a,b,c,d,e,*], Whitney Guthrie, PhD[a,b,d,e,f,g]

KEYWORDS

• Autism spectrum disorder • Screening • Equity • Diagnosis • Artificial intelligence

KEY POINTS

- A variety of screening tools have been developed and tested to identify early signs of autism and aid in early recognition. However, despite long-standing guidance to screen universally for autism, the median age of autism spectrum disorder (ASD) diagnosis is substantially higher than the age at which ASD can reliably be diagnosed, suggesting room for improvements in autism recognition at young ages, when interventions are most beneficial.
- Concerns about screening equity persist with respect to screening completion, screening tool accuracy, and provider and family response to positive autism screens. These inequities may contribute to long-recognized racial, ethnic, income-based, and linguistic disparities in autism prevalence, age of diagnosis, and care.
- Novel approaches to screening through the identification of novel biomarkers, use of technology including artificial intelligence, and implementation of screening in non–health care settings show promise. However, attention to equity is needed to minimize bias in newly developed tools.
- Because no screener can rule out autism with complete accuracy, a child who presents with characteristics of autism should be referred for additional evaluation and intervention even when screens are negative. Conversely, even though many children with a positive screen may not meet criteria for autism, most children with a positive screen have developmental concerns that warrant follow-up care.

Continued

---

[a] Division of Developmental and Behavioral Pediatrics, Children's Hospital of Philadelphia, Philadelphia, PA, USA; [b] Department of Pediatrics, Perelman School of Medicine, University of Pennsylvania, Philadelphia, PA, USA; [c] PolicyLab, Children's Hospital of Philadelphia, Philadelphia, PA, USA; [d] Clinical Futures, Children's Hospital of Philadelphia, Philadelphia, PA, USA; [e] Center for Autism Research, Children's Hospital of Philadelphia, Philadelphia, PA, USA; [f] Department of Child and Adolescent Psychiatry and Behavioral Sciences, Children's Hospital of Philadelphia, Philadelphia, PA, USA; [g] Department of Psychiatry, Perelman School of Medicine, University of Pennsylvania, Philadelphia, PA, USA
* Corresponding author. Roberts Center for Pediatric Research, Room 5362, 2716 South Street, Philadelphia, PA 19146.
E-mail address: wallisk@chop.edu

Pediatr Clin N Am 71 (2024) 127–155
https://doi.org/10.1016/j.pcl.2023.12.003   pediatric.theclinics.com
0031-3955/24/© 2024 Elsevier Inc. All rights reserved.

Continued

- Additional research is needed to demonstrate the benefits and potential harms of universal autism screening. A review of these benefits and risks is being completed by the US Preventive Services Task Force (USPSTF), which may lead to a re-assessment of whether or not USPSTF supports universal autism screening.

INTRODUCTION TO AUTISM SCREENING

In service to the mantra, "the earlier the better," surveillance and screening for autism spectrum disorder (ASD)[a] are designed to support the identification of autism risk as early as possible, when early interventions can have the largest impact on attainment of skills. Although ASD can be diagnosed in children as young as 12 months,[1] the median age of ASD diagnosis remains above 4 years nationally (49 months in 2020).[2] Systematic processes to aid in the early identification of children with autism are imperative, which has led to increased focus on autism screening.

There are many steps along the pathway from identification of general developmental or autism-specific social communication and behavioral concerns, to screening, diagnosis, and accessing general developmental and autism-specific services and therapies. Surveillance refers to the process of systematically identifying risk and should occur within regular and routine health supervision. Surveillance can detect risk of general developmental delays, as well as specific signs of autism. The process of surveillance includes asking caregivers about concerns they have about their child's development or behavior; obtaining, documenting, and maintaining a developmental history; making observations of the child during the clinical visit; identifying risks, strengths, and protective factors; maintaining an accurate record of the surveillance process; and sharing and obtaining information with other professionals (such as child care providers, home visitors, and developmental therapists).[3] Risk factors for autism that can be identified include having a sibling with ASD or having a genetic or medical condition that is associated with autism (for example, Fragile-X or prematurity).[3]

Surveillance alone is not enough, and systematic, universal screening is an additional tool of prevention. A recent analysis of the National Surveys of Children's Health found that developmental monitoring with autism-specific screening, as reported by caregivers, was associated with early identification of autism,[4] as did multiple studies with large populations of children screened in primary care.[5,6]

Screening tools are designed to help identify and report symptoms observed in children who may be showing early signs of autism. Without the use of screening tools, clinical observation alone to detect autism risk has low sensitivity. For example, physician concern alone has an estimated sensitivity of 0.24 (95% CI: 0.17–0.32).[7] This is, in part, because children may not demonstrate signs of autism within a routine, brief clinic visit.[8] Therefore, the American Academy of Pediatrics (AAP) recommends universal screening for developmental delays,[3] as well as autism-specific screening for all young children at 18 and 24 months, regardless of risk factors or results of surveillance efforts. The AAP first issued guidance on early

---

[a] A note on terminology: Autistic self-advocates increasingly appear to prefer the term "autism" instead of autism spectrum disorder. Throughout the text, the authors use the term "autism" except when referring specifically to the diagnosis of autism spectrum disorder (ASD), as ASD is the term used in the Diagnostic and Statistical Manual of Mental Disorders (DSM-5).

identification for autism in 2007,[9] and guidelines were reissued in 2019,[10] which again re-iterated the importance of surveillance, universal screening, and early evaluation. While the AAP guidelines do not delineate between different types of screeners, 3 categories of screeners have been studied and used: broadband screeners ask about developmental milestones or behavioral symptoms; level 1 screeners identify risk in a low-risk, general population; and level 2 screeners can be used with populations already deemed to be at elevated risk for autism (as a result of positive level 1 screening, or other known risk factors).

While the AAP has endorsed screening, it should be noted that questions about the utility and effectiveness of autism screening remain. The US Preventive Services Task Force (USPSTF) released its systematic review and evidence synthesis on screening for autism in young children in 2016 (which included literature published through 2014). At that time, the USPSTF concluded that the evidence was insufficient to determine the harms and benefits of universal screening and that more evidence is needed to examine long-term outcomes for screened versus unscreened children. They also noted that data on the impact of early treatment on children identified through screening versus by usual detection methods was lacking, as was data on the harms of screening.[11] As of this writing, the USPSTF is undertaking a repeat review of the evidence.[12] As other researchers have pointed out, identifying which children are identified and access interventions as a result of universal screening, and which children are diagnosed as a result of caregiver-reported concern/developmental surveillance only, is an important step in considering the benefits and harms of universal screening.[13] Trials are currently undergoing that are attempting to fill these evidence gaps and to link autism-specific interventions to positive screening results.[14]

One of the challenges in screening for autism is that no clear biomarker for the condition has been identified to date that can detect the condition; as of yet, no blood test or physical examination finding that is specific to autism has been found, as there is for anemia or lead poisoning, for example, (although the authors describe in the following paragraphs some promising leads that may serve as screening biomarkers in the future). Therefore, screening tools are used to identify the developmental and specific behavioral features of autism. While general developmental screeners and milestones checklists may identify delays in other streams of development (eg, speech/language, gross and fine motor, cognitive/adaptive), autism-specific screening tools are based on early signs of differences in social communication, interaction, or play, and on the presence of restricted or repetitive behaviors or interests that comprise the core features of autism. It should also be noted that because signs of autism may become more apparent over time as social communication demands and expectations increase with age, children who screen negative or who are not initially diagnosed with autism should continue to be monitored and referred for (repeat) evaluation as appropriate.

Selecting a Screening Tool: Context Matters

As described earlier, there are 3 types of screening tools that have been tested and implemented. A broadband screener usually relies on caregivers to report on a child's behaviors and skills. Autism-specific screening tools can be classified as level 1 or level 2. Level 1 screeners are used universally to identify risk in a low-risk, general population, and many rely on caregiver report to identify features or risk factors. Level 1 screeners are usually what clinicians think about for implementation in primary care pediatrics. Level 2 screeners are deployed among populations already deemed to be at elevated risk for autism, either because of a positive screen at level 1 or a

		Autism Spectrum Disorder		
		Positive ASD Diagnosis	Negative ASD Diagnosis	
Screening Tool Result	Screening Tool Positive	A True Positive	B False Positive	Positive Predictive Value = A/A+B
	Screening Tool Negative	C False Negative	D True Negative	Negative Predictive Value = D/C+D
		Sensitivity = A/ A+C	Specificity = D/ B+D	

Fig. 1. Psychometric calculations of an autism screening tool.

condition that confers elevated risk. Many level 2 screeners are implemented by trained clinicians. Some primary care practices are using level 2 screeners to give a provisional or "best-estimate" ASD diagnosis to help children obtain services[15] In some settings, clinicians are specifically trained in administration of a level 2 screener and are allotted additional time in visits for performing this enhanced screening/diagnostic evaluation. These clinicians may be pediatricians with additional training in autism, or can include psychologists, speech-language pathologists, or other clinicians with training in the evaluation of autism and/or other neuro-developmental disabilities. As the subspecialty workforce of developmental-behavioral pediatricians and other diagnosticians stagnates,[16] there will be an increasing need for multi-disciplinary collaborations between primary care and autism diagnosticians to keep pace with the growing demand for autism evaluations.

When selecting a screening tool, primary care pediatricians should consider their clinical population as selection of a screening tool can be tailored depending on the clinical context. General pediatric practices will likely want to select a level 1 screener to implement in a universal manner. Other clinical settings serving children with higher levels of risk (for example, neonatal intensive care unit [NICU] follow-up clinics) might consider using level 2 screeners more frequently as a way to identify autism risk more specifically.

Clinicians should consider a tool's psychometric properties and the clinical population in which the tool is to be implemented. For example, if the pre-test probability of a child having autism is low (eg, the prevalence of autism is low in the given population), the screening tool will have lower ability to detect autism, in part due to the effect of the underlying population prevalence (base rate) on psychometric properties. Application of the same screening tool in a population with higher autism prevalence will have better functionality.[17] The relevant psychometric properties of a screening tool include the tool's sensitivity (the ability of the screener to identify all children with autism), specificity (the ability to correctly identify all children without autism), positive predictive value (the proportion of children with a positive screen who have autism), and negative predictive value (the likelihood that an individual with a negative screening result does not have autism). See Fig. 1 for graphic depiction of these values.

For practical reasons, many studies of screening tools are only able to follow children who screen positive and are unable to follow children who screen negative for autism; when accounting for this lack of complete follow-up, studies suggest lower accuracy for these tools than previously reported.[18] This makes it harder for a pediatric clinic implementing a screening program to understand the true accuracy of the tool. Importantly, it also highlights that individual clinicians should not minimize emerging signs of autism in a child who has previously screened negative; the negative screen should not outweigh caregiver or clinician concern, and the clinician should pursue diagnostic evaluation and intervention services, as appropriate.

There may be important reasons for clinical teams to decide to select a tool with different psychometric properties. For example, in some situations, it may be worthwhile to choose a tool with higher sensitivity, so that no children are incorrectly missed (false negatives). This may be the case in some primary care settings, where universal detection of risk is important to connect children with early intervention services. In others, the harms of falsely screening positive may be emphasized, and so a tool with higher specificity may be preferred. For example, in settings with fewer diagnostic or intervention resources, clinics may want to select a more specific tool to minimize unnecessary stress and anxiety while caregivers await evaluation. Thus, the clinical context and estimates of population risk level matter.

It is also critical for clinicians to consider the population that they intend to implement the screening tool in and assess how that compares to the population(s) that the tool has been validated in. For example, screening tools will perform differently in low-risk and high-risk populations,[19] and as noted earlier, the prevalence of autism in a population has strong effects on psychometric properties. In addition, performance of screening tools may also vary based on setting, geographic location, and whether the tool is administered universally or only to a selected subset of a population. Importantly, many screening tools have been validated in primarily White, higher-income samples, which do not represent the average child in this country. While clinics might think about using different tools with different populations based on differential estimates of risk and the socio-demographic characteristics of children in the practice, this is likely impractical in busy pediatric settings. There is evidence that combining tools and measures may improve the accuracy of screening.[20] However, the additional value compared to the burden must be weighed. A practice should select a screening tool that optimizes the psychometric characteristics that best meet clinical needs.

Various autism-specific screening tools have been used and validated for different ages. Some screeners have been found to identify autism risk in children as early as 12 months.[21] A systematic review of screening tools available for use in primary care was published in 2020,[22] many of which were also described in the AAP practice guidelines for identification of ASD.[10] The authors conducted a literature review to identify additional studies since the Levy and colleagues systematic review was published in 2020, to identify a comprehensive list of tools and updated validation studies. In **Table 1**, the authors included all papers published since 2020 that focus on screening tools developed and validated for North American-based populations. We discuss studies of screening tools in non-US countries and additional settings in the following paragraphs. The authors describe broad-band screeners with subscales examining ASD concerns, level 1 screeners, and level 2 screeners. The complete list of screening tools, characteristics, and published data on their psychometric properties appear in **Table 1**, followed by a discussion of some commonly used and promising tools. Across screening tools, there is wide heterogeneity in administration, tasks, time, and psychometric values, which can also help guide clinicians in selecting a feasible tool for their intended clinical population.

The Modified Checklist for Autism in Toddlers

While the authors present a variety of screening tools that practices may wish to consider for implementation, the most widely used and studied screening tool is the Modified Checklist for Autism in Toddlers (M-CHAT) along with its revised version (M-CHAT-R), and revised version with follow-up (M-CHAT-R/F).[7] It has more than

Table 1
Screening tools and characteristics

Tool	Description	Validated Age Range	Psychometric Properties	Notes/Keys References
Broadband Screeners				
Ages & Stages Questionnaires: Social Emotional, 2nd Edition (ASQ:SE)	Caregiver-completed questionnaires for specific age ranges (18, 24, 30, 36, 48 mo), social emotional subscale includes up to 9 items per age.	18–48 mo	Referred sample of 60 individuals used for validation, 37 with ASD. Estimated sensitivity among a referred sample is 1.00, and specificity is 0.96. (calculated by author KEW)	Dolata, Sanford-Keller, & Squires,[23] 2020
Child Behavior Checklist: 1½-5	Caregiver-completed questionnaire, broadband screener with subscale scores for pervasive development problems.	3–5 y	In a study of 2413 children, identified children with ASD (n = 656) from those with developmental delay or population controls with sensitivity 0.80, and specificity of 0.50–0.93 depending on comparison group.	Levy et al,[24] 2019
Infant/Toddler Checklist	Caregiver-completed questionnaire with 24 items that screens for language delay, estimated to take 15 min to complete	9–24 mo	5,385 children screened, and 978 participated in behavior samples. Positive and negative predictive values > 0.70 for all children > 9 mo.	Pierce et al,[25] 2011; A. M. Wetherby, Brosnan-Maddox, Peace, & Newton,[26] 2008
Level 1 Screeners				
Autism Spectrum Rating Scales	6-item caregiver-completed questionnaire.	6–18 y	Goldstein: Community sample of 201 children. Sensitivity estimated at 0.91, specificity 0.92,	Goldstein,[27] 2009; Hong et al,[28] 2022

Instrument	Description	Age	Findings	Reference
BABY-Baby and Infant Screen for Children with aUtIsm Traits BISCUIT	6-item caregiver-completed questionnaire based on a modified subset of items from BISCUIT.	17–39 mo	A sample of 504 high-risk infants and toddlers participating in early intervention were included, 17–39 mo. Sensitivity was estimated at 0.82, specificity of 0.96, positive predictive value (PPV) 0.92 and negative predictive value (NPV) 0.91. Hong et al: 490 children referred for evaluation. Using cutoff of 60, sensitivity estimated at 0.89, specificity 0.18, PPV 0.72, and NPV 0.394.	Matson et al,[29] 2022
Developmental Check-In	Caregiver-completed questionnaire that uses pictures instead of written descriptions of behavior with 28 photographs to reduce literacy demands.	24–60 mo	376 children, including high-risk children referred for developmental evaluation and 88 low-risk children recruited from community daycare centers (of whom 214 were diagnosed with ASD). Across groups, sensitivity was 0.66, sensitivity was 0.76.	Janvier et al,[30] 2019
Early Screening for Autism and	Caregiver-completed questionnaire with 47 items currently available	12–36 mo	Sample size = 471, sensitivity estimated between 0.86 and 0.92	Wetherby et al,[31] 2021

(continued on next page)

Table 1
(continued)

Communication Disorders		as a research tool, estimated to take 10–15 min to complete	and specificity estimated between 0.74 and 0.85.	
First-Year Inventory	12 mo	Caregiver-completed questionnaire with 63 items, estimated to take about 10 min to complete. Currently only available for research purposes.	Sample size = 96 infants, 71 of whom were at higher risk of ASD by having ASD in an older sibling. Psychometric values not reported.	Rowberry et al,[32] 2015
Modified Checklist for Autism in Toddlers, Revised with Follow-up (M-CHAT-R/F)	16–30 mo	Caregiver-completed questionnaire with 20 items, estimated to take 5–10 min to complete. A clinician-administered follow-up interview is required to reduce false-positive results. 80 versions available in >50 languages.	Pooled analysis across 51 samples including >277,000 children. Estimated Sensitivity Range 0.22 (95% CI 0.10–0.38) – 1.00 (95% CI 0.85–1.00); pooled estimate 0.83 (95% CI 0.77–0.88); Estimated Specificity Range 0.27 (95% CI 0.12–0.46) – 1.00 (95% CI 0.98–1.00); pooled estimate 0.94 (95% CI 0.89–0.97);	Systematic review and meta-analysis published in 2023, pooled psychometric values presented. Wieckowski et al,[19] 2023
Psychological Development Questionnaire-1	18–36 mo	Caregiver-completed questionnaire with 10 items, estimated to take about <2 min to complete, and <2 min to score.	Diverse, low-risk population of 2007 children screened. Sensitivity estimated at 0.85 and specificity at 0.99, PPV 0.88.	Zahorodny et al,[33] 2018

	Description	Age range	Evidence	References
Parent's Observations of Social Interactions	Caregiver-completed questionnaire with 7 items, estimated to take about 5 min to complete, included as part of the Survey of Well-being of Young Children	16–36 mo	Study 1: 217 children referred for developmental evaluation, aged 18–48 mo. Sensitivity estimated at 0.89, specificity 0.54. Study 2: 232 children in primary care and subspecialty settings aged 16–36 mo. Sensitivity estimated at 0.83, specificity 0.75.[34] Study 3: 524 children referred for developmental evaluation, aged 16–48 mo. Sensitivity estimated at 0.94 for 16–30 mo and 0.75 for 31–48 mo. Specificity estimated at 0.41 for 16–30 mo and 0.48 for 31–48 mo[35]	Salisbury et al,[34] 2018; Smith et al,[35] 2013
Social Communication Questionnaire (SCQ)	Caregiver-completed questionnaire with 40 items, estimated to take fewer than 10 min to complete	4 y or older, with estimated mental age of 2 y or more	590 children included. Sensitivity is reported as 0.71–0.78 and specificity is reported as 0.71.[36]	Snow,[37] 2013 Evans, Boan, Bradley, & Carpenter,[38] 2019
Level 2 Screeners				
Autism Detection in Early Childhood	Direct, play-based observational screening tool of 16 behaviors.	12–36 mo	Sample of 270 children, of whom 106 had ASD. Estimated sensitivity of	Nah et al,[39] 2019, Nevill et al,[40] 2019

(continued on next page)

Table 1
(continued)

	Administration takes about 10–15 min.		0.81, specificity of 0.78, positive predictive value of 0.81, and negative predictive value of 0.78.	
(BISCUIT)	A 3-component assessment battery, consisting of caregiver-completed questionnaire with 62 items in part 1, 71 items in part 2, and 17 items in part 3. Estimated to take about 20–30 min.	17–37 mo	Reported to have sensitivity of 0.93, specificity of 0.87, and PPV of 0.89.	Matson et al,[41] 2010
Evaluation of early social responsiveness (ESR)	4-minute, interactive assessment that provides a system for documenting real-time observations of early social responsiveness such as eye contact, smiling, pointing across 5 play activities. Instructions are given and behaviors are scored at the time of administration of the task	13–24 mo	Study included 157 children. Sensitivity ranged 0.77–0.91, specificity ranged 0.83–0.93, PPV ranged 0.08–0.83, and NPV ranged from 0.096–0.998.	Factor et al,[42] 2022

Tool	Description	Age	Findings	Reference
Rapid Interactive Screening Test for Autism in Toddlers	Clinician-administered interactive observation measure with 9 items, which requires clinician training for administration, estimated to take 20–30 min to complete	12–36 mo	61 toddlers assessed, 23 of whom received ASD diagnosis and 19 who received a diagnosis of another developmental delay. Sensitivity 0.96, specificity 0.84, PPV 0.88, NPV 0.94.	Choueiri & Wagner,[43] 2015 Choueiri et al,[44] 2021
Systematic Observation of Red Flags	Naturalistic video-recorded home observation measure with 22 items, which included written and verbal instructions to caregivers to interact with their children in everyday activities.	18–24 mo	Study included 228 toddlers, of whom 84 were diagnosis with ASD and 82 with developmental delay. Estimated sensitivity of 0.77, specificity of 0.72, PPV of 0.62, and NPV of 0.84.	Dow et al,[45] 2020
Screening Tool for Autism in Toddlers and Young Children (STAT)	Clinician-directed, interactive observation measure with 12 items, which requires clinician training for administration, estimated to take about 20 min to complete.	24–35 mo	52 children deemed at risk. Estimated sensitivity of 0.92, specificity of 0.85, PPV 0.86, NPV 0.92.	Stone et al,[46] 2000; Stone et al,[47] 2004
Toddler Autism Symptom Inventory	Semi-structured caregiver interview with 37 items and a table designed to assess the presence and absence of skills and symptoms, including sensory differences, which takes about 40 min to administer and score.	12–36 mo	336 interviews were completed. Sensitivity was estimated at 0.89 and specificity at 0.68–0.81 (across 2 samples).	Coulter et al,[48] 2021

80 versions available in more than 50 languages (https://mchatscreen.com/). One reason for the widespread usage of the M-CHAT and its related versions is that it is fairly easy to implement, relying on caregivers to answer 20 yes/no questions about their child's skills and behaviors. While the tool's sensitivity has been found to vary across studies, this tool is appealing to practices because use of the follow-up interview can reduce the false-positive rate and thus improve the tool's specificity[22]; the follow-up interview for positive questionnaires added nearly 8 times the diagnostic accuracy.[49]

However, a recent meta-analysis noted significant variation in psychometrics across individual studies.[19] As noted earlier, the M-CHAT(-R)/F's psychometric values (positive predictive value [PPV] and negative predictive value [NPV]) vary based on the population prevalence of autism within the studied cohort. Additionally, the ability to calculate critical psychometric properties (sensitivity, specificity, and NPV) depends upon the ability to follow up on autism diagnostic outcomes for all children—those who screen negative as well as those who screen positive. To that end, studies that report on clinical samples rather than research samples tend to have lower estimates of screening accuracy as they also report on false- negative screens and do not benefit from research support to facilitate and confirm diagnoses for screen-positive populations.[5,6] This highlights the challenge and importance of evaluating real-world practice.[50] Furthermore, numerous studies have found that repeated screening (eg, at both 18 and 24 months) can improve the sensitivity of the screener, such that children who screen negative at 18 months may screen positive and be detected at 24 months.[21,51]

The M-CHAT-R/F remains a widely used tool, and it is feasible to implement in a busy clinic's workflow. It is often embedded into a clinic's electronic health record (EHR). Given that overhauling the EHR is a monumental task, the M-CHAT-R/F is unlikely to be quickly replaced without strong evidence for alternative tools.

CONSIDERATIONS FOR OTHER SCREENING TOOLS

While the authors developed **Table 1** to be inclusive of published studies, it is worth noting that to the authors' knowledge, few if any primary care pediatric practices have chosen to use broadband screeners alone to identify autism risk. These tools are sometimes used as part of a larger battery of tools to generally identify needs (for example, other developmental or behavioral concerns) that warrant additional attention.

From **Table 1**, several additional level 1 screening tools are worth highlighting. The Parent Observations of Social Interactions (POSI) is a shorter, 7-item tool based on the M-CHAT. Generally, the tool's sensitivity is high (but it is less specific than other tools), so clinics may consider implementing the POSI as a quick tool that can identify elevated risk of autism to help connect children with intervention services as quickly as posisble.[34,35]

An additional tool worth highlighting is the Developmental Check-In (DCI). While the DCI is newer and has not yet been widely implemented or studied, this pictorial-based tool shows promise for families with lower literacy levels. The pictures depict target behaviors to help reduce literacy demands.[30,52] If evidence accrues for its accuracy, practices may consider broader use of the DCI.

Some tools, such as the social communication questionnaire (SCQ), have been used in subspecialty clinics to help elicit additional information about autism concerns, including by having teachers and other specialists share information about their observations of the child.[37,38] However, few, if any, primary care practices are using the SCQ universally, in part, because forms must be purchased from a publisher.

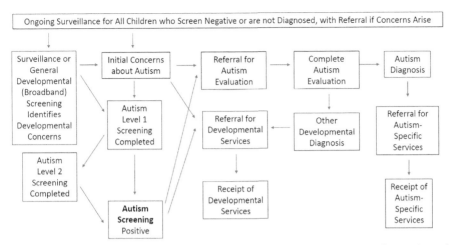

Fig. 2. Steps along the process of autism spectrum disorder (ASD) screening, diagnosis, and service access.

Most other level 1 tools listed in **Table 1** have only been used or tested in select populations. To the authors' knowledge, many of these tools have not been implemented widely in primary care settings at this time and would need further testing before they are considered. As noted earlier, level 2 tools are generally not appropriate for widespread use in primary care settings, but workflows to use level 2 tools with higher risk populations can be considered and adopted as appropriate with training and additional time and resources.

SCREENING PROCESSES AND ADHERENCE TO GUIDELINES

Over time, rates of screening for young children have increased significantly.[53] Nonetheless, barriers to screening remain, including related to ongoing provider knowledge of screening recommendations and self-efficacy related to how to screen.[54] A variety of strategies to support screening uptake, completion, and actions have been developed. For example, training providers and using electronic versions of screening tools can support provider implementation of screening.[5,55–58]

Screening is a unique process from diagnosis. Therefore, once a child is determined to be at risk for a diagnosis of ASD, timely referral for a diagnostic evaluation and for early intervention is indicated. Additional steps along the screening, referral, and diagnostic evaluation process can impact diagnostic rates and care for children who ultimately meet criteria for ASD (**Fig. 2**).[59] For example, many children with a positive screen in primary care are not ultimately referred for diagnostic evaluation or early intervention (EI), limiting the utility of the screening tool.[60–62] The reasons for these non-referrals are numerous. Many clinicians describe factors that impact their ability to identify and provide care for children with autism risk including family factors, reluctance to discuss autism with families, frustration with navigating multiple care systems, feeling of disempowerment from acting upon concerns about autism, long wait times for diagnostic evaluations, limited time in primary care visits, and limited knowledge about autism-related care systems.[63]

Nonetheless, current evidence demonstrates that screening tools have been shown to increase connection with EI for children at risk in a timely fashion.[64] Family navigators and parent partners have been used to further this goal of connecting children with appropriate services, but with somewhat mixed results.[65,66] Research studies that have boosted coordination within systems to support the connection between screening and community providers of autism-specific services are promising.[67–69] Addressing what clinicians can do upon having a patient screen positive—through the provision of a standard set of recommendations and resources to families—is an integral part of screening program implementation.

SCREENING AT-RISK POPULATIONS

As described earlier, screening high-risk populations (those with higher prevalence of autism and thus higher pre-test probability) is more likely to yield positive results and thus have higher estimates of sensitivity and PPV.[17] Many screening tools are therefore initially developed and evaluated in high-risk populations, including infant siblings of children with an ASD diagnosis,[70–74] infants with prematurity or neonatal intensive care history,[75] and children with other medical diagnoses (eg, neonatal encephalopathy).[76] Some studies of younger siblings have examined screening and identification of early signs in children as young as 9 months.[77,78] Studies of very young high-risk children seek to aid in identification of reliable, early signs of autism. However, the extent to which the results of studies of tools developed in high-risk populations generalize to lower risk groups needs further attention. Some high-risk settings, such as NICU follow-up,[79] genetic, or neurodevelopmental clinics for children with critical congenital heart disease,[80,81] where children have higher rates of developmental delays and other neuro-developmental disabilities, might consider using level 2 screeners as a way to identify autism risk more rapidly and specifically. Some very high-risk clinical settings may bypass screening entirely and consider more universal diagnostic assessments; however, the resources for implementing evaluations at scale are substantial.

SCREENING TOOLS USED IN GLOBAL CONTEXTS

Autism is present in all cultures. As such, attention to early identification of autism through screening is not purely a US endeavor. However, there may be variability in the differences with which core features of autism manifest or are recognized across cultures, which suggests that screening tools may need to be tailored to particular populations and cultural contexts.[82] For example, a recent analysis of the M-CHAT in 10 countries found differences in frequency of item endorsement, although items related to joint attention, social engagement, and language comprehension were more similarly endorsed across countries.[83] Nonetheless, screening and identification of developmental disorders and autism are critical as a first step toward quantifying and addressing the need for services for children across the globe, including in low-income and middle-income countries (LMIC). A recent review identified 6 promising tools for screening for autism in LMIC.[84] The authors reviewed literature published since that review was completed and identified a number of studies examining ASD screening in non-US countries. In **Table 2**, the authors list the countries, regions, or languages in which the study took place, and the screening tools used. Many of the screening tools studied in global settings are the same tools from **Table 1**, some of which were modified or adapted. Screening tools need to be continuously adapted to specific populations and contexts, and rigorously evaluated to ensure they function appropriately in the intended population before widespread implementation. Given the multi-ethnic and multi-cultural populations served by many North American clinics, recognizing that additional tools have been developed and/or validated in other countries may offer clinics considerations for adopting additional tools to better serve some immigrant populations.

Table 2
Studies examining autism spectrum disorder screening in countries outside of North America

Country/Region/ Language	Screening Tool Name(s)	References
Arabic (Qatar and Saudi Arabia)	Arabic version of the SCQ	Aldosari et al,[85] 2019
Australia	Social Attention and Communication Surveillance (SACS) tool	Barbaro et al,[86] 2022; Barbaro and Yaari[87] 2020
	Social Attention and Communication Surveillance-Revised (SACS-R)	
	SACS-Preschool (SACS-PR)	
	Autism Observation Scale for Infants (AOSI)	Hudry et al,[88] 2021
Chile	Modified Checklist for Autism in Toddlers, Revised with Follow-Up (M-CHAT-R/F)	Coelho-Medeiros etal,[89] 2019
China	Autism-Spectrum Quotient-Child	Wong[90] 2021
	Autism-Spectrum Quotient-Adolescent	
	Chinese Parent Version of the Autism Spectrum Rating Scale	Yan et al,[91] 2021
	Chinese Version of Autism Spectrum Rating Scale	Zhou et al,[92] 2019
	Chinese Version of Modified Checklist for Autism in Toddlers, Revised with Follow-Up (M-CHAT-R/F)	Guo et al,[93] 2019
	Chinese Version of the SCQ	Liu et al,[94] 2022
	First Year Inventory	Li[95] 2019
Colombia	Qualitative Checklist for Autism in Toddlers (Q-CHAT)	Gutiérrez-Ruiz[96] 2019
French	Autism Discriminative Tool (ADT)	Carlier et al,[97] 2019
	French Version of the Social Responsiveness Scale (SRS)	
Georgia	Autism Spectrum Screening Questionnaire (ASSQ)	Zirakashvili et al,[98] 2022
Iceland	Modified Checklist for Autism in Toddlers, Revised with Follow-up (M-CHAT-R/F)	Jonsdottir[99] 2022
Iran	Modified Checklist for Autism in Toddlers (M-CHAT)	Faraji Goodarzi[100] 2019
	Quantitative Checklist for Autism in Toddlers (Q-CHAT)	Mohammadi[101] 2020
Iraq	Gilliam Autism Rating Scale-3 (GARS-3)	Samadi et al,[102] 2022; Samadi et al,[103] 2022
Israel	Global Developmental Screening (GDS)	Kerub[104] 2020
	Modified Checklist for Autism in Toddlers, Revised with Follow-up (M-CHAT-R/F)	

(continued on next page)

Table 2 (continued)		
Country/Region/ Language	Screening Tool Name(s)	References
Italy	Quantitative Checklist for Autism in Toddlers (Q-CHAT)	Ruta et al,[105] 2019; Rutaa et al,[106] 2019
Kerala, India	Concern-9	Babu et al,[107] 2022
Morocco	Modified Checklist for Autism in Toddlers, Revised with Follow-up (M-CHAT-R/F) in Moroccan Arabic dialect	Tabril et al,[108] 2023
South Korea	Behavior Development Screening for Toddlers	Bong et al,[109] 2019; Bongetal et al,[110] 2021
Spain	Modified Checklist for Autism in Toddlers, Revised (M-CHAT-R)	Magán-Maganto et al,[111] 2020
Taiwan	Child Behavior Checklist	Iao[112] 2020
	Screening Tool for Autism in Two-Year-Olds	Wu et al,[113] 2021; Wu et al,[114] 2020
	Modified Checklist for Autism in Toddlers, Revised with Follow-Up (M-CHAT-R/F)	Tsai et al,[115] 2019
Turkey	Modified Checklist for Autism in Toddlers, Revised with Follow-Up (M-CHAT-R/F)	Oner and Munir[116] 2020
Vietnamese	Modified Checklist for Autism in Toddlers, Revised with Follow-Up- (M-CHAT-R/F) Vietnamese	HyeKyeung[117] 2022
	Social Responsiveness Scale (SRS)	Nguyen et al,[118] 2019

DISCUSSION
Equity Issues Related to Screening

As noted earlier, the fact that many tools developed in the United States have been adapted for use in different populations internationally is evidence of the need for cultural adaptation. Nonetheless, across the United States, populations are diverse and culturally varied, and may have different developmental expectations, preferences, caregiving structures, languages, and health literacy. Finding a screening tool that accounts for this abundant diversity with sufficient accuracy to identify autism can be challenging. While some screening tools are linguistically translated, few if any have undergone a rigorous cultural adaptation process that would be needed to account for some of this variety.[119]

Autism-screening tools are developed, tested, and validated in particular samples (often convenience samples), which may not be representative of the broader population. Thus, screening tools developed in one sample are likely to have different performance when applied to distinct populations. For example, subsequent testing in real-world, racially-diverse and ethnically-diverse samples identified that the M-CHAT-R/F performs less well among non-White populations and children from lower-income families.[5,6] However, other studies have found fewer differences in psychometric properties among Black and White children[120] and among White, Black, and Latine children.[121] (This latter study did find that there were item-level differences across groups, but no differences in overall results across the test.)

Among populations who prefer a language other than English (PLOE), screening rates and accuracy have also been found to be lower.[6] A review of autism-screening tools used in Spanish-speaking populations similarly found that sensitivity was lower in the Spanish versions of these tools.[122] Ongoing efforts to improve the reliability of autism-screening tools for PLOE families are needed. Despite the ongoing need for cultural adaptation of many screening tools,[119] linguistic translation alone is important as screening a child directly in a family's preferred language is associated with higher likelihood of being diagnosed with autism among children who screen positive.[123] Thus, both linguistic translation and cultural adaptation of tools are needed to improve screening accuracy and accessibility.

The challenge of screening children from populations who have historically been under-represented in studies does not diminish the importance of screening among these groups. Instead, clinicians should be alert to the possibility that using tools that have not been specifically tested or validated may differentially identify autism in children from these groups. Therefore, clinicians should use their own judgment when responding to screening, especially when they have concerns that are not being detected on a screen (false negative). However, clinicians should be cautious when overriding screening results because of the difficulty in identifying autism in brief clinical encounters and the possibility that implicit biases in which White boys have long been considered more likely to have autism may lead to under-recognition of autism in non-White children and girls.[124]

In addition to screening tool performance and accuracy among certain populations, these same populations (children from minoritized racial and ethnic groups, lower-income, and from families with PLOE) also appear less likely to be screened in routine clinical care.[5,6] When they are screened and have a positive result, they are less likely to be referred for additional evaluation and intervention than children from White, higher-income, and English-speaking families.[62] These inequities in screening completion, screening tool accuracy, and response to positive autism screens may contribute to long-recognized racial, ethnic, income-based, and linguistic disparities in autism prevalence, age of diagnosis,[125–128] and care.[129] Thus, increasing equity in autism-screening processes is of critical importance as we seek to close those gaps.

Another group that requires additional attention with respect to autism screening is older children (>36 months) as screening tools that have been validated for older children are lacking.[130] This is an important concern that may contribute to worsening disparities among minoritized racial and ethnic groups, as children who identify as Black, Latine, or Asian tend to come to clinical attention later than their White peers,[126] at older ages when there are fewer validated screening tools available to aid in recognition of autistic features. Some researchers have tried to expand the upward the age of screening, including in school-based settings.[131] Others have argued that continuing to screen older preschool children is important to ensure that children who are missed at younger ages have the opportunity to be identified.[130] At this time, two tools have been used in older populations, with the Autism Spectrum Rating Scales approved for use up to age 18[27,28] and the SCQ used for individuals 4 years or older.[37,38]

Family Impacts of Screening

While early identification of autism has been valued as a worthwhile goal, autism screening is not without potential harms that should also be acknowledged and accounted for. Research that identifies potential harms of screening is recommended by the USPSTF review.[11] Harms of screening may include physical, psychological, social, logistical/financial, opportunity costs, attrition, and exacerbation of disparities.[132]

The harm of having a child falsely screen positive may increase parental stress. However, it should be noted that even among children who screen positive and are not diagnosed with autism, the large majority (78%–95%) are diagnosed with another developmental delay that would also merit clinical attention.[6,7] Parents do perceive this as a benefit of the tool. For example, a qualitative study of caregivers of a child who falsely screened positive for autism reported that the screening and evaluation process was still beneficial in that caregivers increased their knowledge, had concerns validated, and improved their child's connection with needed services. However, wait times for developmental evaluation resulted in anxiety.[133] Additional qualitative work examining families' experiences in screening identified that engagement in the process helped sensitize them to recognize autism symptoms, use an autism diagnosis to understand their child's behavior, and engage in shared decision-making.[134]

Potential harms of screening should continue to be evaluated and addressed, and attention paid to processes and information that may minimize those concerns. For example, minimizing false-positive screens, such as through more consistent administration of M-CHAT Follow-Up Interview items, may help reduce unnecessary anxiety for children without autism or developmental risk.

Novel Approaches to Autism Screening

To this point, most of the referenced studies evaluate screening tools that rely on caregiver report and/or clinical observation. Novel tools that rely on assessment of biomarkers or use novel technologies and/or artificial intelligence (AI) are being developed and tested. For example, a study reports on identification of abrupt head circumference acceleration and the absence of the head tilt reflex by 9 months as a biomarker that can identify children at risk of autism.[135] Multiple tools are under development that use features such as eye-tracking or gaze-monitoring,[136–140] analysis of cry or vocal characteristics,[141,142] or AI[143–147] to improve autism detection in young ages. Tools that rely on objective measurement may help improve equity of ASD diagnosis by bypassing human implicit biases. However, as with all AI technology, biased data inputs can produce biased results, and so particular attention to training AI on diverse samples is needed to achieve equity.[148]

Novel Locations for Screening

While pediatric primary care settings are considered highly accessible and one of the places in which to "capture" the highest number of young children, we are increasingly recognizing that some children may still be missed by limiting screening to health care settings. To better meet the needs of some children and families, researchers and autism care providers are looking to additional locations at which to conduct screening to better identify children. For example, early childcare providers and preschools,[52,149,150] as well as elementary schools[131] are being considered as additional sites for autism screening. To better meet family's diverse and varied needs, some researchers are looking outside of educational settings to settings such as Special Supplemental Nutrition Program for Women, Infants, and Children (WIC) offices.[151] Novel approaches and processes are needed to continue to promote equity in autism identification.

Incorporating Universal Screening into Primary Care Practices

As recommended by the AAP, universal screening for autism aims to identify risk and connect families with services and supports as early as possible. A team-based approach including members of the clinical office at all levels—from schedulers, front desk staff, medical assistants, nurses, and clinicians—has been effective with practices that have implemented universal screening programs.[152] It is important to develop buy-in across the enterprise to recognize the resources, time, and continuous training and monitoring that will be needed to successfully implement a screening program.

In addition to selecting a level 1 tool, the team must consider how the screen will be delivered (on paper or electronically?), when (before the visit, in the waiting room, while obtaining patient vitals?), and by whom (front desk staff, medical staff, etc.?). Can the tool be integrated into EHR systems, in a way that can facilitate caregiver completion, scoring, and flagging for clinicians? Additionally, team members must be assigned to ensure the screen is complete, collect paper screens, score the screening tool (if not done electronically), and determine how families will be notified of the result. The clinical team must develop a process for how to uniformly respond to positive screens, and so should have processes in place to facilitate referral to early intervention and for autism diagnostic evaluations.

Lastly, teams must consider how they are going to monitor these processes; often quality improvement approaches can assist with identifying opportunities to boost completion and appropriate follow-up or referral.[57] An essential component of these quality improvement initiatives should be to disaggregate data by race, ethnicity, family language, and socio-economic status to ensure that processes are being implemented in an equitable manner that do not introduce or contribute to the widening of disparities.

Individual clinicians should take some additional considerations into account when engaging in autism screening. Given the variability in screening tools' performance even under optimal circumstances (eg, in supported research settings), clinicians should use screening not only as a way to identify autism risk, but to engage families in conversations about child developmental and autism specifically. Clinicians should consider the possibility that a screen may under-identify or over-identify autism risk in a particular child; false-positive and false- negative results may be more likely in traditionally under-diagnosed populations, including girls, non-White children, and children from families who speak languages other than English. Importantly, even when a screening tool does not accurately identify autism, the vast majority (89% across studies[153]) of children with a positive screen are found to have other developmental delays that warrant attention. Therefore, clinicians may still be appropriate in recommending developmental services and/or additional evaluation to support patients' vast developmental needs.

SUMMARY

Over the last nearly 20 years since the AAP first issued guidance recommending universal screening for autism in pediatric primary care, screening rates and autism prevalence estimates have greatly increased.[125] However, given that the median age of autism diagnosis remains much higher than the usual recognition of first signs of autism (especially among minoritized racial and ethnic groups, low-income children, and those from families who prefer a language other than English), additional work is needed to promote equity in autism identification. Novel screening approaches are being developed, but reliance on technology will require ongoing attention to ensure bias is not perpetuated. As we await publication of the repeat comprehensive, systematic review and pursuant guidance by the USPSTF, children and families are in need of ongoing support, attention, and services to address autism-related concerns. Screening is just one piece of that puzzle.

CLINICS CARE POINTS

- Ongoing developmental surveillance to identify developmental and ASD concerns should take place in all clinical visits.
- Screening for autism should occur whenever there is concern identified and routinely at 18 and 24 months as part of primary care practice for all children.
- A variety of screening tools have been developed and tested to identify early signs of autism and aid in early recognition. These include broadband screeners, level 1 tools (that usually rely on caregiver report), and level 2 tools (that usually utilize clinical observation and are designed to be used after risk has been identified).
- Selection of a screening tool should be tailored depending on the clinical context and population, including the prevalence of autism in the intended population, how it is administered, and psychometric properties of the tool.
- Despite long-standing guidance to screen for autism, the median age of autism diagnosis is higher than the age at which autism can reliably be diagnosed, suggesting room for improvements in autism recognition at young ages, when interventions are most beneficial.
- Concerns about screening equity persist with respect to screening completion, screening tool accuracy, and response to positive autism screens. These inequities may contribute to long-recognized racial, ethnic, income-based, and linguistic disparities in autism prevalence, age of diagnosis, and care.
- Novel approaches to screening through the identification of biomarkers, use of technology including AI, and implementation of screening in non–health care settings show promise. However, as new screening methods are developed, attention to equity is needed to minimize bias.
- Additional research is needed to demonstrate the benefits and potential harms of universal autism screening. A review of these benefits and risks is being completed by the USPSTF, which may lead to a re-assessment of whether or not USPSTF supports universal autism screening.

ACKNOWLEDGMENTS

The authors would like to thank Jennifer Lege-Matsuura, MSLIS, AHIP, medical research librarian at University of Pennsylvania Libraries for assisting with literature review.

DISCLOSURE

No financial disclosures.

REFERENCES

1. Pierce K, Gazestani VH, Bacon E, et al. Evaluation of the diagnostic stability of the early autism spectrum disorder phenotype in the general population starting at 12 months. JAMA Pediatr 2019;173(6):578–87.
2. Maenner MJ, Warren Z, Williams AR, et al. Prevalence and characteristics of autism spectrum disorder among children aged 8 years - autism and developmental disabilities monitoring network, 11 sites, united states, 2020. Morb Mortal Wkly Rep - Surveillance Summ 2023;72(2):1–14.
3. Lipkin PH, Macias MM, COUNCIL ON CHILDREN WITH DISABILITIES, SECTION ON DEVELOPMENTAL AND BEHAVIORAL PEDIATRICS. Promoting optimal development: identifying infants and young children with developmental

disorders through developmental surveillance and screening. Pediatrics 2020; 145(1):e20193449.

4. Barger B, Rice C, Benevides T, et al. Are developmental monitoring and screening better together for early autism identification across race and ethnic groups? J Autism Dev Disord 2022;52(1):203–18.

5. Carbone PS, Campbell K, Wilkes J, et al. Primary care autism screening and later autism diagnosis. Pediatrics 2020;e20192314. https://doi.org/10.1542/peds.2019-2314.

6. Guthrie W, Wallis K, Bennett A, et al. Accuracy of autism screening in a large pediatric network. Pediatrics 2019;144(4). https://doi.org/10.1542/peds.2018-3963.

7. Robins DL, Casagrande K, Barton M, et al. Validation of the modified checklist for Autism in toddlers, revised with follow-up (M-CHAT-R/F). Pediatrics 2014; 133(1):37–45.

8. Gabrielsen TP, Farley M, Speer L, et al. Identifying autism in a brief observation. Pediatrics 2015;135(2):e330–8.

9. Johnson CP, Myers SM, American Academy of Pediatrics Council on Children With Disabilities. Identification and evaluation of children with autism spectrum disorders. Pediatrics 2007;120(5):1183–215.

10. Hyman SL, Levy SE, Myers SM, et al. Identification, evaluation, and management of children with autism spectrum disorder. Pediatrics 2019;e20193447. https://doi.org/10.1542/peds.2019-3447.

11. McPheeters M, Weitlauf A, Vehorn A, et al. Screening for autism spectrum disorder in young children: a systematic evidence review for the u.s. preventive services task force. Vol. AHRQ Publication No. 13-05185-EF-1. 2016:691-6. 0098-7484. Feb 16. https://doi.org/10.1001/jama.2016.0018

12. Final Research Plan: Screening for autism spectrum disorder in young children. Accessed July 17, 2021. https://uspreventiveservicestaskforce.org/uspstf/document/final-research-plan/autism-spectrum-disorder-young-children-1

13. Hickey E, Sheldrick RC, Kuhn J, et al. A commentary on interpreting the United States preventive services task force autism screening recommendation statement. Autism: The International Journal of Research and Practice 2021;25(2): 588–92.

14. McClure LA, Lee NL, Sand K, et al. Connecting the Dots: a cluster-randomized clinical trial integrating standardized autism spectrum disorders screening, high-quality treatment, and long-term outcomes. Trials 2021;22(1):319.

15. McNally Keehn R, Swigonski N, Enneking B, et al. Diagnostic accuracy of primary care clinicians across a statewide system of autism evaluation. Pediatrics 2023. https://doi.org/10.1542/peds.2023-061188.

16. Bridgemohan C, Bauer NS, Nielsen BA, et al. A workforce survey on developmental-behavioral pediatrics. Pediatrics 2018;141(3):e20172164.

17. Groen WB, Swinkels SH, van der Gaag RJ, et al. Finding effective screening instruments for autism using bayes theorem. Arch Pediatr Adolesc Med 2007; 161(4):415–6.

18. Sheldrick RC, Hooker JL, Carter AS, et al. The influence of loss to follow-up in autism screening research: Taking stock and moving forward. J Child Psychol Psychiatry Allied Discip 2023. https://doi.org/10.1111/jcpp.13867.

19. Wieckowski AT, Williams LN, Rando J, et al. Sensitivity and specificity of the modified checklist for autism in toddlers (original and revised): a systematic review and meta-analysis. JAMA Pediatr 2023. https://doi.org/10.1001/jamapediatrics.2022.5975.

20. Christopher K, Bishop S, Carpenter LA, et al. The implications of parent-reported emotional and behavioral problems on the modified checklist for autism in toddlers. J Autism Dev Disord 2021;51(3):884–91.

21. Wieckowski AT, Hamner T, Nanovic S, et al. Early and repeated screening detects autism spectrum disorder. J Pediatr 2021;234:227–35.

22. Levy SE, Wolfe A, Coury D, et al. Screening tools for autism spectrum disorder in primary care: a systematic evidence review. Pediatrics. Apr 2020;145(Suppl 1): S47–59.

23. Dolata JK, Sanford-Keller H, Squires J. Modifying a general social-emotional measure for early autism screening. Int J Dev Disabil 2020;66(4):296–303.

24. Levy SE, Rescorla LA, Chittams JL, et al. ASD screening with the child behavior checklist/1.5-5 in the study to explore early development. J Autism Dev Disord 2019;49(6):2348–57.

25. Wetherby AM, Brosnan-Maddox S, Peace V, et al. Validation of the Infant-Toddler Checklist as a broadband screener for autism spectrum disorders from 9 to 24 months of age. Autism : The International Journal of Research and Practice 2008;12(5):487–511.

26. Pierce K, Carter C, Weinfeld M, et al. Detecting, studying, and treating autism early: the one-year well-baby check-up approach. J Pediatr 2011;159(3): 458–65, e1-6.

27. Hong JS, Perrin J, Singh V, et al. Psychometric evaluation of the autism spectrum rating scales (6–18 years parent report) in a clinical sample. J Autism Dev Disord 2022/12/26 2022. https://doi.org/10.1007/s10803-022-05871-x.

28. Goldstein S, & Naglieri, J. A. . Autism Spectrum Rating Scales (ASRS™). . 2009.

29. Matson JL, Callahan MM, Montrenes JJ. Development and initial testing of the BABY-BISCUIT in an at-risk population. Dev Neurorehabil. Aug 2022;25(6):361–9.

30. Janvier YM, Coffield CN, Harris JF, et al. The Developmental Check-In: Development and initial testing of an autism screening tool targeting young children from underserved communities. Autism : The International Journal of Research and Practice 2019;23(3):689–98.

31. Wetherby AM, Guthrie W, Hooker JL, et al. The early screening for autism and communication disorders: field-testing an autism-specific screening tool for children 12 to 36 months of age. Autism : The International Journal of Research and Practice 2021. https://doi.org/10.1177/13623613211012526. 13623613211012526.

32. Rowberry J, Macari S, Chen G, et al. Screening for autism spectrum disorders in 12-month-old high-risk siblings by parental report. J Autism Dev Disord 2015; 45(1):221–9.

33. Zahorodny W, Shenouda J, Mehta U, et al. Preliminary evaluation of a brief autism screener for young children. J Dev Behav Pediatr : JDBP (J Dev Behav Pediatr) 2018;39(3):183–91.

34. Smith NJ, Sheldrick RC, Perrin EC. An abbreviated screening instrument for autism spectrum disorders. Infant Ment Health J 2013;34(2):149–55.

35. Salisbury LA, Nyce JD, Hannum CD, et al. Sensitivity and specificity of 2 autism screeners among referred children between 16 and 48 months of age. J Dev Behav Pediatr : JDBP. Apr 2018;39(3):254–8.

36. Corsello C, Hus V, Pickles A, et al. Between a ROC and a hard place: decision making and making decisions about using the SCQ. J Child Psychol Psychiatry Allied Discip 2007;48(9):932–40.

37. Snow A. Social communication questionnaire. In: Volkmar FR, editor. Encyclopedia of autism spectrum disorders. New York: Springer; 2013. p. 2893–5.

38. Evans SC, Boan AD, Bradley C, et al. Sex/gender differences in screening for autism spectrum disorder: implications for evidence-based assessment. J Clin Child Adolesc Psychol 2019;48(6):840–54.
39. Nah YH, Young RL, Brewer N. Development of a brief version of the Autism Detection in Early Childhood. Autism: The International Journal of Research and Practice 2019;23(2):494–502.
40. Nevill RE, Hedley D, Uljarević M. Brief report: replication and validation of the brief autism detection in early childhood (BADEC) in a clinical sample. J Autism Dev Disord 2019;49(11):4674–80.
41. Matson JL, Boisjoli JA, Hess JA, et al. Factor structure and diagnostic fidelity of the Baby and Infant Screen for Children with aUtIsm Traits–Part 1 (BISCUIT–part 1). Dev Neurorehabil 2010/01/01 2010;13(2):72–9.
42. Factor RS, Arriaga RI, Morrier MJ, et al. Development of an interactive tool of early social responsiveness to track autism risk in infants and toddlers. Dev Med Child Neurol 2022;64(3):323–30.
43. Choueiri R, Wagner S. A new interactive screening test for autism spectrum disorders in toddlers. J Pediatr 2015;167(2):460–6.
44. Choueiri R, Lindenbaum A, Ravi M, et al. Improving Early Identification and Access to Diagnosis of Autism Spectrum Disorder in Toddlers in a Culturally Diverse Community with the Rapid Interactive screening Test for Autism in Toddlers. J Autism Dev Disord 2021;51(11):3937–45.
45. Dow D, Day TN, Kutta TJ, et al. Screening for autism spectrum disorder in a naturalistic home setting using the systematic observation of red flags (SORF) at 18-24 months. Autism Res 2020;13(1):122–33.
46. Stone WL, Coonrod EE, Turner LM, et al. Psychometric properties of the STAT for early autism screening. J Autism Dev Disord 2004;34(6):691–701.
47. Stone WL, Coonrod EE, Ousley OY. Brief report: screening tool for autism in two-year-olds (STAT): development and preliminary data. J Autism Dev Disord 2000; 30(6):607–12.
48. Coulter KL, Barton ML, Boorstein H, et al. The Toddler Autism Symptom Inventory: Use in diagnostic evaluations of toddlers. Autism : The International Journal of Research and Practice 2021;25(8):2386–99.
49. Lipkin PH. Screening Success in the Age of Autism. JAMA Pediatr 2023. https://doi.org/10.1001/jamapediatrics.2022.5972.
50. Wallis KE, Guthrie W. Identifying Autism Spectrum Disorder in Real-World Health Care Settings. Pediatrics 2020;146(2). https://doi.org/10.1542/peds.2020-1467.
51. Dai YG, Miller LE, Ramsey RK, et al. Incremental utility of 24-month autism spectrum disorder screening after negative 18-month screening. J Autism Dev Disord 2020;50(6):2030–40.
52. Janvier YM, Harris JF, Coffield CN, et al. Screening for autism spectrum disorder in underserved communities: Early childcare providers as reporters. Autism : The International Journal of Research and Practice 2015.
53. Lipkin PH, Macias MM, Baer Chen B, et al. Trends in Pediatricians' Developmental Screening: 2002–2016. Pediatrics 2020;e20190851. https://doi.org/10.1542/peds.2019-0851.
54. Mazurek MO, Kuhlthau K, Parker RA, et al. Autism and general developmental screening practices among primary care providers. J Dev Behav Pediatr : JDBP (J Dev Behav Pediatr) 2021;42(5):355–62.
55. Jimenez ME, Fiks AG, Shah LR, et al. Factors associated with early intervention referral and evaluation: a mixed methods analysis. Academic pediatrics May--Jun 2014;14(3):315–23.

56. Carbone PS, Norlin C, Young PC. Improving Early Identification and Ongoing Care of Children With Autism Spectrum Disorder. Pediatrics 2016;137(6). https://doi.org/10.1542/peds.2015-1850.

57. Campbell K, Carbone PS, Liu D, et al. Improving Autism Screening and Referrals With Electronic Support and Evaluations in Primary Care. Pediatrics 2021; 147(3). https://doi.org/10.1542/peds.2020-1609.

58. Steinman KJ, Stone WL, Ibañez LV, et al. Reducing Barriers to Autism Screening in Community Primary Care: A Pragmatic Trial Using Web-Based Screening. Academic Pediatrics 2022;22(2):263–70.

59. Wallis KE. The Roadmap to Early and Equitable Autism Identification. Pediatrics 2021;148(Suppl 1):s21–4.

60. Monteiro SA, Dempsey J, Berry LN, et al. Screening and Referral Practices for Autism Spectrum Disorder in Primary Pediatric Care. Pediatrics 2019;144(4). https://doi.org/10.1542/peds.2018-3326.

61. Rea KE, Armstrong-Brine M, Ramirez L, et al. Ethnic Disparities in Autism Spectrum Disorder Screening and Referral: Implications for Pediatric Practice. J Dev Behav Pediatr : JDBP. Sep 2019;40(7):493–500.

62. Wallis KE, Guthrie W, Bennett AE, et al. Adherence to screening and referral guidelines for autism spectrum disorder in toddlers in pediatric primary care. PLoS One 2020;15(5):e0232335.

63. Hamp N, DeHaan SL, Cerf CM, et al. Primary care pediatricians' perspectives on autism care. Pediatrics 2022. https://doi.org/10.1542/peds.2022-057712. e2022057712.

64. Guevara JP, Gerdes M, Localio R, et al. Effectiveness of developmental screening in an urban setting. Pediatrics 2013;131(1):30–7.

65. Badawi DG, Thomas J, Archuleta P, et al. Improving developmental screening and supporting families with paid parent partners. J Dev Behav Pediatr : JDBP (J Dev Behav Pediatr) 2023;44(1):e49–55.

66. DiGuiseppi C, Rosenberg SA, Tomcho MA, et al. Family navigation to increase evaluation for autism spectrum disorder in toddlers: Screening and Linkage to Services for Autism pragmatic randomized trial. Autism : The International Journal of Research and Practice 2021;25(4):946–57.

67. Ibañez LV, Stoep AV, Myers K, et al. Promoting early autism detection and intervention in underserved communities: study protocol for a pragmatic trial using a stepped-wedge design. BMC Psychiatr 2019;19(1):169.

68. Flower KB, Massie S, Janies K, et al. Increasing Early Childhood Screening in Primary Care Through a Quality Improvement Collaborative. Pediatrics 2020; 146(3). https://doi.org/10.1542/peds.2019-2328.

69. McNally Keehn R, Ciccarelli M, Szczepaniak D, et al. A statewide tiered system for screening and diagnosis of autism spectrum disorder. Pediatrics 2020; 146(2). https://doi.org/10.1542/peds.2019-3876.

70. Bradbury K, Robins DL, Barton M, et al. Screening for Autism Spectrum Disorder in High-Risk Younger Siblings. J Dev Behav Pediatr : JDBP (J Dev Behav Pediatr) Oct-Nov 2020;41(8):596–604.

71. Parikh C, Iosif AM, Ozonoff S. Brief Report: Use of the Infant-Toddler Checklist in Infant Siblings of Children with Autism Spectrum Disorder. J Autism Dev Disord 2021;51(3):1007–12.

72. Pasco G, Davies K, Ribeiro H, et al. Comparison of parent questionnaires, examiner-led assessment and parents' concerns at 14 months of age as indicators of later diagnosis of autism. J Autism Dev Disord 2021;51(3):804–13.

73. Raza S, Zwaigenbaum L, Sacrey LR, et al. Brief Report: Evaluation of the Short Quantitative Checklist for Autism in Toddlers (Q-CHAT-10) as a Brief Screen for Autism Spectrum Disorder in a High-Risk Sibling Cohort. J Autism Dev Disord 2019;49(5):2210–8.

74. Zwaigenbaum L, Bryson SE, Brian J, et al. Assessment of autism symptoms from 6 to 18 months of age using the autism observation scale for infants in a prospective high-risk cohort. Child Dev 2021;92(3):1187–98.

75. Scarlytt de Oliveira Holanda N, Delgado Oliveira da Costa L, Suelen Santos Sampaio S, et al. Screening for autism spectrum disorder in premature subjects hospitalized in a neonatal intensive care unit. Int J Environ Res Publ Health 2020; 17(20). https://doi.org/10.3390/ijerph17207675.

76. Karabulut B, Sahbudak B. Autism Spectrum Disorder Screening at 18-36 Months in Infants with Moderate and Severe Neonatal Encephalopathy: Is Routine Screening Required? Psychopharmacol Bull 2020;50(3):8–22.

77. Sacrey LR, Zwaigenbaum L, Bryson S, et al. Screening for Behavioral Signs of Autism Spectrum Disorder in 9-Month-Old Infant Siblings. J Autism Dev Disord 2021;51(3):839–48.

78. Sung S, Fenoglio A, Wolff JJ, et al. Examining the factor structure and discriminative utility of the Infant Behavior Questionnaire-Revised in infant siblings of autistic children. Child Dev 2022;93(5):1398–413.

79. Haffner DN, Bartram LR, Coury DL, et al. The Autism Detection in Early Childhood Tool: Level 2 autism spectrum disorder screening in a NICU Follow-up program. Infant Behav Dev. Nov 2021;65:101650.

80. Loblein HJ, Vukmirovich PW, Donofrio MT, et al. Prevalence of neurodevelopmental disorders in a clinically referred sample of children with CHD. Cardiol Young 2023;33(4):619–26.

81. Ware J, Butcher JL, Latal B, et al. Neurodevelopmental evaluation strategies for children with congenital heart disease aged birth through 5 years: recommendations from the cardiac neurodevelopmental outcome collaborative. Cardiol Young 2020;30(11):1609–22.

82. Wallis KE, Pinto-Martin J. The challenge of screening for autism in a culturally diverse society. Acta Pediatrica 2008 2008;97(5):539–40.

83. Stevanovic D, Robins DL, Costanzo F, et al. Cross-cultural similarities and differences in reporting autistic symptoms in toddlers: A study synthesizing M-CHAT(-R) data from ten countries. Research in Autism Spectrum Disorders 2022;95:1–10.

84. Marlow M, Servili C, Tomlinson M. A review of screening tools for the identification of autism spectrum disorders and developmental delay in infants and young children: recommendations for use in low- and middle-income countries. Autism Res 2019;12(2):176–99.

85. Aldosari M, Fombonne E, Aldhalaan H, et al. Validation of the Arabic version of the Social Communication Questionnaire. Autism: The International Journal of Research and Practice 2019;23(7):1655–62.

86. Barbaro J, Sadka N, Gilbert M, et al. Diagnostic accuracy of the social attention and communication surveillance-revised with preschool tool for early autism detection in very young children. JAMA Netw Open 2022;5(3):e2146415.

87. Barbaro J, Yaari M. Study protocol for an evaluation of ASDetect - a Mobile application for the early detection of autism. BMC pediatrics 2020;20(1):21.

88. Hudry K, Chetcuti L, Boutrus M, et al. Performance of the Autism Observation Scale for Infants with community-ascertained infants showing early signs of

autism. Autism: The International Journal of Research & Practice 2021;25(2): 490–501.

89. Coelho-Medeiros ME, Bronstein J, Aedo K, et al. M-CHAT-R/F Validation as a screening tool for early detection in children with autism spectrum disorder. Rev Chil Pediatr 2019;90(5):492–9. Validación del M-CHAT-R/F como instrumento de tamizaje para detección precoz en niños con trastorno del espectro autista.

90. Wong PP, Wai VC, Chan RW, et al. Autism-spectrum quotient-child and autism-spectrum quotient-adolescent in chinese population: screening autism spectrum disorder against attention-deficit/hyperactivity disorder and typically developing peers. Autism: The International Journal of Research and Practice 2021;25(7): 1913–23.

91. Yan W, Siegert RJ, Zhou H, et al. Psychometric properties of the Chinese Parent Version of the Autism Spectrum Rating Scale: Rasch analysis. Autism: The International Journal of Research and Practice 2021;25(7):1872–84.

92. Zhou H, Li CP, Huang Y, et al. Reliability and validity of the translated Chinese version of Autism Spectrum Rating Scale (2-5 years). World J Pediatr 2019; 15(1):49–56.

93. Guo C, Luo M, Wang X, et al. Reliability and Validity of the Chinese Version of Modified Checklist for Autism in Toddlers, Revised, with Follow-Up (M-CHAT-R/F). J Autism Dev Disord 2019;49(1):185–96.

94. Liu SY, Wang X, Chen Q, et al. The validity and reliability of the simplified Chinese version of the Social Communication Questionnaire. Autism Res. Sep 2022;15(9):1732–41.

95. Li WH, Hu LF, Yuan L, et al. The Application of the First Year Inventory for ASD Screening in China. J Pediatr Nurs 2019;44:e72–8.

96. Gutiérrez-Ruiz K, Delgado AR, Prieto G. Rasch analysis of the Q-CHAT in Colombian toddlers with Autism Spectrum Disorder. Curr Psychol: A Journal for Diverse Perspectives on Diverse Psychological Issues 2019;38(1):116–20.

97. Carlier S, Ducenne L, Leys C, et al. Improving autism screening in French-speaking countries: Validation of the Autism Discriminative Tool, a teacher-rated questionnaire for clinicians' use. Research in Autism Spectrum Disorders 2019;61:33–44.

98. Zirakashvili M, Gabunia M, Mebonia N, et al. Adaptation of autism spectrum screening questionnaire (ASSQ) for use in Georgian school settings. J Publ Ment Health 2022;21(4):309–22.

99. Jonsdottir SL, Saemundsen E, Jonsson BG, et al. Validation of the Modified Checklist for Autism in Toddlers, Revised with Follow-up in a Population Sample of 30-Month-Old Children in Iceland: A Prospective Approach. J Autism Dev Disord 2022;52(4):1507–22.

100. Faraji Goodarzi M, Taee N, Hormozi PA. Evaluation of autistic spectrum disorders screening in children of Khorramabad (West of Iran) between 2015 and 2016. Early Child Dev Care 2019;189(9):1509–14.

101. Mohammadi MR, Zahed G, Zarafshan H. Early Screening of Autism among 18 to 24 months Old Toddlers Using the Quantitative Checklist for Autism in Toddlers (Q-CHAT). Iran J Child Neurol 2020;14(4):55–62.

102. Samadi SA, McConkey R, Nuri H, et al. Screening Children for Autism Spectrum Disorders in Low- and Middle-Income Countries: Experiences from the Kurdistan Region of Iraq. Int J Environ Res Publ Health 2022;19(8). https://doi.org/10.3390/ijerph19084581.

103. Samadi SA, Noori H, Abdullah A, et al. The Psychometric Properties of the Gilliam Autism Rating Scale (GARS-3) with Kurdish Samples of Children with Developmental Disabilities. Children 2022;9(3):434.

104. Kerub O, Haas EJ, Meiri G, et al. A Comparison Between Two Screening Approaches for ASD Among Toddlers in Israel. J Autism Dev Disord 2020;50(5):1553–60.

105. Ruta L, Chiarotti F, Arduino GM, et al. Validation of the Quantitative Checklist for Autism in Toddlers in an Italian clinical sample of young children with autism and other developmental disorders. Front Psychiatr 2019;10:10.

106. Rutaa L, Arduino GM, Gagliano A, et al. Psychometric properties, factor structure and cross-cultural validity of the quantitative CHecklist for Autism in Toddlers (Q-CHAT) in an Italian community setting. Research in Autism Spectrum Disorders 2019;64:39–48.

107. Babu G, Scaria LM, Prasanna GL, et al. A Nine-Item Red Flag Sign Card for Identification of Autism Spectrum Disorder among Toddlers Aged 12 to 18 Months. Indian J Pediatr. Mar 2022;89(3):288–90.

108. Tabril T, Chekira A, Moukhless S, et al. Cultural Adaptation and Validation of the Modified Checklist for Autism in Toddlers, Revised with Follow-up in Moroccan Arabic dialect. Encephale 2023;49(1):15–20.

109. Bong G, Kim JH, Hong Y, et al. The feasibility and validity of autism spectrum disorder screening instrument: behavior development screening for toddlers (BeDevel)-a pilot study. Autism Res 2019;12(7):1112-1128.

110. Bong G, Kim SY, Song DY, et al. Short caregiver interview and play observation for early screening of autism spectrum disorder: Behavior development screening for toddlers (BeDevel). Autism Res 2021;14(7):1472-1483. doi:

111. Magan-Maganto M, Canal-Bedia R, Hernandez-Fabian A, et al. Spanish cultural validation of the modified checklist for autism in toddlers, revised. J Autism Dev Disord 2020;50(7):2412–23.

112. Iao L-S, Yu W-H, Wu C-C. Early screening for autism spectrum disorder in young children with developmental problems using the Chinese version of the Child Behavior Checklist. Research in Autism Spectrum Disorders 2020;70:10.

113. Wu CC, Chiang CH, Chu CL, et al. T-STAT for detecting autism spectrum disorder in toddlers aged 18-24 months. Autism: The International Journal of Research and Practice 2021;25(4):911–20.

114. Wu CC, Chu CL, Stewart L, et al. The utility of the screening tool for autism in 2-year-olds in detecting autism in taiwanese toddlers who are less than 24 months of age: a longitudinal study. J Autism Dev Disord 2020;50(4):1172–81.

115. Tsai JM, Lu L, Jeng SF, et al. Validation of the modified checklist for autism in toddlers, revised with follow-up in Taiwanese toddlers. Res Dev Disabil 2019;85:205–16.

116. Oner O, Munir KM. Modified Checklist for Autism in Toddlers Revised (MCHAT-R/F) in an Urban Metropolitan Sample of Young Children in Turkey. Journal of Autism and Developmental Disorders 2020;50(9):3312–9.

117. HyeKyeung S, Bui J, San P. Screening Vietnamese Children in the United States for Autism Risk: Examination of the Modified Checklist for Autism in Toddlers–Revision With Follow-Up Vietnamese. Perspectives of the ASHA Special Interest Groups 2022;7:2027–38.

118. Nguyen PH, Ocansey ME, Miller M, et al. The reliability and validity of the social responsiveness scale to measure autism symptomology in Vietnamese children. Autism Res 2019;12(11):1706–18.

119. Bevan SL, Liu J, Wallis KE, et al. Screening Instruments for Developmental and Behavioral Concerns in Pediatric Hispanic Populations in the United States: A Systematic Literature Review. J Dev Behav Pediatr 2020;41(1):71–80.

120. Dai YG, Porto KS, Skapek M, et al. Comparison of the Modified Checklist for Autism in Toddlers, Revised with Follow-Up (M-CHAT-R/F) Positive Predictive Value by Race. J Autism Dev Disord 2021;51(3):855–67.

121. McClain MB, Harris B, Schwartz SE, et al. Differential Item and Test Functioning of the Autism Spectrum Rating Scales: A Follow-Up Evaluation in a Diverse, Nonclinical Sample. J Psychoeduc Assess 2021;39(2):247–57.

122. Alonso-Esteban Y, Marco R, Hedley D, et al. Screening instruments for early detection of autism spectrum disorder in Spanish speaking communities. Psicothema 2020;32(2):245–52.

123. Kuhn J, Levinson J, Udhnani MD, et al. What Happens After a Positive Primary Care Autism Screen Among Historically Underserved Families? Predictors of Evaluation and Autism Diagnosis. J Dev Behav Pediatr 2021. https://doi.org/10.1097/dbp.0000000000000928.

124. Wallis KE, Buttenheim AM, Mandell DS. Insights from Behavioral Economics: A Case of Delayed Diagnosis of Autism Spectrum Disorder. J Dev Behav Pediatr 2021;42(2):109–13.

125. Maenner MJ, Bakian AV, Bakian AV, et al. Prevalence and Characteristics of Autism Spectrum Disorder Among Children Aged 8 Years — Autism and Developmental Disabilities Monitoring Network, 11 Sites, United States, 2018. MMWR Surveill 2021;70(No. SS-11):1–16.

126. Wiggins LD, Durkin M, Esler A, et al. Disparities in documented diagnoses of autism spectrum disorder based on demographic, individual, and service factors. Autism Res 2019. https://doi.org/10.1002/aur.2255.

127. Shenouda J, Barrett E, Davidow AL, et al. Prevalence and Disparities in the Detection of Autism Without Intellectual Disability. Pediatrics 2023;151(2). https://doi.org/10.1542/peds.2022-056594.

128. Constantino JN, Abbacchi AM, Saulnier C, et al. Timing of the Diagnosis of Autism in African American Children. Pediatrics 2020;146(3). https://doi.org/10.1542/peds.2019-3629.

129. Smith KA, Gehricke J-G, Iadarola S, et al. Disparities in Service Use Among Children With Autism: A Systematic Review. Pediatrics 2020;145(Supplement 1):S35–46.

130. Zuckerman KE, Broder-Fingert S, Sheldrick RC. To reduce the average age of autism diagnosis, screen preschoolers in primary care. Autism : The International Journal of Research and Practice 2021;25(2):593–6.

131. Wright B, Konstantopoulou K, Sohal K, et al. Systematic approach to school-based assessments for autism spectrum disorders to reduce inequalities: a feasibility study in 10 primary schools. BMJ Open 2021;11(1):e041960.

132. Petruccelli M, Ramella L, Schaefer AJ, et al. A Taxonomy of Reported Harms in Pediatric Autism Spectrum Disorder Screening: Provider and Parent Perspectives. J Autism Dev Disord 2022;52(2):647–73.

133. Eilenberg JS, Kizildag D, Blakey AO, et al. Implications of Universal Autism Screening: Perspectives From Culturally Diverse Families With False-Positive Screens. Academic Pediatrics 2022;22(2):279–88.

134. Mackie TI, Schaefer AJ, Ramella L, et al. Understanding how parents make meaning of their child's behaviors during screening for autism spectrum disorders: a longitudinal qualitative investigation. J Autism Dev Disord 2021;51(3):906–21.

135. Samango-Sprouse CA, Stapleton EJ, Aliabadi F, et al. Identification of infants at risk for autism spectrum disorder and developmental language delay prior to 12 months. Autism: The International Journal of Research and Practice 2015; 19(3):327–37.
136. Ghosh S, Guha T. Towards Autism Screening through Emotion-guided Eye Gaze Response. Annu Int Conf IEEE Eng Med Biol Soc 2021;2021:820–3.
137. Jensen K, Noazin S, Bitterfeld L, et al. Autism Detection in Children by Combined Use of Gaze Preference and the M-CHAT-R in a Resource-Scarce Setting. J Autism Dev Disord 2021;51(3):994–1006.
138. Ozdemir S, Akin-Bulbul I, Kok I, et al. Development of a visual attention based decision support system for autism spectrum disorder screening. Int J Psychophysiol 2022;173:69–81.
139. Han J, Jiang G, Ouyang G, et al. A Multimodal Approach for Identifying Autism Spectrum Disorders in Children. IEEE Trans Neural Syst Rehabil Eng 2022;30: 2003–11.
140. Jiang M, Francis SM, Srishyla D, et al. Classifying Individuals with ASD Through Facial Emotion Recognition and Eye-Tracking. Annu Int Conf IEEE Eng Med Biol Soc 2019;2019:6063–8.
141. Khozaei A, Moradi H, Hosseini R, et al. Early screening of autism spectrum disorder using cry features. PLoS One 2020;15(12):e0241690.
142. VanDam M, Yoshinaga-Itano C. Use of the LENA Autism Screen with Children who are Deaf or Hard of Hearing. Medicina (Kaunas). 2019;55(8). https://doi.org/10.3390/medicina55080495.
143. Corona LL, Wagner L, Wade J, et al. Toward Novel Tools for Autism Identification: Fusing Computational and Clinical Expertise. J Autism Dev Disord 2021; 51(11):4003–12.
144. Mujeeb Rahman KK, Monica Subashini M. A Deep Neural Network-Based Model for Screening Autism Spectrum Disorder Using the Quantitative Checklist for Autism in Toddlers (QCHAT). J Autism Dev Disord 2022;52(6):2732–46.
145. Romero-García R, Martínez-Tomás R, Pozo P, et al. A robotic approach to autism screening in toddlers. J Biomed Inform 2021;118:103797.
146. Scott AJW, Wang Y, Abdel-Jaber H, et al. Improving screening systems of autism using data sampling. Technol Health Care 2021;29(5):897–909.
147. Shahamiri SR, Thabtah F. Autism AI: A new autism screening system based on artificial intelligence. Cognitive Computation 2020;12(4):766–77.
148. Parikh RB, Teeple S, Navathe AS. Addressing Bias in Artificial Intelligence in Health Care. JAMA 2019;322(24):2377–8.
149. Au AH, Shum KK, Cheng Y, et al. Autism spectrum disorder screening in preschools. Autism : The International Journal of Research and Practice 2021; 25(2):516–28.
150. Brewer L. Community-based screening and referrals for autism. J Occup Ther Sch Early Interv 2020;13(2):147–57.
151. Zuckerman KE, Chavez AE, Reeder JA. Decreasing disparities in child development assessment: identifying and discussing possible delays in the special supplemental nutrition program for women, infants, and children (WIC). J Dev Behav Pediat 2017;38(5):301–9.
152. King TM, Tandon SD, Macias MM, et al. Implementing developmental screening and referrals: lessons learned from a national project. Pediatrics 2010;125(2):350–60.
153. Aishworiya R, Ma VK, Stewart S, et al. Meta-analysis of the modified checklist for autism in toddlers, revised/follow-up for screening. . Pediatrics 2023;151(6). https://doi.org/10.1542/peds.2022-059393.

Differential Diagnosis of Autism and Other Neurodevelopmental Disorders

Lindsay Olson, PhD[a], Somer Bishop, PhD[a], Audrey Thurm, PhD[b],*

KEYWORDS

- Autism • Autism diagnosis • Differential diagnosis • Neurodevelopmental disorders

KEY POINTS

- The diagnosis of autism spectrum disorder (ASD) is complex, with different challenges depending on the chronologic age and developmental level of the child or adolescent.
- Clear understanding of an individual's developmental level and associated developmental expectations are critical for differentiating ASD from other conditions that may show significant symptom overlap with ASD.
- Pediatricians play a key role in providing surveillance and screening for ASD, as well as in facilitating appropriate and timely referrals. Some pediatricians may receive specialized training to directly participate in the diagnostic assessment process.
- Comprehensive assessment and management of individuals with ASD should include evaluation of genetic, medical, and mental health conditions that commonly occur in youth with ASD at different points in development.

The diagnostic criteria for autism spectrum disorder (ASD) have changed considerably over time.[1] Here, we present the current criteria as they are outlined in both the Diagnostic and Statistical Manual of Mental Disorders, fifth edition, text revision (DSM-5-TR),[2] as well as in the International Classification of Diseases, 11th version (ICD-11).[3]

As shown in **Box 1**, the DSM-5-TR has substantial overlap but not complete alignment, with the ICD-11, both in terms of diagnostic coding and description of diagnoses. In the DSM-5-TR, ASD is 1 of 7 different categories of neurodevelopmental disorders (NDDs), along with intellectual developmental disorder (which includes 6 different codes), communication disorders (including 5 different diagnoses), attention-deficit hyperactivity disorder (with 5 presentation codes), specific learning disorder (with 3 separate designations for specific impairments), motor disorders (with 2 separate

[a] Department of Psychiatry and Behavioral Sciences, UCSF Weill Institute for Neurosciences, University of California, 675 18th Street, San Francisco, CA 94143, USA; [b] Intramural Research Program, Neurodevelopmental and Behavioral Phenotyping Service, National Institute of Mental Health, 10 Center Drive, Room 1C250, MSC 1255, Bethesda, MD 20892, USA
* Corresponding author.
E-mail address: athurm@mail.nih.gov

Pediatr Clin N Am 71 (2024) 157–177
https://doi.org/10.1016/j.pcl.2023.12.004
0031-3955/24/Published by Elsevier Inc.

pediatric.theclinics.com

Box 1
Diagnostic Criteria for ASD in the DSM-5-TR and ICD-11

DSM-5-TR (APA, 2022)

A. Persistent deficits in social communication and social interaction across multiple contexts, as manifested by the following, currently or by history (examples are illustrative, not exhaustive, see text; APA, 2022):
  • Deficits in social-emotional reciprocity, ranging, for example, from abnormal social approach and failure of normal back-and-forth conversation; to reduced sharing of interests, emotions, or affect; to failure to initiate or respond to social interactions.
  • Deficits in nonverbal communicative behaviors used for social interaction, ranging, for example, from poorly integrated verbal and nonverbal communication; to abnormalities in eye contact and body language or deficits in understanding and use of gestures; to a total lack of facial expressions and nonverbal communication.
  • Deficits in developing, maintaining, and understanding relationships, ranging, for example, from difficulties adjusting behavior to suit various social contexts; to difficulties in sharing imaginative play or in making friends; to absence of interest in peers.

B. Restricted, repetitive patterns of behavior, interests, or activities, as manifested by at least two of the following, currently or by history (examples are illustrative, not exhaustive, see text):
  • Stereotyped or repetitive motor movements, use of objects, or speech (eg, simple motor stereotypes, lining up toys or flipping objects, echolalia, idiosyncratic phrases).
  • Insistence on sameness, inflexible adherence to routines, or ritualized patterns of verbal or nonverbal behavior (eg, extreme distress at small changes, difficulties with transitions, rigid thinking patterns, greeting rituals, need to take same route or eat same food every day).
  • Highly restricted, fixated interests that are abnormal in intensity or focus (eg, strong attachment to or preoccupation with unusual objects, excessively circumscribed or perseverative interests).
  • Hyperreactivity or hyporeactivity to sensory input or unusual interest in sensory aspects of the environment (eg, apparent indifference to pain/temperature, adverse response to specific sounds or textures, excessive smelling or touching of objects, visual fascination with lights or movement).

C. Symptoms must be present in the early developmental period (but may not become fully manifest until social demands exceed limited capacities, or may be masked by learned strategies in later life).

D. Symptoms cause clinically significant impairment in social, occupational, or other important areas of current functioning.

E. These disturbances are not better explained by ID (intellectual developmental disorder) or global developmental delay. ID and ASD frequently co-occur; to make comorbid diagnoses of ASD and ID, social communication should be below that expected for general developmental level.

ICD-11 (WHO, 2019):

Persistent deficits in initiating and sustaining social communication and reciprocal social interactions that are outside the expected range of typical functioning given the individual's age and level of intellectual development. Specific manifestations of these deficits vary according to chronologic age, verbal and intellectual ability, and disorder severity. Manifestations may include limitations in the following:
  • Understanding of, interest in, or inappropriate responses to the verbal or non-verbal social communications of others.
  • Integration of spoken language with typical complimentary non-verbal cues, such as eye contact, gestures, facial expressions and body language. These non-verbal behaviors may also be reduced in frequency or intensity.
  • Understanding and use of language in social contexts and ability to initiate and sustain reciprocal social conversations.

- Social awareness, leading to behavior that is not appropriately modulated according to the social context.
- Ability to imagine and respond to the feelings, emotional states, and attitudes of others.
- Mutual sharing of interests.
- Ability to make and sustain typical peer relationships.

diagnoses), and tic disorders.[2] The "other neurodevelopmental disorders" section includes 2 additional codes, "other specific neurodevelopmental disorder" and "unspecified neurodevelopmental disorder," which can be used when full criteria are not met for ASD and a specific reason is described, or not described, respectively. One additional diagnosis in the ICD-11 is secondary neurodevelopmental syndrome (code 6E60), which is included in the section on secondary mental or behavioral syndromes associated with disorders or diseases classified elsewhere. This is a diagnosis that may be used when symptoms of ASD develop after the early developmental period, such as in the case of autoimmune encephalitis, or when criteria person meets some but not all criteria for ASD and/or another NDD, such as in the context of a specific genetic condition.[3]

NDDs are generally conceptualized as representing qualitative impairments resulting from the extreme ends of developmental domains, such as social communication, cognition, and attention, as examples. NDDs share several overlapping features, which can make differential diagnosis challenging. Thus, it may be particularly challenging to determine when symptoms of a second or third NDD are subthreshold or meet criteria for an additional diagnosis. In relation to ASD specifically, other NDDs are prevalent among the many co-occurring conditions that are often present.[4]

Due to the complexities of ASD diagnosis, its behavioral nature, its many diagnostic differentials (see later discussion), comorbidities, and its early childhood onset, diagnosis of ASD requires a thorough, systematic assessment by a trained expert.[5] Such a professional (or team) must be well versed in the use of diagnostic instruments, their limitations, and how to apply them to individuals with different characteristics that may influence administration and/or interpretation.[6] Pediatricians play a critical role in ASD surveillance, and mounting evidence underscores the importance of active screening practices for facilitating timely referrals.[7] Some pediatricians may also seek additional, specialized training in diagnostic assessment of ASD but this requires training beyond what is provided in pediatric residency. Further, given the complexities of differential diagnosis (see later discussion), even those with additional training may not feel equipped to make or rule out diagnoses of ASD (and/or other NDDs) in all cases. Although this article will not delve into the full listing of tests available nor details of all of the best practices for diagnosis, we refer the reader to other training materials, including several provided by the American Academy of Pediatrics.[8–12] We will also not provide an exhaustive review of factors that may affect diagnostic assessment of ASD—these include chronologic age, developmental and language level, sex and gender, cultural and linguistic differences, and other societal influences, including access to diagnosticians and services. However, we will try to highlight a few and provide exemplars of issues to consider.

Those involved in making diagnoses of ASD or other NDDs must acquire deep understanding of typical child development, manifestations of autism across development, and commonly co-occurring conditions. However, general practitioners and pediatric providers can develop the skills to discern when cases should be referred for specialty assessment.[13] Indeed, equipping some pediatric providers with necessary training to identify children at particularly high likelihood for ASD could significantly reduce wait times and increase timely access to diagnostic services, thereby opening the doorway to appropriate supports and interventions.[13] In addition to consulting the aforementioned training materials provided by the AAP, and the information presented in this article, pediatricians should consider seeking training programs or shadowing seasoned diagnosticians in order to increase their competencies in the diagnostic arena.[13] Training models such as ECHO Autism[14] have also been developed with the specific purpose of increasing capacity among pediatricians to identify likely ASD cases and are quickly gaining popularity across the United States and abroad.[15]

When should a child be evaluated for ASD? Before answering this, we will discuss when a child should receive surveillance and screening for ASD, which should lead a child and family down a path toward a diagnostic evaluation if results of screeners indicate concern. Surveillance is the process of monitoring children to be able to identify those showing developmental concerns.[16] Screening is an active process that should occur at certain timepoints. Screening should assess for general developmental concerns, followed by ASD-specific concerns, per instruction of the American Academy of Pediatrics.[16] Screening results may necessitate a referral for a diagnostic evaluation. Although this process has mostly been studied and promoted with respect to young children,[17] it is increasingly apparent that there are many autistic adolescents and adults who were not diagnosed as children.[18,19] As such, a variation on this process may also be relevant for older children and adolescents presenting with concerns in social-communication and/or other developmental domains.[20]

The American Academy of Pediatrics recommends that in addition to general developmental screening at 9, 18, and 30 months of age, pediatricians use validated instruments to screen children for ASD specifically at 18 and 24 months of age.[21] Screening can also occur at any age when concerns develop. One reason for the repeated screenings is that, for some children, regression or loss of skills may be a feature of autism symptom onset, so a child may "pass" an earlier screener but fail a later one. Caregiver questionnaires and interviews are often used as "level 1" screeners but pediatricians may also be trained in "level II" screeners that can involve brief and often structured direct observation measures, which require reliability training for coding. In particular, providers could seek training in level II screeners such as the Rapid Interactive Screening Test for Autism in Toddlers or the Screening Tool for Autism in Toddler and Young Children to support implementation of models where those who fail these screeners are expedited for referrals for comprehensive evaluations.[22]

Once a child is referred for comprehensive diagnostic evaluation of ASD, best practices include several elements: a parent/caregiver interview to determine history and pervasiveness of symptoms; an in-person portion with direct observation and interaction with the individual; and outside corroboration of the impaired functioning (eg, collateral information from teachers).[5] The developmental history is critical for ascertaining whether Criterion C are met, that is, that symptoms are present in the early developmental period (ie, before 5 years of age). In addition, cognitive or developmental testing is necessary to determine whether any observed deficits in social-communication and/or play are beyond what would be expected based on an individual's developmental level (ie, to consider all criteria, including Criterion E of DSM-5 criteria for ASD).[23] The best-practice components of an assessment may be carried out by a sole provider, or as part of a multidisciplinary team (eg, including pediatric providers, speech-language pathologists, psychologists, and others). As opposed to many other diagnoses that pediatric providers make, the diagnosis of ASD or any other NDD cannot be made based on results from any particular test.[1,6] There are no definitive diagnostic biomarkers, and there is no behavioral test that is sufficiently accurate on its own to diagnose ASD. Further, individuals present with extremely variable constellations of symptoms, which also change within individuals over time, meaning that clinical expertise is another critical component of the diagnostic assessment process.[6] The process of administering standardized diagnostic instruments can improve diagnostic decision-making by eliciting diagnostically salient information to inform expert clinical judgment.[6] However, misuse of these instruments, including overreliance on scores and classifications, likely contributes to high rates of misdiagnosis,[24] especially because sensitivity and specificity of these instruments varies significantly based on developmental and behavioral factors.[25]

Because of the extreme phenotypic heterogeneity characteristic of ASD, a major focus of the comprehensive assessment is to describe the individual's profile in sufficient detail to meaningfully inform treatment planning. Thus, the DSM-5-TR includes specifiers to encourage clinicians to go beyond the simple consideration of whether ASD is present, which could be the case for individuals with any level of language or cognitive ability or other differences. Specifiers are a convention of the DSM to define subgroups within a disorder for individuals who share features. There are several specifiers available in the ASD diagnosis, including indication for intellectual and/or language impairment. However, even within these specifiers, there is huge variability. Specifiers are also used to indicate whether there are known medical and/or genetic factors, and/or co-occurring diagnoses (including other NDDs). Importantly, although, clinicians should also assign independent diagnoses whenever applicable. This means that even in an individual diagnosed with ASD with accompanying intellectual impairment or language impairment, an additional DSM-5 diagnosis of intellectual disability (ID) and/or language disorder might also be appropriate.

The DSM-5 further includes specifiers to indicate the level of support required for core ASD-related impairments (ie, social-communication deficits and restricted and repetitive behaviors).[2] This represents another attempt to explicitly acknowledge the wide range of symptom severity among people with ASD. These categorical designations include level 1: requiring support, level 2: requiring substantial support, and level 3: requiring very substantial support. Unfortunately, these categories were neither field-tested nor there is any evidence regarding their validity or reliability. Based on studies of other measures of ASD "severity," it is unlikely that such designations provide meaningful information beyond what can be conveyed by an individual's current developmental and language level.[26,27] By developmental level, we generally mean nonverbal mental age, which can be gleaned from developmental tests or cognitive tests, or estimated based on knowledge of the individual's adaptive functioning in various developmental areas. Given the degree of intraindividual change, especially in young children with ASD, it is also not clear what, if any, prognostic value these designations have. Without more explicit guidance about how they should be operationalized (ie, to capture symptom severity beyond what is attributable to cognitive and/or language level), or at what point in development they can be reliably assigned, these severity levels are unlikely to provide meaningful information to providers or families. Further, they may have the potential to do more harm than good (eg, if insurance providers attempt to limit coverage for individuals with "level 1 ASD").[1,28,29] There is also no comparable metric in the ICD-11.

In contrast to the DSM-5 support specifiers and other potentially misleading terms for describing an individual with ASD (eg, "low" vs "high" functioning),[30] detailed information about an individual's specific profile across developmental and behavioral domains is much more helpful for treatment planning. This includes language, attention, motor function, as well as various areas of cognition, including memory and executive functioning, and the broader context of psychiatric symptoms that may occur over time. As mentioned above, because "ASD" is used to describe individuals with such a wide range of symptom profiles, the diagnostic label does not convey information about which types of supports are needed for that individual. Specific therapies are often necessary to promote adaptive functioning and allow participation in developmentally appropriate learning opportunities, and these therapies will vary significantly between individuals. Specific therapies may include speech therapy, occupational therapy, or home or center-based behavioral therapies that focus on various aspects of adaptive functioning (eg, communication, daily living skills). Educational support needs will also vary widely, and some individuals with a medical diagnosis of ASD may not meet criteria for an educational classification of autism if their ASD symptoms do not interfere with their ability to access the curriculum. However, even if a child with ASD is excelling academically, it is important to consider whether they require support to improve social functioning in the school setting.[31]

Regardless of the treatment plan developed from a comprehensive diagnostic assessment, it is critical to remember that treatment needs change over time as a function of both age and the degree and rate of developmental progress.[32] In addition, transient or chronic medical, behavioral, psychiatric, and/or educational concerns that arise may require various specialized assessment, management, and treatment services.[33] This underscores the importance of periodic reevaluations, as would be recommended with any chronic condition, to evaluate changes that are needed to the treatment plan.[32,34] Further, as it becomes available, it is important to communicate information to individuals and their families regarding expectations for the future.[35] If applicable, information about co-occurring diagnoses such as ID should also be clearly communicated.[36,37]

Importantly, there is no one behavioral feature that is universal to all individuals with ASD, just as there is no symptom that is entirely specific to ASD.[2] This significantly complicates diagnosis because children with various NDDs or psychiatric diagnoses may present with symptoms that seem very similar to those of ASD. Increasingly, children with social challenges are referred for diagnostic assessment of ASD but as described in more detail in later discussion, children can experience social difficulties for myriad reasons, some of which are not related to ASD. These may include other symptoms of other NDDs, such as inattention or impulsivity, or a variety of other behavioral or emotional issues, or even experiences they are having (eg, bullying and trauma).[38,39] Thus, it is only after careful consideration of a child's complete developmental and behavioral profile that a diagnosis of ASD should be considered.

ASSOCIATED CONDITIONS AND DIFFERENTIAL DIAGNOSES WITH AUTISM

The following sections focus on conditions that show significant symptom overlap with ASD and are also commonly co-occurring. All of these conditions may also need to be considered as differential diagnoses with autism depending on the clinical presentation.

Attention Deficit/Hyperactivity Disorder

Attention deficit/hyperactivity disorder (ADHD) is characterized by attention dysregulation, and/or by the presence of hyperactive and impulsive behaviors that cause impairments in at least 2 settings (eg, school and home).[2] ADHD commonly co-occurs with ASD, with rates as high or higher than 40%, and it may also be mistaken for autism or vice versa.[40,41] Although DSM-IV did not allow for the additional diagnosis of ADHD to be made when ASD was present, this restriction was lifted in DSM-5. This decision was made due to growing recognition that many individuals with ASD do present with additional ADHD symptoms that are not fully accounted for by ASD, and these individuals might benefit from evidence-based treatments for ADHD.[42] Still, the question about whether an additional diagnosis of ADHD is warranted must be considered carefully, especially in children with ASD who are young and/or with global developmental delays or ID. For these individuals, symptoms of inattention, impulsivity, and/or hyperactivity may be largely explained by lower developmental level. Similar to Criterion E for ASD, the DSM-5 diagnostic criteria for ADHD indicate that inattention and hyperactivity must be inappropriate for developmental level in order to be considered symptoms.[2] Related, some children with ASD may seem to be inattentive and/or hyperactive because of social disinhibition and reduced ability to modify behaviors appropriately to the social situation (eg, frequently leaving group classroom activities due to disinterest/lack of engagement; not attending to others' conversational attempts).[43] Thus, providers making diagnoses of ADHD in the context of ASD must be trained in assessment and diagnosis of both conditions.[43]

Differential diagnosis of ASD versus ADHD is also challenging because although social challenges are not a core diagnostic feature of ADHD (as they are in ASD), individuals with ADHD commonly experience social problems. Therefore, especially in verbal school-aged children and adolescents with intact cognitive abilities, it can be unclear whether social difficulties develop from ASD-related and/or ADHD-related symptoms (or both). Further, children with ADHD are likely to receive elevated scores on ASD screening and diagnostic instruments,[44] which underscores the importance of careful attention to and specific training in this complex differential diagnosis.

Deficits in basic social communication skills (such as nonverbal communication) is a key distinguishing factor between ADHD and ASD. However, much like children with ASD, children with ADHD commonly experience rejection by peers, and they tend to have fewer friendships and poorer friendship quality than neurotypical peers.[45] Many of these characteristic social challenges in ADHD are likely attributable to impulsivity and its associated costs (eg, frequent interruption, difficulty waiting one's turn, and so forth).[46] Although children with ASD often lack social knowledge, studies suggest that children with ADHD show intact social knowledge despite difficulty with social interactions and forming friendships.[46,47] As such, identifying specific sources of social difficulties can be useful for distinguishing lack of interest or engagement related to ASD symptoms from difficulty participating successfully in social interactions due to symptoms of ADHD (or if both apply).

Language Disorders

Language disorders are defined by deficits in acquiring and using language (spoken, signed, or written)[2] due to reduced vocabulary, limited sentence structure (ie, putting words together according to rules of grammar), and impairments in discourse (ie, having conversations or describing topics).[2] To qualify for a language disorder diagnosis, language abilities must be below age expectations, and there must be evidence of functional impairments in communication, socialization, academic achievement, or occupational performance. Onset of symptoms must occur early in development and language difficulties cannot be attributable to sensory impairment, motor dysfunction, another neurologic condition, or ID.[2]

The estimated prevalence of language disorders in school age children is ~7.5% (not including children with language delays in the presence of other NDDs).[48] For children with other NDDs such as ASD or ADHD, the prevalence of language disorder is estimated at 30% to 50%.[48–50] In order to distinguish between ASD and language disorder, it is necessary to consider aspects of social communication that are not associated with language level.[51] Communication behaviors including showing, directing attention, and coordinating gaze, facial expressions, and gestures, do not depend on language level and are, by definition, limited or absent in ASD.[2,51] Thus, a child with language disorder in the absence of ASD would be expected to show many such compensatory communication strategies. Further, symptoms such as lack of imitation and limitations in pretend play are much more prevalent in ASD than language disorder.[52–55] Additionally, when differentiating between ASD and language disorder in early childhood, parent report indicating delays in social and self-help skills may be more indicative of concern for ASD than language disorder.[56]

Social Pragmatic Communication Disorder

Social pragmatic communication disorder (SPCD) is defined by deficits in pragmatic language. These encompass social aspects of language including taking turns in conversation, using and understanding figurative language, greeting others, and so forth.[2] To meet diagnostic criteria for SPCD, these pragmatic language deficits cannot be accompanied by the presence of restricted and repetitive behaviors or interests associated with ASD, structural language disorders, or ID.[2] Symptoms of SPCD overlap with some of the social-communication deficits of ASD but are more confined. Although data are limited, the estimated prevalence of SPCD is less than 1%.[57,58] Further, there has been ongoing debate regarding the validity of the SPCD diagnosis because social pragmatic deficits rarely occur in the absence of ASD.[57] Implementation of SPCD diagnosis is challenging due to the lack of established assessment measures and the high rates of overlap between SPCD and other disorders, including ADHD, conduct disorder, and genetic conditions.[59] Given the diagnostic confusion and lack of diagnostic utility, many have argued that challenges associated with SPCD should be considered as a set of symptoms that cuts across multiple NDDs.[59]

Intellectual Developmental Disorder (Intellectual Disability)

ID is defined by deficits in intellectual and adaptive functioning.[2] It can range in severity from mild to profound. These severity levels represent distinct diagnostic entities and are important to designate given their vastly different symptom profiles and associated support needs and prognoses.[60] Individuals with mild ID (the most frequent type) often live and work independently with minimal supports needed at various times, whereas individuals with profound ID continue to require 24-hour supervision throughout their lives given basic support needs.[60,61]

ID also commonly co-occurs with ASD. Earlier studies showed it to be present in the majority of ASD cases,[62] and as a result, issues in differential diagnosis of ID and ASD were historically a focal point of the assessment literature, where discussion was largely focused on how to differentiate whether ASD was present in the context of ID. However, the distribution has shifted such that now a minority of individuals with ASD is diagnosed with ID.[63] Given this shifting prevalence of combined ID and ASD,[64,65] many newly trained clinicians are much less experienced in differential diagnosis of ID and ASD. Consequently, there are growing concerns that ASD may be overdiagnosed in ID, especially in developmentally or medically complex populations such as those with genetic conditions that require special expertise.[24,66,67]

To diagnose ASD in the context of ID, or global developmental delay for younger children, challenges in social communication, and the presence of restrictive/repetitive behaviors/interests, need to be beyond what would be expected for developmental age.[2,66,67] Therefore, developmental or cognitive testing is a critical component of any diagnostic evaluation because it is impossible to evaluate the presence of social communication deficits without establishing an individual's expected level of social communication ability. If direct cognitive or developmental testing is not possible, clinicians may consider using cognitive measures that rely heavily on parent report of cognitive skills (eg, the cognitive subtest of the Developmental Profile or the Developmental Assessment of Young Children, Second Edition).[68–70] However, clinicians should be aware of the limitations of using parent-report measures to estimate cognitive ability, and this method should only be used as a measure of last resort because it does not adhere to recommended best practices in ASD diagnostic assessment.[71] Requesting reports from school Individualized Education Plan evaluations is another strategy for obtaining estimates of developmental level, which can then be used to determine whether observed deficits in social communication are beyond what would be expected based on overall developmental level.

Among children identified as having global developmental delays or ID, assessing for differences in more basic/early emerging social communication behaviors, such as eye contact, joint attention, and showing can help distinguish ASD from ID because these skills are likely to be better developed in individuals without ASD even at very low mental ages.[23] Standardized instruments that quantify these behaviors based on direct observation and parent report are helpful in gathering information about deficits or capacities in basic social communication behaviors but to appropriately interpret results of these tests, the assessor must still exercise judgment about what would be expected for an individual's developmental level. Early development may also hold clues relevant to differential diagnosis. Although some children with ASD show delays from early on, these are often subtle, transient, and not detected without intensive assessment. Further, the majority of children with ASD achieve early motor milestones such as sitting and walking on time, which may contribute to the impression that they are developing normally during the first years of life.[72,73] In contrast, clinically identifiable motor delays are common in children with ID when ASD is not present. Regardless of whether a child is diagnosed with ASD and/or ID, identifiable delays in early motor milestones are likely to signal a potential genetic etiology and should prompt referral for genetic testing.[72,74]

As noted in DSM-5-TR criterion E and ICD-11 diagnostic criteria, the diagnosis of ASD in individuals with ID is particularly difficult, and requires in-depth and sometimes longitudinal assessments.[2,3] Individuals with visual, hearing, and motor impairments, which commonly occur in the context of severe to profound ID and genetic conditions, have been excluded from ASD diagnostic instrument validation samples. This exclusion limits the availability of data on differential diagnosis of ASD and ID within these conditions, as well as the availability of tools that can be validly used for such purposes.[23,75,76] The issue is so complex that Kanner actually excluded these children from his initial descriptions of ASD, claiming that these children's symptoms did not align with other descriptions of ASD.[77] However, to avoid diagnostic overshadowing, it is important to emphasize that an additional diagnosis of ASD *should* be made if skills in social reciprocity and communication are significantly impaired relative to the individual's general level of intellectual ability.[2,3,23]

Anxiety Disorders

Anxiety disorders are generally characterized by excessive fear or worry and avoidance of feared situations or stimuli. Differential diagnosis of autism and anxiety is nuanced and can be difficult. The challenges in differential diagnosis are somewhat related to symptom overlap between autism and anxiety.[78] Autism and anxiety also frequently co-occur.[79,80] Social anxiety disorder (SAD) very commonly co-occurs with ASD.[81–83] SAD is characterized by fear of negative evaluation by others, resulting in avoidance of social situations, possibly impacting school, work, and social life.[2] Both SAD and ASD are characterized by difficulty with social communication, leading some youth with SAD to receive elevated scores and/or score above cutoffs on ASD screening tools.[81] Thus, clinicians must consider not only the sensitivity of ASD screeners (ie, how likely they are to identify ASD in a child diagnosed with ASD) but also their specificity (ie, how likely they are to *not* identify ASD in a child who is not diagnosed with ASD). Age of onset can be useful in distinguishing between SAD and ASD because ASD is present early in the developmental period, whereas SAD more commonly emerges in early adolescence.[81,84] Youth with ASD can be expected to show overall greater generalized impairments in social function compared with youth with SAD.

Youth with selective mutism (SM) are also likely to score above cutoffs on some ASD screeners.[85] Both SM and autism are characterized by communication challenges. SM is an anxiety disorder defined by the lack of speaking in specific settings (eg, school) despite the ability to speak in other settings (eg, home).[2] It commonly co-occurs with other anxiety disorders, and SAD in particular.[86] SM can start at any age, although it most often presents in early childhood.[87] SM cannot currently be diagnosed in the context of ASD, although some argue that the 2 conditions can co-occur.[2,86] One key distinguishing feature between SM and ASD is the pervasiveness of communication difficulties. In contrast to ASD, communication challenges associated with SM are not present in all settings. In addition, whereas symptoms of ASD are present in early childhood, anxiety disorders tend to develop in later childhood and adolescence.[81] Thus, gathering a careful and comprehensive developmental history including detailed information about if, how, and when symptoms present across settings, is necessary for differentiating ASD from SM and other anxiety disorders that may have symptom overlap with ASD.

Obsessive Compulsive Disorder

Obsessive compulsive disorder is defined by the presence of obsessions (ie, intrusive, unwanted thoughts, images, or urges) and compulsions (repetitive behaviors or mental acts).[2,3] The difficulty in differentiating between OCD and ASD typically relates to distinguishing ASD-associated repetitive motor behaviors from compulsions, and distinguishing ASD-associated restricted interests or insistence on sameness from OCD-related obsessions, as they may appear very similar at first glance.[88] Compulsions in the context of OCD typically relieve anxiety caused by obsessive thoughts.[2,89] For example, hand washing is a common compulsion that relieves anxiety associated with contamination-related obsessive thoughts. Although they may bring relief from anxiety, compulsions are generally distressing to people with OCD, whereas repetitive behaviors in the context of ASD are often enjoyed.[90] When differentiating between repetitive thoughts and behaviors that are ASD-related versus OCD-related, it is important to consider that individuals (including children) can lack insight into their symptoms, so this can make it more difficult to assess for the presence of ego dystonic distress associated with symptoms (characteristic of OCD but not ASD).[90]

Depressive Disorders

Depressive disorders, generally, are characterized by persistent feelings of sadness, hopelessness, and lack of interest or pleasure in activities.[2,3] Depressive symptoms can also include changes in sleep and appetite and difficulty concentrating.

Depression has well-documented impacts on social function. In particular, youth with depression may show reduced interest in social activities and can also display flattened facial and vocal affect.[91] As is the case with other differential diagnoses, a detailed clinical and developmental history is helpful for distinguishing whether flattened affect and increased withdrawal from social activities are attributable to depression versus ASD, or depression in the context of ASD. As with anxiety disorders, the age of onset for depressive disorders tends to occur in adolescence or adulthood, differentiating it from ASD's early developmental period onset. Although they can be persistent, depressive disorders are often episodic. Thus, considering one's social behavior in the absence of a mood-related depressive episode will be important for distinguishing between social impairment due to ASD versus depression. Importantly, depression and autism commonly co-occur, especially in adolescence and adulthood, and screening for mood disturbance is important in the context of ASD.[92–94]

Schizophrenia Spectrum Disorders

Schizophrenia and autism have a history of diagnostic confusion. Before the first description of autism by Leo Kanner in 1943, "autism" was a term used to describe a symptom of schizophrenia.[77,95] Autism was not formally recognized as a separate disorder from childhood onset schizophrenia until 1980 with the publication of the DSM III.[95] Schizophrenia spectrum disorder (SSD) is a chronic disorder involving cognitive, behavioral, and emotional symptoms, and perceptual abnormalities associated with psychosis (eg, hallucinations).[2,3] Although not included in the neurodevelopmental disorder section of the DSM, schizophrenia is often considered an NDD.[96] Because SSD typically emerges in late adolescence and/or early adulthood, it has been considered at least nosologically distinct from other NDDs. However, there is increasing evidence that SSD, similar to other childhood NDDs, develops after early neurobiological insults causing perturbations in typical brain developmental patterns.[97] Both ASD and SSD are characterized by impairments in social behavior and cognition but the impairments differ qualitatively.[2,3] Although they have distinguishable features (eg, presence of psychotic features), there is significant phenotypic overlap between SSD and ASD. In addition to phenotypic overlap in social cognition, SSD and ASD also have some shared genetic features.[97]

Although frank symptom onset in SSD typically occurs in late adolescence or early adulthood,[2] individuals later diagnosed with schizophrenia often show atypical early developmental patterns similar to those commonly observed in autism (eg, speech and motor delay, and social impairments).[98] Given that SSD and ASD are both associated with atypical early social development, clinicians may still be unclear regarding the differential between SSD and ASD after obtaining a detailed early developmental history. Additionally, as with most other disorders discussed, ASD and SSD can co-occur.[99] Further, childhood-onset schizophrenia, characterized by onset before 13 years of age, is very rare, although is an appropriate diagnosis for some children (estimated prevalence ∼ 1/40,000).[100]

Symptoms of schizophrenia are divided into 2 categories: negative symptoms refer to the absence of typical social communication behaviors associated with SSD, including flat affect, lack of speech apathy, anhedonia, and inattentiveness; and positive symptoms refer to the presence of atypical symptoms (eg, hallucinations/delusions). Notably, much of the phenotypic overlap between SSD and ASD is in the negative symptoms category (eg, lack of eye contact, reduced use of gesture, limited range of facial expressions), as positive symptoms tend to me more disorder specific.[101] Given the potential behavioral overlap between SSD and ASD, especially in adolescence and adulthood, it is unsurprising that administration of the Autism

Diagnostic Observation Schedule, Second Edition (ADOS-2)[102] in adolescents and adults with schizophrenia results in a high rate of false positives (ie, exceeding cutoffs for an ADOS-2 classification of "ASD").[96,101] This further illustrates the dangers of overreliance on scores for making diagnoses, rather than considering multiple sources of information including expert clinical judgment, especially in situations involving complex differential diagnostic questions.

Stereotypic Movement Disorder

Motor stereotypies are repetitive, nonfunctional motor behaviors that are commonly observed in both autistic and nonautistic youth.[2,3,103] Stereotypic motor movements commonly present before 3 years of age and can continue into adulthood.[2,104] These predictable movements include arm flapping, hand flapping, and rocking back and forth, among many other repetitive movements.[103,104] Although they are most often described in the context of ASD and/or ID, motor stereotypies are also very common in children without other neurodevelopmental conditions.[105] They are also common in typically developing children, with prevalence estimates for simple motor stereotypies such as nail or lip biting and hair twirling ranging from 20% to 70% in children older than 3 years.[104] Motor stereotypies are also commonly observed in children with anxiety, OCD, ADHD, and tic disorders.[104]

In order to meet DSM-5 criteria for stereotypic movement disorder, movements must interfere with daily activities and may result in self-injury.[2,104,106] Stereotypic movement disorder, unlike ASD, is not characterized by the presence of deficits in social communication.[2,3] As such, if stereotypic movements are interfering and unaccompanied by the presence of deficits in social communication, it is more likely the child has stereotypic movement disorder than ASD. There is very little data on the prevalence of stereotypic movement disorder, especially in children without other NDDs. However, the DSM-5 does indicate these types of movements are more common in individuals with ID.

Genetic Conditions

Although the previous differentials described are behaviorally defined diagnoses included in DSM-5-TR, genetic condition are diagnosed based on genetic testing or screening for the presence of characteristic phenotypes. Many genetic syndromes and single gene variants are associated with increased likelihood of ASD[107,108]; however, this is almost always in the context of other neurodevelopmental concerns, often including ID. For instance, in conditions that confer significant risk for ID, such as Fragile X syndrome, Down syndrome, and tuberous sclerosis, individuals are also more likely to have ASD than those in the general population.[109,110] As mentioned above, it can be especially challenging to determine the presence of ASD in the context of a genetic condition and severe to profound ID.[23,111] However, even in the context of mild or moderate ID, it is important for clinicians to carefully consider and ensure that difficulties in social communication and the presence of restricted and repetitive behaviors (RRBs) are not better explained by ID or global developmental delay.[2]

However, as with all individuals with ID and/or complex medical profiles, it is important to avoid diagnostic overshadowing of ASD in the context of a genetic condition. For example, Down syndrome was historically thought to be a clearly contrasting condition to ASD but it is now recognized that a subset of children with Down syndrome does meet criteria for ASD, and it is important that these children are afforded specialized treatment for their relative deficits in social communication. Indeed, recent estimates of prevalence of ASD in the context of Down syndrome range from 16% to 42%.[110,112,113]

For youth with genetic condition who have ID, differential diagnosis is also complicated because of the common presence of RRBs.[114] It is important to consider the degree to which RRBs interfere with social interaction when making a differential diagnosis.[115] Rett syndrome, a genetic condition associated with an NDD caused by variants in the MeCP2 gene, shares some phenotypic overlap with ASD, including hand stereotypies in some cases.[114] Clinically, Rett syndrome is characterized by regression in motor skills, loss of spoken language, gait abnormalities, and hand stereotypies.[116] Although it was previously considered alongside autism as a pervasive developmental disorder in DSM-IV, because a gene was identified and because there are many conditions with similar circumstances, it was removed from DSM-5 except as a potential specifier (eg, ASD with Rett syndrome). It also remains as a medical diagnosis in the ICD-11 along with many other genetic conditions.

Co-occurring Conditions that Accompany Autism Spectrum Disorder

In addition to understanding differential diagnoses, it is important to consider that most individuals diagnosed with ASD are also diagnosed with co-occurring conditions.[117,118] Numerous studies have examined rates, demographics, and potential reasons for the generally high comorbidity rates found in individuals with ASD.[4] Moreover, multimorbidities may be described as the rule, rather than the exception, for NDDs generally.[119] Diagnoses already discussed in this article are among the most frequently co-occurring for youth with ASD, with ADHD currently considered the most prevalent.[4]

Given the co-occurring mental health and behavioral needs among youth with ASD, it is very important for clinicians to screen for the presence of mental health concerns and consider these needs when developing treatment plans.[117] As mentioned, it is important that clinicians be aware of diagnostic overshadowing, which could cause them to overlook co-occurring disorders (eg, attributing emotional symptoms to an established ASD diagnosis rather than the possible presence of a co-occurring mood disorder).[117] The presence of mental health concerns that do not fit clearly within the bounds of ASD as defined in DSM-5 (eg, anxiety, depression, obsessions/compulsions, and so forth) should be considered by clinicians as additional diagnostic questions during comprehensive evaluations. Screening for mental health concerns, especially in adolescents and adults with ASD, is extremely important given the high rates of suicide among individuals with autism.[120] Suicide is estimated to be at least 3 times as common among individuals with autism as compared with the general population. Suicidal ideation is also thought to occur at very high rates in adult population with autism ($\sim$66%).[121] Given the increased risk of suicide among people with autism, including children and adolescents, it is recommended that all people with autism be screened for suicidal ideation and previous attempts.[122]

In addition to mental health, it is also important to consider medical comorbidities among autistic youth. Youth with autism show higher rates of many medical conditions than nonautistic youth, including seizures, eczema, asthma, food allergies, sleep difficulties, and gastrointestinal problems.[4,123] At the time of diagnosis, and certainly if behavioral changes occur later, it is important to consider potential medical contributors and additional diagnoses, especially for younger and/or minimally verbal or nonspeaking autistic youth who may not communicate about their pain verbally. Co-occurring medical conditions could exacerbate symptoms associated with autism and can also contribute to other behavioral challenges.[124] For example, self-injury can reflect underlying medical problems or pain, in some cases.[125]

SUMMARY

Autism is a behaviorally defined condition with multiple etiologies and heterogeneous clinical presentation. Thus, accurate diagnosis requires expertise in autism and common rule-out conditions. Often an autism diagnosis merits consideration of genetic testing to determine if there is a genetic condition causing or contributing to autism symptoms, especially in the context of co-occurring ID. Additionally, autistic youth and their families should be offered ongoing monitoring and periodic reevaluations to identify updated support needs throughout development.

CLINICS CARE POINTS

- The diagnosis of ASD is complex, with different challenges depending on the chronologic and developmental age of the child or adolescent
- Autism is a behaviorally defined condition associated with many different etiologies, including rare genetic conditions; therefore, practitioners need to be aware of the importance of genetic and medical assessment in addition to psychodiagnostic evaluation
- Pediatricians play a key role in providing surveillance and screening for ASD in all children; practitioners who wish to participate in the ASD diagnostic assessment process require additional, specialized training
- Needs and diagnoses for autistic youth can change across time; therefore, it is important for youth to have continued monitoring and reevaluation across different developmental periods
- Even after an ASD diagnosis has been established, clinicians must consider other important elements of management, including the diagnosis of co-occurring medical, genetic, and/or psychiatric conditions that can present at various points throughout development
- Characteristics associated with ASD can be observed in several other conditions. Some of the most challenging differential diagnoses from Autism include the following (most of which can also co-occur with ASD):
  - ADHD
  - Language disorders
  - SPCD
  - ID
  - Anxiety disorders
  - Depressive disorders
  - SSDs
  - Stereotypic movement disorder
  - Genetic conditions
- Diagnosis of ASD requires a thorough, systematic assessment by a trained expert. A diagnostic evaluation includes both direct observation of the child as well as detailed developmental history obtained from the youth's caregiver. Clinicians must have both expertise in autism and ample experience in identifying commonly co-occurring conditions
- It is important that clinicians working with autistic youth understand the limitations of current assessment measures especially when evaluating children with genetic conditions and/or other medical issues or sensory differences (eg, hearing or visual impairments)

DISCLOSURE

This article was written as part of Audrey Thurm's official duties as a Government employee. The views expressed in this article do not necessarily represent the views of the National Institutes of Health (NIH), Department of Health and Human Services

(HHS), or the United States Government. S. Bishop receives royalties for sales of the Autism Diagnostic Observation Schedule, Second Edition (ADOS-2).

REFERENCES

1. Lord C, Charman T, Havdahl A, et al. The Lancet Commission on the future of care and clinical research in autism. Lancet 2022;399(10321):271–334.
2. American Psychiatric Association. Diagnostic and Statistical Manual of Mental Disorders. Diagnostic and Statistical Manual of Mental Disorders 2022. https://doi.org/10.1176/APPI.BOOKS.9780890425787.
3. World Health Organization. International Statistical Classification of Diseases and Related Health Problems. 11th ed.; 2019. Available at: https://icd.who.int/en. Accessed May 7, 2023.
4. Khachadourian V, Mahjani B, Sandin S, et al. Comorbidities in autism spectrum disorder and their etiologies. Transl Psychiatry 2023;13(1):1–7.
5. Duvall S, Armstrong K, Shahabuddin A, et al. A road map for identifying autism spectrum disorder: Recognizing and evaluating characteristics that should raise red or "pink" flags to guide accurate differential diagnosis. Clin Neuropsychol 2022;36(5):1172–207.
6. Bishop SL, Lord C. Commentary: Best practices and processes for assessment of autism spectrum disorder – the intended role of standardized diagnostic instruments. J Child Psychol Psychiatry 2023. https://doi.org/10.1111/JCPP.13802.
7. Self TL, Parham DF, Rajagopalan J. Autism Spectrum Disorder Early Screening Practices 2014;36(4):195–207.
8. Developmental Screening/Testing Coding Fact Sheet for Primary Care Pediatricians. Available at: https://downloads.aap.org/AAP/PDF/coding_factsheet_developmentalscreeningtestingandEmotionalBehvioraassessment.pdf.
9. Hyman SL, Levy SE, Myers SM, et al. Identification, evaluation, and management of children with autism spectrum disorder. Pediatrics 2020;145(1). https://doi.org/10.1542/PEDS.2019-3447.
10. Autism Toolkit | AAP Toolkits | American Academy of Pediatrics. Available at: https://publications.aap.org/toolkits/pages/Autism-Toolkit?_ga=2.81406549.354996877.1684853451-984848857.1679074220. Accessed May 22, 2023.
11. Pediatrics AA of. Standardized Screening/Testing Coding Fact Sheet for Primary Care Pediatricians: Developmental/Behavioral/Emotional. Published online October 3, 2019. Available at: https://publications.aap.org/toolkits/book/338/chapter/5732104/Standardized-Screening-Testing-Coding-Fact-Sheet. Accessed May 23, 2023.
12. American Academy of Pediatrics. Tools and Resources for pediatricians. Published 2021. Available at: https://www.aap.org/en/patient-care/autism/tools-and-resources-for-pediatricians/. Accessed October 3, 2023.
13. Guan X, Zwaigenbaum L, Sonnenberg LK, et al. Building Capacity for Community Pediatric Autism Diagnosis: A Systemic Review of Physician Training Programs. Journal of Developmental and Behavioral Pediatrics 2022;43(1):44–54. Available at: http://links.lww.com/JDBP/A339. Accessed October 3, 2023.
14. Nowell KP, Christopher K, Sohl K. Equipping Community Based Psychologists to Deliver Best Practice ASD Diagnoses Using The ECHO Autism Model. Child Health Care 2020;403–24. https://doi.org/10.1080/02739615.2020.1771564.
15. Mazurek MO, Curran A, Burnette C, et al. ECHO Autism STAT: Accelerating Early Access to Autism Diagnosis. J Autism Dev Disord 2019;49(1):127–37.

16. Lipkin PH, Macias MM, Hyman SL, et al. Promoting Optimal Development: Identifying Infants and Young Children With Developmental Disorders Through Developmental Surveillance and Screening. Pediatrics 2020;145(1). https://doi.org/10.1542/PEDS.2019-3449.
17. Guthrie W, Wallis K, Bennett A, et al. Accuracy of Autism Screening in a Large Pediatric Network. Pediatrics 2019;144(4). https://doi.org/10.1542/PEDS.2018-3963.
18. Davidovitch M, Levit-Binnun N, Golan D, et al. Late diagnosis of autism spectrum disorder after initial negative assessment by a multidisciplinary team. J Dev Behav Pediatr 2015;36(4):227–34.
19. Avlund SH, Thomsen PH, Schendel D, et al. Factors Associated with a Delayed Autism Spectrum Disorder Diagnosis in Children Previously Assessed on Suspicion of Autism. J Autism Dev Disord 2021;51(11):3843–56.
20. Hirota T, So R, Kim YS, et al. A systematic review of screening tools in non-young children and adults for autism spectrum disorder. Res Dev Disabil 2018; 80:1–12.
21. Hyman SL, Levy SE, Myers SM, et al. Executive summary: Identification, evaluation, and management of children with autism spectrum disorder. Pediatrics 2020;145(1). https://doi.org/10.1542/PEDS.2019-3448/37021.
22. Choueiri R, Garrison WT, Tokatli V, et al. The RITA-T (Rapid Interactive Screening Test for Autism in Toddlers) Community Model to Improve Access and Early Identification of Autism in Young Children. Child Neurol Open 2023;10. https://doi.org/10.1177/2329048X231203817.
23. Thurm A, Farmer C, Salzman E, et al. State of the Field: Differentiating Intellectual Disability From Autism Spectrum Disorder. Front Psychiatry 2019;10. https://doi.org/10.3389/FPSYT.2019.00526.
24. Fombonne E. Editorial: Is autism overdiagnosed? JCPP (J Child Psychol Psychiatry) 2023;64(5):711–4.
25. Havdahl KA, Hus Bal V, Huerta M, et al. Multidimensional Influences on Autism Symptom Measures: Implications for Use in Etiological Research. J Am Acad Child Adolesc Psychiatry 2016;55(12):1054–63.e3.
26. Bishop S, Farmer C, Kaat A, et al. The need for a developmentally based measure of social-communication skills. J Am Acad Child Adolesc Psychiatry 2019; 58(6):555.
27. Weitlauf AS, Gotham KO, Vehorn AC, et al. Brief report: DSM-5 "levels of support:" a comment on discrepant conceptualizations of severity in ASD. J Autism Dev Disord 2014;44(2):471–6.
28. Rice CE, Carpenter LA, Morrier MJ, et al. Defining in Detail and Evaluating Reliability of DSM-5 Criteria for Autism Spectrum Disorder (ASD) Among Children. J Autism Dev Disord 2022;52(12):5308.
29. Gardner LM, Campbell JM, Keisling B, et al. Correlates of DSM-5 Autism Spectrum Disorder Levels of Support Ratings in a Clinical Sample. J Autism Dev Disord 2018;48(10):3513–23.
30. Bal VH, Farmer C, Thurm A. Describing function in ASD: Using the DSM-5 and other methods to improve precision. J Autism Dev Disord 2017;47(9):2938.
31. Ruble LA, Dalrymple NJ, McGrew JH. The Effects of Consultation on Individualized Education Program Outcomes for Young Children With Autism: The Collaborative Model for Promoting Competence and Success. J Early Interv 2010; 32(4):286.

32. Elias R, Lord C. Diagnostic stability in individuals with autism spectrum disorder: insights from a longitudinal follow-up study. J Child Psychol Psychiatry 2022; 63(9):973.
33. Hirota T, King BH. Autism Spectrum Disorder: A Review. JAMA 2023;329(2): 157–68.
34. Simonoff E, Kent R, Stringer D, et al. Trajectories in Symptoms of Autism and Cognitive Ability in Autism From Childhood to Adult Life: Findings From a Longitudinal Epidemiological Cohort. J Am Acad Child Adolesc Psychiatry 2020; 59(12):1342–52.
35. Pickles A, Anderson DK, Lord C. Heterogeneity and plasticity in the development of language: a 17-year follow-up of children referred early for possible autism. J Child Psychol Psychiatry 2014;55(12):1354–62.
36. Thurm A, Srivastava S. On Terms: What's in a Name? Intellectual Disability and "Condition," "Disorder," "Syndrome," "Disease," and "Disability.". Am J Intellect Dev Disabil 2022;127(5):349–54.
37. Cohen E, Houtrow A. Disability Is Not Delay: Precision Communication about Intellectual Disability. J Pediatr 2019;207:241–3.
38. Bishop SL, Zheng S, Kaat A, et al. Dr. Bishop et al. Reply. J Am Acad Child Adolesc Psychiatry 2020;59(11):1200–2.
39. Lord C, Bishop SL. Let's Be Clear That "Autism Spectrum Disorder Symptoms" Are Not Always Related to Autism Spectrum Disorder. Am J Psychiatry 2021; 178(8):680–2.
40. Lyall K, Croen L, Daniels J, et al. The Changing Epidemiology of Autism Spectrum Disorders. Annu Rev Public Health 2017;38:81–102.
41. Zablotsky B, Bramlett MD, Blumberg SJ. The co-occurrence of autism spectrum disorder in children with ADHD HHS Public Access. J Atten Disord 2020;24(1): 94–103.
42. Taurines R, Schwenck C, Westerwald E, et al. ADHD and autism: differential diagnosis or overlapping traits? A selective review. Atten Defic Hyperact Disord 2012;4(3):115–39.
43. Harkins CM, Handen BL, Mazurek MO. The Impact of the Comorbidity of ASD and ADHD on Social Impairment. J Autism Dev Disord 2022;52(6):2512–22.
44. Guttentag S, Bishop S, Doggett R, et al. The utility of parent-report screening tools in differentiating autism versus attention-deficit/hyperactivity disorder in school-age children. Autism 2021;26(2):473–87.
45. Mikami AY, Normand S. The Importance of Social Contextual Factors in Peer Relationships of Children with ADHD. Curr Dev Disord Rep 2015;2(1):30–7.
46. Antshel KM, Russo N. Autism Spectrum Disorders and ADHD: Overlapping Phenomenology, Diagnostic Issues, and Treatment Considerations. Curr Psychiatry Rep 2019;21(5):1–11.
47. Aduen PA, Day TN, Kofler MJ, et al. Social Problems in ADHD: Is it a Skills Acquisition or Performance Problem? J Psychopathol Behav Assess 2018; 40(3):440–51.
48. Paul R. Language disorders. Handb Clin Neurol 2020;174:21–35.
49. Tager-Flusberg H, Joseph RM. Identifying neurocognitive phenotypes in autism. Phil Trans Biol Sci 2003;358(1430):303.
50. Mueller KL, Tomblin JB. Examining the comorbidity of language disorders and ADHD. Top Lang Disord 2012;32(3):228.
51. Lord C, Pickles A. Language level and nonverbal social-communicative behaviors in autistic and language-delayed children. J Am Acad Child Adolesc Psychiatry 1996;35(11):1542–50.

52. Charman T, Swettenham J, Baron-Cohen S, et al. Infants with autism: an investigation of empathy, pretend play, joint attention, and imitation. Dev Psychol 1997;33(5):781–9.

53. Charman T, Swettenham J, Baron-Cohen S, et al. Michigan Association for Infant Mental Health. Infant Ment Health J 1998;19(2):260–75.

54. Charman T, Baird G. Practitioner review: Diagnosis of autism spectrum disorder in 2- and 3-year-old children. J Child Psychol Psychiatry 2002;43(3):289–305.

55. Mayes L, Volkmar F, Hooks M, et al. Differentiating pervasive developmental disorder not otherwise specified from autism and language disorders. J Autism Dev Disord 1993;23(1):79–90.

56. Richard AE, Hodges EK, Carlson MD. Differential Diagnosis of Autism Spectrum Disorder Versus Language Disorder in Children Ages 2 to 5 Years: Contributions of Parent-Reported Development and Behavior. Clin Pediatr (Phila) 2019; 58(11–12):1232–8.

57. Saul J, Griffiths S, Norbury CF. Prevalence and functional impact of social (pragmatic) communication disorders. J Child Psychol Psychiatry 2023;64(3):376–87.

58. Kim YS, Fombonne E, Koh YJ, et al. A Comparison of DSM-IV PDD and DSM-5 ASD Prevalence in an Epidemiologic Sample. J Am Acad Child Adolesc Psychiatry 2014;53(5):500.

59. Norbury CF, Holloway R. Practitioner Review: Social (pragmatic) communication disorder conceptualization, evidence and clinical implications. JCPP (J Child Psychol Psychiatry) 2014;55(3):204–16.

60. McKenzie K, Milton M, Smith G, et al. Systematic Review of the Prevalence and Incidence of Intellectual Disabilities: Current Trends and Issues. Curr Dev Disord Rep 2016;3(2):104–15.

61. Srour M, Shevell M. Genetics and the investigation of developmental delay/intellectual disability. Arch Dis Child 2014;99(4):386–9.

62. Fombonne E, Psych FRC. Epidemiology of Autistic Disorder and Other Pervasive Developmental Disorders. J Clin Psychiatry 2005;66(suppl 10): 6490. Available at: https://www.psychiatrist.com/jcp/psychiatry/epidemiology-autistic-disorder-pervasive-developmental. Accessed May 9, 2023.

63. Maenner MJ, Warren Z, Williams AR, et al. Prevalence and Characteristics of Autism Spectrum Disorder Among Children Aged 8 Years — Autism and Developmental Disabilities Monitoring Network, 11 Sites, United States, 2020. MMWR Surveillance Summaries 2023;72(2):1–14.

64. Polyak A, Kubina RM, Girirajan S. Comorbidity of intellectual disability confounds ascertainment of autism: implications for genetic diagnosis. Am J Med Genet Part B: Neuropsychiatric Genetics 2015;168(7):600–8.

65. Baio J, Wiggins L, Christensen DL, et al. Prevalence of Autism Spectrum Disorder Among Children Aged 8 Years — Autism and Developmental Disabilities Monitoring Network, 11 Sites, United States, 2014. MMWR Surveillance Summaries 2018;67(6):1.

66. Jenner L, Richards C, Howard R, et al. Heterogeneity of Autism Characteristics in Genetic Syndromes: Key Considerations for Assessment and Support. Curr Dev Disord Rep 2023;10(2):132.

67. Hepburn SL, Moody EJ. Diagnosing Autism in Individuals with Known Genetic Syndromes: Clinical Considerations and Implications for Intervention. Int Rev Res Dev Disabil 2011;40(1):229–59.

68. Swartzmiller MD. Test Review: Developmental Assessment of Young Children–Second Edition (DAYC-2). J Psychoeduc Assess 2014;32(6):577–80.

69. Voress JK, Maddox T. Developmental assessment of young children. 2nd edition. Austin, TX: PRO-ED; 2013.

70. Wetherby AM, Allen L, Cleary J, et al. Validity and Reliability of the Communication and Symbolic Behavior Scales Developmental Profile With Very Young Children. J Speech Lang Hear Res 2002;45(6):1202–18.

71. Lee CM, Green Snyder L, Carpenter LA, et al. Agreement of parent-reported cognitive level with standardized measures among children with autism spectrum disorder. Autism Res 2023;16:1210–24.

72. Wickstrom J, Farmer C, Green Snyder LA, et al. Patterns of delay in early gross motor and expressive language milestone attainment in probands with genetic conditions versus idiopathic ASD from SFARI registries. JCPP (J Child Psychol Psychiatry) 2021;62(11):1297–307.

73. Bishop SL, Thurm A, Farmer C, et al. Autism Spectrum Disorder, Intellectual Disability, and Delayed Walking. Pediatrics 2016;137(3). https://doi.org/10.1542/PEDS.2015-2959.

74. Bishop SL, Farmer C, Bal V, et al. Identification of Developmental and Behavioral Markers Associated With Genetic Abnormalities in Autism Spectrum Disorder. Am J Psychiatry 2017;174(6):576–85.

75. Risi S, Lord C, Gotham K, et al. Combining Information From Multiple Sources in the Diagnosis of Autism Spectrum Disorders. J Am Acad Child Adolesc Psychiatry 2006;45(9):1094–103.

76. Moss J, Howlin P, Oliver C. The Assessment and Presentation of Autism Spectrum Disorder and Associated Characteristics in Individuals with Severe Intellectual Disability and Genetic Syndromes. The Oxford Handbook of Intellectual Disability and Development 2011. https://doi.org/10.1093/OXFORDHB/9780195305012.013.0018.

77. Harris J. Leo Kanner and autism: a 75-year perspective. Int Rev Psychiatry 2018;30(1):3–17.

78. White SW, Oswald D, Ollendick T, et al. Anxiety in children and adolescents with autism spectrum disorders. Clin Psychol Rev 2009;29(3):216–29.

79. Gotham K, Bishop SL, Hus V, et al. Exploring the relationship between anxiety and insistence on sameness in autism spectrum disorders. Autism Res 2013; 6(1):33–41.

80. Kerns CM, Rump K, Worley J, et al. The Differential Diagnosis of Anxiety Disorders in Cognitively-Able Youth With Autism. Cogn Behav Pract 2016;23(4): 530–47.

81. Capriola-Hall NN, McFayden T, Ollendick TH, et al. Caution When Screening for Autism among Socially Anxious Youth. J Autism Dev Disord 2021;51(5):1540–9.

82. Kuusikko S, Pollock-Wurman R, Jussila K, et al. Social anxiety in high-functioning children and adolescents with autism and Asperger syndrome. J Autism Dev Disord 2008;38(9):1697–709.

83. Spain D, Sin J, Linder KB, et al. Social anxiety in autism spectrum disorder: A systematic review. Res Autism Spectr Disord 2018;52:51–68.

84. De Lijster JM, Dierckx B, Utens EMWJ, et al. The age of onset of anxiety disorders: A meta-analysis. Can J Psychiatr 2017;62(4):237–46.

85. Cholemkery H, Mojica L, Rohrmann S, et al. Can autism spectrum disorders and social anxiety disorders be differentiated by the social responsiveness scale in children and adolescents? J Autism Dev Disord 2014;44(5):1168–82.

86. Muris P, Ollendick TH. Selective Mutism and Its Relations to Social Anxiety Disorder and Autism Spectrum Disorder. Clin Child Fam Psychol Rev 2021;24(2): 294–325.

87. Kristensen H. Selective mutism and comorbidity with developmental disorder/ delay, anxiety disorder, and elimination disorder. J Am Acad Child Adolesc Psychiatry 2000;39(2):249–56.

88. Jiujias M, Kelley E, Hall L. Restricted, Repetitive Behaviors in Autism Spectrum Disorder and Obsessive-Compulsive Disorder: A Comparative Review. Child Psychiatry Hum Dev 2017;48:944–59.

89. Starcevic V, Berle D, Brakoulias V, et al. Functions of Compulsions in Obsessive–Compulsive Disorder. Aust N Z J Psychiatry 2011;45(6):449–57.

90. Wu MS, Rudy BM, Storch EA. Obsessions, compulsions, and repetitive behavior: Autism and/or OCD. Handbook of autism and anxiety 2014;107–20.

91. Pezzimenti F, Han GT, Vasa RA, et al. Depression in Youth with Autism Spectrum Disorder. Child Adolesc Psychiatr Clin N Am 2019;28(3):397–409.

92. Howlin P. Outcomes in Autism Spectrum Disorders. Handbook of Autism and Pervasive Developmental Disorders 2005;201–20. https://doi.org/10.1002/9780470939345.CH7.

93. Uljarević M, Hedley D, Rose-Foley K, et al. Anxiety and Depression from Adolescence to Old Age in Autism Spectrum Disorder. J Autism Dev Disord 2020;50(9):3155–65.

94. Wigham S, Barton S, Parr JR, et al. A systematic review of the rates of depression in children and adults with high-functioning autism spectrum disorder. J Ment Health Res Intellect Disabil 2017;10(4):267–87.

95. Rosen NE, Lord C, Volkmar FR. The Diagnosis of Autism: From Kanner to DSM-III to DSM-5 and Beyond. J Autism Dev Disord 2021;51(12):4253.

96. Stachowiak MK, Kucinski A, Curl R, et al. Schizophrenia: A neurodevelopmental disorder — Integrative genomic hypothesis and therapeutic implications from a transgenic mouse model. Schizophr Res 2013;143(2–3):367–76.

97. Owen MJ, O'Donovan MC. Schizophrenia and the neurodevelopmental continuum:evidence from genomics. World Psychiatr 2017;16(3):227–35.

98. Niemi LT, Suvisaari JM, Tuulio-Henriksson A, et al. Childhood developmental abnormalities in schizophrenia: evidence from high-risk studies. Schizophr Res 2003;60(2–3):239–58.

99. Zheng Z, Zheng P, Zou X. Association between schizophrenia and autism spectrum disorder: A systematic review and meta-analysis. Autism Res 2018;11(8):1110–9.

100. Gochman P, Miller R, Rapoport JL. Childhood-onset schizophrenia: the challenge of diagnosis. Curr Psychiatry Rep 2011;13:321–32.

101. Trevisan DA, Foss-Feig JH, Naples AJ, et al. Autism Spectrum Disorder and Schizophrenia Are Better Differentiated by Positive Symptoms Than Negative Symptoms. Front Psychiatry 2020;11:548.

102. Lord C, Rutter M, Dilavore P, et al. Autism diagnostic observation schedule, second edition (ADOS-2) manual (Part I): modules 1–4. Torrance, CA: Western Psychological Services; 2012.

103. McCarty MJ, Brumback AC. Rethinking Stereotypies in Autism. Semin Pediatr Neurol 2021;38:100897.

104. Katherine M. Stereotypic Movement Disorders. Semin Pediatr Neurol 2018;25:19–24.

105. Péter Z, Oliphant ME, Fernandez TV. Motor stereotypies: A pathophysiological review. Front Neurosci 2017;11:171.

106. Singer HS. Stereotypic movement disorders. Handb Clin Neurol 2011;100:631–9.

107. Sanders SJ, He X, Willsey AJ, et al. Insights into Autism Spectrum Disorder Genomic Architecture and Biology from 71 Risk Loci. Neuron 2015;87(6): 1215–33.
108. Satterstrom FK, Kosmicki JA, Wang J, et al. Large-scale exome sequencing study implicates both developmental and functional changes in the neurobiology of autism. Cell 2020;180(3):568–84.
109. Geschwind DH. Genetics of Autism Spectrum Disorders. Trends Cogn Sci 2011; 15(9):409.
110. Hamner T, Hepburn S, Zhang F, et al. Cognitive Profiles and Autism Symptoms in Comorbid Down Syndrome and Autism Spectrum Disorder. J Dev Behav Pediatr 2020;41(3):172–9.
111. Soorya L, Leon J, Trelles MP, et al. Framework for assessing individuals with rare genetic disorders associated with profound intellectual and multiple disabilities (PIMD): the example of Phelan McDermid Syndrome. Clin Neuropsychol 2018; 32(7):1226–55.
112. Moss J, Howlin P. Autism spectrum disorders in genetic syndromes: implications for diagnosis, intervention and understanding the wider autism spectrum disorder population. J Intellect Disabil Res 2009;53(10):852–73.
113. Reilly C. Autism spectrum disorders in Down syndrome: A review. Res Autism Spectr Disord 2009;3(4):829–39.
114. Goldman S, Temudo T. Hand stereotypies distinguish Rett syndrome from autism disorder. Movement Disorders 2012;27(8):1060–2.
115. Nunnally AD, Nguyen V, Anglo C, et al. Symptoms of Autism Spectrum Disorder in Individuals with Down Syndrome. Brain Sci 2021;11(10).
116. Neul JL. The relationship of Rett syndrome and MECP2 disorders to autism. Dialogues Clin Neurosci 2022;14(3):253–62.
117. Rosen TE, Mazefsky CA, Vasa RA, et al. Co-occurring psychiatric conditions in autism spectrum disorder. Int Rev Psychiatry 2018;30(1):40–61.
118. Mosner MG, Kinard JL, Shah JS, et al. Rates of Co-occurring Psychiatric Disorders in Autism Spectrum Disorder using the Mini International Neuropsychiatric Interview. J Autism Dev Disord 2019;49(9):3819.
119. Thapar A, Rutter M. Genetic Advances in Autism. J Autism Dev Disord 2021; 51(12):4321–32.
120. South M, Costa AP, McMorris C. Death by Suicide Among People With Autism: Beyond Zebrafish. JAMA Netw Open 2021;4(1):e2034018.
121. Cassidy S, Bradley P, Robinson J, et al. Suicidal ideation and suicide plans or attempts in adults with asperger's syndrome attending a specialist diagnostic clinic: A clinical cohort study. Lancet Psychiatr 2014;1(2):142–7.
122. Mayes SD, Gorman AA, Hillwig-Garcia J, et al. Suicide ideation and attempts in children with autism. Res Autism Spectr Disord 2013;7(1):109–19.
123. Al-Beltagi M. Autism medical comorbidities. World J Clin Pediatr 2021;10(3):15.
124. Symons FJ, Harper VN, McGrath PJ, et al. Evidence of increased non-verbal behavioral signs of pain in adults with neurodevelopmental disorders and chronic self-injury. Res Dev Disabil 2009;30(3):521–8.
125. Summers J, Shahrami A, Cali S, et al. Self-Injury in Autism Spectrum Disorder and Intellectual Disability: Exploring the Role of Reactivity to Pain and Sensory Input. Brain Sci 2017. https://doi.org/10.3390/brainsci7110140.

Etiologic Evaluation of Children with Autism Spectrum Disorder

Steven M. Lazar, MD, MEd[a],*, Thomas D. Challman, MD[b],
Scott M. Myers, MD[b]

KEYWORDS

- Autism • Genetics • Metabolic • Etiology • Evaluation

KEY POINTS

- Autism spectrum disorder (ASD) is clinically and etiologically heterogeneous.
- A causal genetic variant can be identified in approximately 20% to 25% of affected individuals with currently available clinical genetic testing, and all patients with an ASD diagnosis should be offered genetic etiologic evaluation.
- We suggest that exome sequencing with copy number variant coverage should be the first-line etiologic evaluation for ASD. Neuroimaging, neurophysiologic, metabolic, and other biochemical evaluations can provide insight into the pathophysiology of ASD but should only be recommended in the appropriate clinical circumstances.

INTRODUCTION

When formulating neurodevelopmental diagnoses and counseling families, etiologic factors (Why does my child have this diagnosis?), categorical disorders or symptom-cluster syndromes (What is the diagnosis?), and specific impairments and their interventions must be considered (What does this mean for my child/What can be done?).[1] Autism spectrum disorder (ASD) is a categorical disorder defined by a set of specific, reproducible symptom clusters. A diagnosis of ASD describes the presence of core specific impairments in social communication, repetitive behaviors, and restricted interests within an atypical pattern of neurodevelopmental delays, dissociations, and deviance.[2] This descriptive diagnosis, although, does not account for the myriad etiologic factors that can lead to a diagnosis of ASD and does not imply a

[a] Section of Pediatric Neurology and Developmental Neuroscience, Meyer Center for Developmental Pediatrics & Autism, Baylor College of Medicine – Texas Children's Hospital, 6701 Fannin Street Suite 1250, Houston, TX 77030, USA; [b] Geisinger Autism & Developmental Medicine Institute, Geisinger Commonwealth School of Medicine, 120 Hamm Drive, Suite 2A, Lewisburg, PA 17837, USA
* Corresponding author.
E-mail address: Steven.Lazar@bcm.edu

Pediatr Clin N Am 71 (2024) 179–197
https://doi.org/10.1016/j.pcl.2023.12.002
0031-3955/24/© 2024 Elsevier Inc. All rights reserved.
pediatric.theclinics.com

specific etiology. Similarly, an etiologic diagnosis can neither fully confirm nor refute a clinical diagnosis of ASD but only provide explanatory factors and determination of relative risk for those who do not currently have a diagnosis of ASD (**Fig. 1**).

An etiologic evaluation for individuals with ASD can be quite important to the individual, family, and broader societal context. A categorical diagnosis of ASD, coupled with the profiling of an individual's specific impairments, is often critical to planning behavioral, education, and pharmacologic treatments. An etiologic diagnosis can guide the identification of associated medical problems, prognostication and family planning, and has emerging treatment implications. Broadly speaking, ASD can be conceptualized alongside other neurodevelopmental disorders as a product of developmental brain dysfunction (see Moreno De Luca and colleagues for review[3]) that leads to atypical behaviors and development.

The origins of this dysfunction range from genetic, cellular, structural, and functional neuroanatomy to environmental agents as well as complex multifactorial interactions. Even some of the earliest likely descriptions of ASD in folkloric traditions (changelings) and feral children (Wild Boy of Aveyron) have tried to uncover and understand the causes of atypical neurodevelopment in children.[4] The twentieth century provided scientific descriptions of ASD in the 1920s: Grunya Sukhareva,[5,6] Lauretta Bender (childhood schizophrenia),[7] Leo Kanner,[8] and Hans Asperger[9] in the mid-twentieth century. Etiologic study focusing on genetic evaluation has had the most substantial clinical impact; current clinically available genetic testing can account at least 25% of ASD.[10]

A wide range of neuroanatomic, neurophysiologic, and environmental or acquired (ie, infectious, inflammatory, and traumatic) causes has been proposed. A single, consolidated ASD-specific etiology or pathogenesis is unlikely to be found.[11] Given

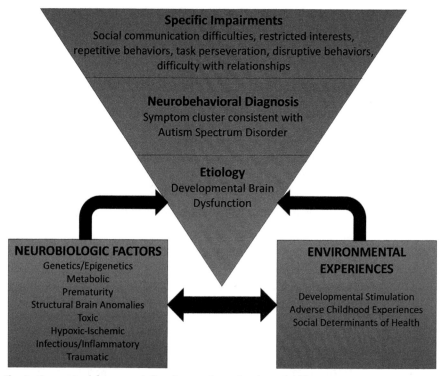

Fig. 1. Conceptual framework for diagnostic evaluation of ASD.

this, ASD is best characterized as one of the many symptom cluster presentations of developmental brain dysfunction more broadly, and etiologic investigations should be based on individualized history and examination.

Overall, the goal of this article is to provide a practical overview of the clinical etiologic evaluation of ASD with an emphasis on genetic evaluation. Clinically, etiologic evaluation focuses primarily on genetic evaluation. Upcoming research-based neuroimaging, neurophysiologic, and advanced genetic techniques may have potential to find early biomarkers, treatment response targets, and pre-/early symptomatic identification of individuals at risk for a diagnosis of ASD although they are not currently clinically applicable for an individual patient. Ideal biomarkers should be readily available, and affordable, tools for early identification, diagnostic certainty, symptom monitoring, and/or treatment response to objectively measure and monitor the effectiveness of various supports and interventions.[12,13]

As with the clinical diagnosis of ASD, the etiologic evaluation should be driven by neurodevelopmental history (including medical, social, family, academic, and developmental) and examination (dysmorphology, comprehensive physical examination including detailed neurologic examination, and developmental assessment).[14,15] **Table 1** provides an overview of components of the neurodevelopmental history and examination that can help guide etiologic evaluation.

ETIOLOGY FACTORS AND EVALUATION
Genetic Testing and Autism Spectrum Disorder

Pathogenic (causative) genetic associations with ASD include single nucleotide variants, copy number variants (CNVs; microdeletions and duplications), chromosomal aneuploidy (abnormal numbers of chromosomes), trinucleotide repeat expansions, imprinting/methylation disorders, and polygenic-multifactorial genetic alterations.[16,17] There is no single genetic test that can accurately capture all potential etiologic associations with ASD. Evidence-based, clinically oriented decisions must be made to recommend the most appropriate cost-effective and clinically relevant genetic testing. Clinically available genetic testing methods, their indications, and pros and cons are summarized in **Table 2**.

Through evaluation of twin and family aggregate studies, ASD heritability ranges from 60% to 90%.[18] Commonly ordered testing in ASD include chromosomal microarray (CMA; diagnostic yield of at least 5%–10%), exome sequencing (ES; also known was whole exome sequencing [WES][19]; diagnostic yield of at least 15%), and fragile X *FMR1* CGG repeat analysis (diagnostic yield of at least 0.5%). Increasing diagnostic yield is noted with lower IQ, neurologic comorbidities (such as epilepsy and motor dysfunction), dysmorphic features, and congenital anomalies with an overall diagnostic yield of at least 20% to 25% of individuals with ASD.[10] The remainder of missing heritability is thought to be due to yet-undescribed genetic causes, whether they be undiscovered gene associations or more complex genetic pathogenesis that is not able to be addressed with current technology.[20]

Current clinical pathways and society recommendations exist on the most appropriate stepwise use of genetic testing for ASD—and other neurodevelopmental disorders more broadly—with an emphasis on first-line testing with CMA and fragile X analysis.[14,21–23] Professional society recommendations often lag considerably behind the evidence base but ES (with CNV coverage) or genome sequencing (GS; also known as whole genome sequencing[19]) is expected to become a first-tier recommendation for individuals with ASD, similar to the existing recommendation for intellectual developmental disorder, global developmental delay, or congenital anomalies.[10,24,25]

Table 1
The neurodevelopmental assessment of autism spectrum disorder and etiologic implications

Component of the Neurodevelopmental Evaluation	Findings that Guide Etiologic Evaluation	Possible Evaluation
Chief complaint and history of present illness	Clinical events concerning for seizures (unresponsive shaking, staring spells without ability to regain attention) Difficulty responding to verbal cues Asymmetric movement or weakness Acute or intermittent decompensations, cyclic vomiting	EEG Audiology Brain MRI Metabolic testing
Developmental and academic history	Developmental regression	Brain MRI, Metabolic testing, Sleep-capture EEG
Birth history	Maternal history of miscarriages; maternal medications; prenatal toxic exposures; gestational hypertension/preeclampsia; gestational age; birthweight; other risk factors for neurologic impairment	Genetic testing
Medical history	Neurologic co-occurring disorders such as epilepsy Decompensation with minor illness, cyclic vomiting, failure to thrive	EEG and/or Brain MRI Metabolic testing
Family history	Family history of ASD or other neurodevelopmental disorders	Genetic/metabolic testing
Social history	Adverse childhood experiences; social determinants of health	
Physical/neurodevelopmental examination	Macro/microcephaly Significant abnormal neurologic examination findings (ataxia, spasticity/rigidity, asymmetric weakness) Neurocutaneous syndrome skin findings Abnormal movements (chorea, dystonia, rigidity/spasticity) Dysmorphic features	Brain MRI, Genetic/metabolic testing

Table 2
Genetic tests and their indications, pros, cons, and limitations

Genetic Test	Common Clinical Indications	Pros/Pathology Tested	Cons/Limitations
Karyotype	Specific dysmorphic features History of multiple miscarriages in mother	Trisomies, including mosaic Large chromosomal deletions Balanced chromosomal rearrangements, rings	Does not detect microdeletions, microduplications, or single nucleotide variants.
Chromosomal microarray (CMA)	Dysmorphic features Multiple congenital anomalies Associated developmental delay Nonspecific phenotype	Microdeletions/duplications Single nucleotide polymorphism arrays detect regions of homozygosity and uniparental disomy	Does not detect small deletions or insertions Does not detect balanced rearrangements Variants of unknown significance
Special testing: repeat expansion/methylation analysis	Specific disorder and gene	Specific testing not covered by CMA or ES	Disorder specific testing (eg, fragile X-related *FMR1* CGG repeats, Angelman/Prader Willi methylation analysis)
Gene panel/targeted single gene sequencing	Limited and variable evaluation of specific phenotypes (eg, autism/intellectual disability, cerebral palsy, epilepsy, and neuromuscular disorders)	May have better coverage of specific genes than ES in certain cases Sequencing and CNVs of limited genes included	Limited number of genes covered, may miss newly described or candidate genes Reanalysis is limited to genes included in original panel
Exome sequencing (ES) (+mtDNA genome)	Nonspecific phenotype: specific phenotype but possibility of gene discovery	Broad coverage of genes Some laboratories provide CNV calling on reports* Medically actionable secondary findings (not related to current phenotype) Higher yield than selective gene panels Reanalysis can be done to include new information, including new gene-disease relationships	Variants of unknown significance Some laboratories do not provide CNV calling Does not detect tandem repeat expansions

(continued on next page)

Table 2
(continued)

Genetic Test	Common Clinical Indications	Pros/Pathology Tested	Cons/Limitations
Mitochondrial DNA (mtDNA) sequencing	Mitochondrial DNA specific conditions	Specific coverage of the mitochondrial genome	Variants of unknown significance Decreased yield in heteroplasmy Overall low yield in ASD
Genome sequencing (GS)	Nonspecific phenotype; specific phenotype but possibility of novel gene discovery/ association	Detect single base pair changes, CNVs, and repeat expansions Able to detect promotor region and terminal chromosomal pathogenic variants	Insurance coverage Newly available clinically Variants of unknown significance

*Newer technologies have allowed improved and accurate CNV calling on ES with implications of ES as a first-line evaluation of CNVs.[14]
Adapted from Genetic Testing and Counseling in Child Neurology, Sadat and Emrick (2021), Neurologic Clinics. ©Elsevier.[23]

Metabolic Testing and Autism Spectrum Disorder

As with genetic testing, metabolic testing encompasses a vast array of tests that range from nonspecific screening of multiple conditions (eg, lactate in mitochondrial disorders), to categorical groups of disorders (eg, plasma amino acids for urea cycle disorders and urine organic acids for organic acidemias), and evaluation of individual disorders (specific lysosomal enzyme function for lysosomal disorders).[26] More recently, untargeted metabolomic assays that measure hundreds to thousands of small molecule metabolites across numerous metabolic pathways have become clinically available.[27–29] See **Table 3** for a description of common metabolic tests and the conditions they help to evaluate.

Genetic and biochemical evidence implicates a wide variety of inborn errors of metabolism, including mitochondrial disorders, in the pathogenesis of a small subset (~5%) of children with ASD.[30,31] Several studies have suggested that the yield of routine metabolic testing in patients with ASD is very low, particularly in those without metabolic-specific findings on history and physical.[32] Although inborn errors of metabolism are uncommon causes of ASD, there are major implications for treatment and recurrence risk when one is uncovered.[30,33]

The availability of "wide-net" nonspecific serologic and biochemical markers of metabolomics have demonstrated initial promise as a potential screening tool for biomarker development in ASD.[29,33–36] However, although there are group-level case-control differences using these techniques, they have not yet demonstrated clinical utility at the level of the individual patient and will require larger longitudinal and confirmatory studies before being validate for routine clinical application.[29,36,37]

Genetic Testing in Practice

When performing genetic testing for ASD or any other reason, pretest counseling is paramount to successful clinical care. As with any intervention, the risks, benefits, and limitations of the test should be outlined for families to make informed decisions about which tests to pursue. Specific areas that should be discussed in pretest counseling include the test selected, possible results, limitations of the findings, implications for the patient based on possible results, implications for other family members,[26] and privacy considerations (**Table 4**). Full interpretation of abnormal or equivocal results may require referral to an appropriate subspecialist. Potential outcomes include one or more pathogenic or likely pathogenic (causative) variants, one or more variants of uncertain significance, one or more secondary, or incidental but medically actionable pathogenic variants (not necessarily related to the reported clinical phenotype), any combination of or none of the above.[38,39]

Posttest counseling is required when testing identifies variants that are pathogenic, likely pathogenic, of uncertain clinical significance, or incidental to the indication for testing but medically actionable (secondary findings). The issue of secondary findings, or incidental but medically actionable pathogenic variants, is particularly relevant in the case of broad-range testing, including ES and GS; the American College of Medical Genetics and Genomics has specifically recommended that informed consent for testing that discusses this possible outcome be obtained.[38]

Given the currently available evidence, and considering the decreasing costs/greater availability of broad-range testing such as ES, we suggest the following approach to genetic testing in all children with an ASD diagnosis (**Box 1**).[10]

Metabolic Testing in Practice

Metabolic disorders associated with ASD are most commonly autosomal recessive disorders that present early in life with symptoms such as acute or intermittent

Table 3
Common metabolic tests and the conditions they evaluate

Metabolic Tests	Conditions Evaluated
Serum	
Ammonia	Urea cycle disorders[a] and Organic acidemias[a]
Lactate	Mitochondrial disorders[a]
Pyruvic acid	Pyruvate metabolism disorders
Plasma amino acids	Urea cycle disorders,[a] phenylketonuria,[a] Maple syrup urine disease (branched chain ketoacid dehydrogenase kinase deficiency[a]), organic acidemias, and nonketotic hyperglycinemia
Acylcarnitine profile	Fatty acid oxidation disorders,[a] glutaric aciduria, and mitochondrial disorders
Homocysteine	Disorders of cobalamin synthesis and metabolism (homocystinuria[a])
Creatine/Guanidinoacetate	Creatine synthesis disorders[a]
Carbohydrate deficient transferrin assay	Congenital disorders of glycosylation N and O type
Metabolomics	Broad screening for small molecule metabolism/synthesis disorders (semiquantitative)
Lysosomal enzymes	Specific enzymes based on the disorder (Sanfilippo syndrome—mucopolysaccharidosis type III[a])
Biotinidase enzyme	Biotinidase deficiency[a]
Copper and ceruloplasmin	Menkes, Wilson disease
Cerebrospinal fluid (CSF)	
CSF amino acids	Nonketotic hyperglycemia, serine biosynthesis disorders, alanine—mitochondrial disorders
CSF neurotransmitters	Pyridoxine responsive epilepsy, adenylosuccinate lyase deficiency, biopterin, and folinic acid gamma-aminobutyric acid (GABA)-transaminase deficiency if GABA included
CSF glucose/plasma glucose	Glucose transport defect—(GLUT1 deficiency)
Urine	
Urine organic acids	Organic acidurias[a] and cobalamin disorders
Creatine/guanidinoacetate	Creatine transporter[a]
Urine glycosaminoglycans	Lysosomal disorders—mucopolysaccharidoses[a]
Oligosaccharides	Lysosomal disorders[a]—oligosaccharidosis; some gangliosidoses
Alpha aminoadipic semialdehyde	Pyridoxine-responsive seizures and folinic acid-responsive seizures, Molybdenum cofactor deficiency
Sulfocysteine	Molybdenum cofactor deficiency, sulfite oxidase deficiency
Purine and pyrimidine panel	Disorders of purine and pyrimidine metabolism[a] (Adenylosuccinate lyase deficiency, hypermethionemia due to adenosine kinase deficiency, and beta-ureidopropionase deficiency)

[a] Nonexhaustive examples of disorders rarely associated with an ASD phenotype.[10,11,27]

Table 4
Pretest counseling in genetic evaluation

Topic	Sample Questions	Possible Answers	Clinical Considerations
Test Selection	What does the test cover? How is the sample collected?	Single/multiple genes, whole exome (all protein coding genes), whole genome (the entirety of DNA), and segments of DNA Saliva, buccal swab, and blood/serum	Test selection can be tailored to the clinical phenotype and associated findings on neurodevelopmental evaluation and history Saliva and buccal swab samples may be less traumatic for patients than venipuncture
Possible results	What are the possible results that the test can show?	Diagnostic results: Pathogenic variant(s) (disease/disorder causing changes) Likely pathogenic variant(s) Variant(s) of unknown significance (genetic changes that may be benign or pathogenic) Nondiagnostic results: Likely benign variant(s) Benign variant(s) No reported results	Some results will necessitate further testing to either clarify results, expand the coverage of testing, or help determine familial risk and potentially other affected family members
Limitations	What are the limitations of the test?	No one single test accounts for all possible genetic variants associated with ASD. Multiple rounds and types of testing may be required to complete a genetic evaluation	
Impact on the patient	How will this test affect the patient and family?	The possibility of altering treatment recommendations, connecting with social and support groups related to a pathogenic finding Identifying risk for medical comorbidities that could be present at the time of diagnosis or deve op later in life, refining recurrence risk counseling for the family to inform reproductive decision-making, avoiding avoid unnecessary diagnostic tests	There may be opportunities to be more specific in prognostication and outcomes based on others with similar genetic findings. Social supports can provide a community of others with similar conditions related to etiology and expand connections to resources and etiology-based therapies and research

(continued on next page)

Table 4
(continued)

Topic	Sample Questions	Possible Answers	Clinical Considerations
Risks	What are the risks associated with testing?	Parental and familial guilt around a genetic (inherited) disorder, insurance coverage and costs Findings of nonpaternity or biologic relationship between parents Unexpected incidental findings	As part of a pedigree development and family history, the biologic relationship between family members should be discussed and the potential for unknown or undisclosed findings such as potential nonpaternity or biologic relationship between parents should be discussed

---

Box 1
Clinical approach to genetic etiologic evaluation in ASD, IDD, and GDD (reproduced [CC BY 4.0], © 2021 Savatt and Myers)[10]

1. Complete physical examination and collect developmental, medical, and family history.
   - If a specific etiology is suspected, pursue the appropriate specific genetic testing (eg, *PTEN* sequencing and deletion/duplication analysis, *MECP2* sequencing and deletion/duplication analysis, *FMR1* CGG repeat analysis)
   - If a specific etiology is not suspected, proceed to step 2.

2. Pursue broad examination for causal exonic sequence variants and CNVs.
   - This is most efficiently achieved through ES with CNV coverage.
   - If insurance restrictions or laboratory offerings dictate a stepwise approach to CNV analysis and WES, CMA and WES can be pursued individually. WES should be pursued as the initial evaluation when possible.
   - WES should be performed using a trio analysis, when possible, to decrease the number of candidate variants and inform variant classification.
   - If an etiology is not determined, proceed to step 3.

3. Complete periodic reanalysis of reported variants and exome data; consider additional genetic testing (eg, genome sequencing, *FMR1* CGG repeat analysis if not already done, cytogenetic testing, if warranted, based on WES/CMA results and clinical findings) and/or referral for medical genetics evaluation if indicated.

---

decompensation and neurodevelopmental regression, lethargy, seizures, failure to thrive, and multisystem organ dysfunction (**Box 2**).[26,40] At this time, based on the available evidence, no metabolic tests are routinely recommended for all children with ASD.[14,15] Although metabolic disorders are uncommon causes of ASD, the potential impact is substantial because of high recurrence risk and the possibility of targeted treatment and, as such, clinical findings such as those listed in **Box 2** should increase the level of suspicion of an inborn error of metabolism. Those planning to recommend metabolic testing should take similar considerations on pretest and posttest counseling as well as risks and benefits as detailed in the genetic testing section above.

Box 2
Potential indications for clinical metabolic testing

- Acute or intermittent decompensations
- Neurodevelopmental regression
- Lethargy
- Seizures
- Extrapyramidal movement disorder
- Severe hypotonia
- Ataxia
- Hearing loss
- Cyclic vomiting
- Failure to thrive
- Multisystem organ dysfunction (eg, cardiac, hepatic, and renal).

Neuroimaging and Autism Spectrum Disorder

MRI has allowed researchers to evaluate anatomic images of the brain noninvasively, with increasingly higher spatial resolution as techniques advance. MRI studies have tended to focus on brain volumetrics, cortical surface measures, and metrics of white-matter integrity. The number of anatomic neuroimaging studies has grown exponentially during the last few decades, although the clinical applicability of these findings is limited.[41] Some clinical cohort MRI studies have found that neuroradiologic abnormalities are more common in children with ASD compared with typical controls,[41,42] whereas others have not found a significant difference.[43] Similarly, the majority of reported neuroradiologic abnormalities reported in ASD cohorts were incidental (unexpected findings that are however typically asymptomatic in presentation) and without clear clinical implications. Incidental findings overall are quite common in children undergoing brain MRIs for any reason.[44]

Although structural neuroimaging research has identified case-control morphometric differences (primarily in cortical surface area and thickness, gray matter volume, and white matter connectivity including the frontal cortex, temporal cortex, and amygdala),[45] reliable markers at the individual level for diagnosis or clinical subtyping have not been identified, and clinical neuroimaging is therefore not recommended for all individuals with ASD.[15,46] However, the presence of comorbid seizures, headaches, or abnormalities on neurologic examination is associated with higher likelihood of finding definite and actionable pathology on MRI than when the indication for imaging is simply ASD diagnosis.[47,48]

Alongside structural neuroimaging, functional MRI (fMRI) is a technique that records an indirect measure of brain activity related to regional blood oxygen levels. Research-based studies have identified functional differences between children with ASD and typical controls during tasks highlighting such ASD-relevant psychological constructs as facial recognition (amygdala and anterior frontal cortex), reward (frontal-striatum and lateral frontal cortex), and social cognition (amygdala, superior temporal sulcus, and ventrolateral prefrontal cortex).[49] Although these findings may help elucidate regional-level and network-level functional differences between children with ASD and typical controls, the evidence for utility in diagnosis and predictive value is currently limited and will require larger, longitudinal studies before these complex computational studies can be applied to individuals for diagnostic or predictive use.[50]

Neuroimaging in Practice

High-resolution structural and functional neuroimagings such as MRI and fMRI are not recommended for the etiologic evaluation of all children with a diagnosis of ASD.

The decision to perform structural MRI should be guided by clinical history and examination regardless of a diagnosis of ASD; restated, MRI should be ordered in autistic patients mostly under the same circumstances in which one would order an MRI in any other child, while recognizing that some of these indications are more common in ASD than in the general population. Clinical reasons for obtaining a brain MRI for a child with ASD (or, for that matter, without ASD) include, but are not limited to the following: focal neurologic findings (ie, spasticity, ataxia, focal weakness or sensory loss), skin findings suggestive of neurocutaneous syndromes, signs of elevated intracranial pressure, micro/macrocephaly, developmental regression, or historical evidence of acquired brain injury (severe traumatic brain injury, meningitis/encephalitis, prematurity, and associated complications such as intraventricular hemorrhage; **Box 3**). Abnormal findings on MRI can further contribute to the planning of etiologic

Box 3
Potential indications for brain MRI in a child with autism spectrum disorder

- Focal neurologic findings (eg, spasticity, ataxia, focal weakness, or sensory loss)
- Skin findings suggestive of neurocutaneous syndromes
- Genetic diagnosis with recognized central nervous system (CNS) abnormalities
- Epilepsy
- Signs of elevated intracranial pressure
- Unexplained micro/macrocephaly
- Developmental regression
- Historical evidence of an acquired brain injury

workup in children with ASD, such as targeted genetic or metabolic testing or suggest findings of in utero infections (eg, congenital cytomegalovirus).

Clinical use of fMRI is currently limited to language mapping and planning for epilepsy surgery and other forms of neurosurgery. Currently, there is not enough evidence to recommend the use of fMRI for either diagnostic or etiologic evaluation of ASD.[50]

Pretest counseling and the weighing of benefits and risks is also needed for appropriate use of neuroimaging because it is in genetic testing. Families and patients should be counseled on the potential outcomes including a normal study, possibility of incidental findings, and pathologic changes. A normal structural MRI does not preclude an underlying metabolic or genetic disorder, and follow-up is necessary to determine if repeated imaging or more advanced studies are necessary. Incidental findings, however, are quite common and can cause significant distress to families even if they are considered benign and not related to the child's neurodevelopmental diagnosis. Additional risks that may be related to neuroimaging include the likely need for sedation/anesthesia to complete the study and high costs associated with the test.

Electroencephalography and Autism Spectrum Disorder

Electroencephalography (EEG) is a noninvasive test that records the electrical activity of the outermost layer of the cerebral cortex.[51] EEG is used in 2 different contexts: research applications, which often use a large number of sensors (electrodes) as well as advanced signal processing analyses, and clinical EEG, which uses a smaller number of electrodes and is interpreted via visual inspection of the waveforms by a specially trained neurologist. EEG has been used in research studies with the hope of providing insight into the neural networks relevant to the behavioral manifestations of ASD.

EEG technology has been used to help quantitatively measure differences in sensory perception and processing through the study of event-related potentials (ERPs), a research EEG technique. ERPs are quantitative measures of electrical brain responses to sensory stimuli or motor acts. Children with ASD, at the group level, have decreased amplitudes and increased latencies of specific ERP components during specific task conditions.[52] Some of these findings have extended to high-risk infants and toddlers and have been proposed as presymptomatic or early symptomatic biomarkers for ASD.[53,54] EEG findings in ASD have also implicated a relationship between altered functional connectivity in brain networks at rest that is related to measures of the severity of restricted interests and repetitive behaviors.[53] As with the earlier discussion on advanced neuroimaging techniques, these research and population-based findings have been useful in determining the neurobiological underpinnings of ASD but are not readily applicable to the individual outside of the appropriate clinical context.

Clinical EEGs, typically used for the diagnosis of epilepsy, have reported a range of abnormal findings in case-control studies of autism, some which are, in the general population, indicative of an increased risk for epilepsy, and some which nonspecifically indicate other types of brain dysfunction. Even without a history of epilepsy, abnormalities occur in ASD samples at a rate of 4% to 80%.[55] However, because these findings are not specific to ASD, the clinical EEG cannot currently be used to aid in the diagnosis of ASD. Similarly to MRI, clinical EEG is currently used in autism care primarily under the same circumstances as when it would be used for nonautistic children: when epilepsy is suspected or needs further evaluation (eg, definition of epilepsy type/syndrome/localization). An exception to this rule is when a developmental epileptic encephalopathy is suspected, as described in the following paragraph. Approximately 5% to 46% of children with ASD are diagnosed with epilepsy,[56] compared with about 1% in nonautistic children.[57]

Developmental epileptic encephalopathies (DEEs) are a group of disorders in which there is a presumed causative relationship between epilepsy and developmental disorders (including intellectual developmental disability [IDD] and ASD), although the common etiologic underpinnings are likely at the genetic and brain structure level.[58] Many but not all children with DEEs also have convulsive seizures; the others have epileptic brain activity that contributes to autistic-like cognitive/behavioral features and is in the differential diagnosis of idiopathic autism. Behavioral features may resolve in some cases with appropriate antiseizure medication.

Electroencephalography in Practice

Based on the available evidence, an EEG is not routinely indicated for all children with ASD but is recommended when seizures or epileptic encephalopathies are suspected clinically (**Box 4**).[54,59]

A primary goal of the clinical EEG is to assist in the determination of the presence of seizures, which may be on the differential diagnosis of staring spells or unusual movements (eg, stereotypies).[60] However, evidence suggests that even when children with ASD are evaluated for episodes of staring and reduced responsiveness, the yield of significant interictal (background or EEG recording between clinical events) EEG findings on routine EEG is low[61]; however, if a generalized epilepsy (eg, childhood absence epilepsy) is suspected, the sensitivity and specificity of the EEG is quite high. Furthermore, the high baseline prevalence of epileptiform abnormalities in the EEGs of autistic children (including in the absence of co-occurring epilepsy) means that the EEG is not always informative, if positive, when evaluating an autistic child for co-occurring epilepsy. Moreover, certainly a positive (ie, epileptiform) EEG in the absence of clinical concern for epilepsy would not prompt antiseizure medication use, except in specific circumstances not described here.

Box 4
Potential indications for electroencephalography in autism spectrum disorder

- Clinical concern for seizures
- Developmental regression (notably regression in expressive and receptive language)
- Cortical CNS malformations

Pediatric health-care providers should discuss the increased risk and the signs and symptoms of seizures with the families of children diagnosed with ASD, maintain a high index of clinical suspicion for seizures, and refer to a pediatric neurologist when concerned about the possibility of seizures.[15,62] Although the evidence is mixed, unexplained developmental regression, especially involving language, may warrant an EEG with appropriate sampling of slow-wave sleep, preferably an overnight study.[62,63] This is to determine the presence of DEEs and specifically the syndrome of electrical status epilepticus in slow-wave sleep (ESES) and related language regression, eponymously known as Landau-Kleffner syndrome, or the ESES-related clinical syndrome of continuous spike-waves during slow-wave sleep associated with global regression.[64] Landau-Kleffner syndrome is typically distinguished from classic "autistic regression" in that Landau-Kleffner syndrome tends to occur in older children and encompasses a significant loss of prior mastered language skills (ie, loss of full functional conversative speech as opposed to loss of babbling and nonmastered early linguistic development in late infancy). Outside of known DEEs, the overall association between autism with developmental regression and abnormal EEG findings and epilepsy is relatively weak.[65]

Before ordering an EEG, families and patients should be counseled on the potential outcomes including a normal study, possibility of incidental findings, and pathologic changes that could affect management. Additionally, behavioral difficulties and sensory sensitivities in child some children with ASD and communication difficulties can lead to stress on the patient and affect the setup, monitoring, and recording of the EEG. Moreover, it is particularly important when discussing the utility of EEG that a normal EEG does not rule out seizures or epilepsy and epileptic abnormalities do not directly affirm the diagnosis, given the high prevalence of abnormalities in individuals without seizures or epilepsy.[55,59,66]

SUMMARY

In this article, we have described the etiologic (causative) evaluation process of ASD under a guiding framework of developmental brain dysfunction. Based on the current evidence available, all children with an ASD diagnosis should be offered genetic etiologic evaluation with ES with CNV coverage or combined ES and CMA for the highest diagnostic year. Metabolic testing, neuroimaging, and electrophysiologic testing should be offered in the appropriate clinical context and not routinely for all children with an ASD diagnosis.

Advanced neuroimaging and electrophysiologic techniques, particularly with the use of advanced computational models and machine learning methods,[67,68] are emerging technologies that can help derive biomarkers for the early identification and risk stratification of ASD diagnosis, although they are not readily applicable to individual patients at this time. Similarly, broad range metabolic testing is emerging as a tool to find emerging biomarkers and insights into the pathogenesis of ASD but without current clinical utilization for individual patients.

CLINICS CARE POINTS

- Etiologic evaluation of ASD can provide a framework of family support, including advocacy and etiology-based networking, family planning, surveillance of other associated medical issues, improved prognostication, and potential for targeted interventions.

- Positive or inconclusive etiologic investigations into ASD do not affirm or refute a clinical diagnosis of ASD.

- Clinically available genetic testing including ES with CNV coverage or combined ES and chromosomal microarray (CMA) have the highest yield for etiologic evaluation in ASDs.
- The etiologic evaluation of ASD should be driven by clinical judgment through a formal neurodevelopmental history and examination.
- Although electroencephalography (EEG, brain MRI, serum, spinal fluid, and urine metabolic markers may provide insight into the pathophysiology of ASD, they are recommended only in the appropriate clinical context.

DISCLOSURE

None of the authors report any financial conflicts of interests as they pertain to the subject of this article.

REFERENCES

1. Myers SM. Diagnosing developmental disabilities. In: Batshaw ML, Roizen NJ, Pellegrino L, editors. *Children with disabilities.* 8th edition. Baltimore, MD: Brooks Publishing; 2019. p. 199–224.
2. American Psychiatric Association. Diagnostic and statistical manual of mental disorders: DSM-5-Text Revision. 5th edition, Text Revision. Washington, DC: American Psychiatric Association (APA); 2022.
3. Moreno-De-Luca A, Myers SM, Challman TD, et al. Developmental brain dysfunction: Revival and expansion of old concepts based on new genetic evidence. Lancet Neurol 2013;12(4):406–14.
4. Wing L. The History of Ideas on Autism: Legends, Myths and Reality. Autism 1997;1(1):13–23.
5. Wolff S, Ssucharewa GE. The First Account of the Syndrome Asperger Described? Translation of a Paper Entitled "Die Schizoiden Psychopathien Im Kindesalter." Vol 5. Q Steinkopff Verlag; 1996.
6. Sher DA, Gibson JL. Pioneering, prodigious and perspicacious: Grunya Efimovna Sukhareva's life and contribution to conceptualising autism and schizophrenia. Eur Child Adolesc Psychiatr 2021. https://doi.org/10.1007/s00787-021-01875-7.
7. Faretra G. Lauretta bender on autism: A review. Child Psychiatr Hum Dev 1979; 10(2):118–29.
8. Kanner L. Autistic disturbances of affective contact. Nervous child 1943;2(3):217–50.
9. Asperger H. 'Autistic psychopathy' in childhood. Autism and Asperger Syndrome 1991;37–92.
10. Savatt JM, Myers SM. Genetic Testing in Neurodevelopmental Disorders. Front Pediatr 2021;9(February):1–24.
11. Myers SM, Challman TD, Bernier R, et al. Insufficient Evidence for "Autism-Specific" Genes. Am J Hum Genet 2020;106(5):587–95.
12. Ewen JB, Sweeney JA, Potter WZ. Conceptual, Regulatory and Strategic Imperatives in the Early Days of EEG-Based Biomarker Validation for Neurodevelopmental Disabilities. Front Integr Neurosci 2019;13. Available at: https://www.frontiersin.org/articles/10.3389/fnint.2019.00045.
13. Ewen JB, Potter WZ, Sweeney JA. Biomarkers and neurobehavioral diagnosis. Biomark Neuropsychiatry 2021;4:100029.
14. Schaefer GB, Mendelsohn NJ. Clinical genetics evaluation in identifying the etiology of autism spectrum disorders: 2013 guideline revisions. Genet Med 2013; 15(5):399–407.

15. Hyman SL, Levy SE, Myers SM, et al. Identification, evaluation, and management of children with autism spectrum disorder. Pediatrics 2020;145(1).
16. Manoli DS, State MW. Autism spectrum disorder genetics and the search for pathological mechanisms. Am J Psychiatr 2021;178(1):30–8.
17. Havdahl A, Niarchou M, Starnawska A, et al. Genetic contributions to autism spectrum disorder. Psychol Med 2021;51(13):2260–73.
18. Sandin S, Lichtenstein P, Kuja-Halkola R, et al. The Heritability of Autism Spectrum Disorder. JAMA 2017;318(12):1182.
19. Jarvik GP, Evans JP. Mastering genomic terminology. Genet Med 2017;19(5): 491–2.
20. Dominguez-Alonso S, Carracedo A, Rodriguez-Fontenla C. The non-coding genome in Autism Spectrum Disorders. Eur J Med Genet 2023;66(6):104752.
21. Moeschler JB, Shevell M, Saul RA, et al. Comprehensive evaluation of the child with intellectual disability or global developmental delays. Pediatrics 2014; 134(3):e903–18.
22. Miller DT, Adam MP, Aradhya S, et al. Consensus statement: chromosomal microarray is a first-tier clinical diagnostic test for individuals with developmental disabilities or congenital anomalies. Am J Hum Genet 2010;86(5):749–64.
23. Michelson DJ, Shevell MI, Sherr EH, et al. Evidence report: Genetic and metabolic testing on children with global developmental delay: report of the Quality Standards Subcommittee of the American Academy of Neurology and the Practice Committee of the Child Neurology Society. Neurology 2011;77(17):1629–35.
24. Srivastava S, Love-Nichols JA, Dies KA, et al. Meta-analysis and multidisciplinary consensus statement: exome sequencing is a first-tier clinical diagnostic test for individuals with neurodevelopmental disorders. Genet Med 2019;21(11):2413–21.
25. Manickam K, McClain MR, Demmer LA, et al. Exome and genome sequencing for pediatric patients with congenital anomalies or intellectual disability: an evidence-based clinical guideline of the American College of Medical Genetics and Genomics (ACMG). Genet Med 2021;23(11):2029–37.
26. Sadat R, Emrick L. Genetic Testing and Counseling in Child Neurology. Neurol Clin 2021;39(3):705 17.
27. Alseekh S, Aharoni A, Brotman Y, et al. Mass spectrometry-based metabolomics: a guide for annotation, quantification and best reporting practices. Nat Methods 2021;18(7):747–56.
28. Clish CB. Metabolomics: an emerging but powerful tool for precision medicine. Cold Spring Harb Mol Case Stud 2015;1(1):a000588.
29. Glinton KE, Elsea SH. Untargeted Metabolomics for Autism Spectrum Disorders: Current Status and Future Directions. Front Psychiatr 2019;10:450894.
30. Žigman T, Petković Ramadža D, Šimić G, et al. Inborn Errors of Metabolism Associated With Autism Spectrum Disorders: Approaches to Intervention. Front Neurosci 2021;15:673600.
31. Zecavati N, Spence SJ. Neurometabolic disorders and dysfunction in autism spectrum disorders. Curr Neurol Neurosci Rep 2009;9(2):129–36.
32. Campistol J, Díez-Juan M, Callejón L, et al. Inborn error metabolic screening in individuals with nonsyndromic autism spectrum disorders. Dev Med Child Neurol 2016;58(8):842–7.
33. Smith AM, King JJ, West PR, et al. Amino Acid Dysregulation Metabotypes: Potential Biomarkers for Diagnosis and Individualized Treatment for Subtypes of Autism Spectrum Disorder. Biol Psychiatr 2019;85(4):345–54.
34. Rangel-Huerta OD, Gomez-Fernández A, de la Torre-Aguilar MJ, et al. Metabolic profiling in children with autism spectrum disorder with and without mental

regression: preliminary results from a cross-sectional case–control study. Metabolomics 2019;15(7):1–11.

35. Timperio AM, Gevi F, Cucinotta F, et al. Urinary Untargeted Metabolic Profile Differentiates Children with Autism from Their Unaffected Siblings. Metabolites 2022;12(9):797.

36. Qureshi F, Hahn J. Towards the development of a diagnostic test for autism spectrum disorder: Big data meets metabolomics. Can J Chem Eng 2023;101(1):9–17.

37. Smith AM, Natowicz MR, Braas D, et al. A Metabolomics Approach to Screening for Autism Risk in the Children's Autism Metabolome Project. Autism Res 2020; 13(8):1270–85.

38. Directors AB of. ACMG policy statement: updated recommendations regarding analysis and reporting of secondary findings in clinical genome-scale sequencing. Genet Med 2015;17(1):68–9.

39. Richards S, Aziz N, Bale S, et al. Standards and Guidelines for the Interpretation of Sequence Variants: A Joint Consensus Recommendation of the American College of Medical Genetics and Genomics and the Association for Molecular Pathology. Genet Med 2015;17(5):405.

40. Manzi B, Loizzo AL, Giana G, et al. Autism and Metabolic Diseases. J Child Neurol 2008;23(3):307–14.

41. Ambrosino S, Elbendary H, Lequin M, et al. In-depth characterization of neuroradiological findings in a large sample of individuals with autism spectrum disorder and controls. Neuroimage Clin 2022;35. https://doi.org/10.1016/j.nicl.2022.103118.

42. Rochat MJ, Distefano G, Maffei M, et al. Brain magnetic resonance findings in 117 children with autism spectrum disorder under 5 years old. Brain Sci 2020; 10(10):1–15.

43. Monterrey JC, Philips J, Cleveland S, et al. Incidental brain MRI findings in an autism twin study. Autism Res 2017;10(1):113–20.

44. Dangouloff-Ros V, Roux CJ, Boulouis G, et al. Incidental brain MRI findings in children: A systematic review and meta-analysis. Am J Neuroradiol 2019;40(11): 1818–23.

45. Li X, Zhang K, He X, et al. Structural, Functional, and Molecular Imaging of Autism Spectrum Disorder. Neurosci Bull 2021;37(7):1051–71.

46. Myers L, Ho ML, Cauvet E, et al. Actionable and incidental neuroradiological findings in twins with neurodevelopmental disorders. Sci Rep 2020;10(1).

47. Zeglam AM, Al-Ogab MF, Al-Shaftery T. MRI or not to MRI! Should brain MRI be a routine investigation in children with autistic spectrum disorders? Acta Neurol Belg 2015;115(3):351–4.

48. Cooper AS, Friedlaender E, Levy SE, et al. The Implications of Brain MRI in Autism Spectrum Disorder. J Child Neurol 2016;31(14):1611–6.

49. Rafiee F, Rezvani Habibabadi R, Motaghi M, et al. Brain MRI in Autism Spectrum Disorder: Narrative Review and Recent Advances. J Magn Reson Imag 2022; 55(6):1613–24.

50. Hiremath CS, Sagar KJV, Yamini BK, et al. Emerging behavioral and neuroimaging biomarkers for early and accurate characterization of autism spectrum disorders: a systematic review. Transl Psychiatry 2021;11(1):1–12.

51. Tivadar RI, Murray MM. A Primer on Electroencephalography and Event-Related Potentials for Organizational Neuroscience. Organ Res Methods 2019;22(1): 69–94.

52. McPartland JC, Bernier RA, Jeste SS, et al. The Autism Biomarkers Consortium for Clinical Trials (ABC-CT): Scientific Context, Study Design, and Progress Toward Biomarker Qualification. Front Integr Neurosci 2020;14.

53. Clairmont C, Wang J, Tariq S, et al. The Value of Brain Imaging and Electrophysiological Testing for Early Screening of Autism Spectrum Disorder: A Systematic Review. Front Neurosci 2022;15.
54. Boutros NN, Lajiness-O'Neill R, Zillgitt A, et al. EEG changes associated with autistic spectrum disorders. Neuropsychiatr Electrophysiol 2015;1(1).
55. Precenzano F, Parisi L, Lanzara V, et al. Electroencephalographic Abnormalities in Autism Spectrum Disorder: Characteristics and Therapeutic Implications. Medicina (Kaunas) 2020;56(9):1–13.
56. Milovanovic M, Grujicic R. Electroencephalography in Assessment of Autism Spectrum Disorders: A Review. Front Psychiatr 2021;12:686021.
57. Liu X, Sun X, Sun C, et al. Prevalence of epilepsy in autism spectrum disorders: A systematic review and meta-analysis. Autism 2022;26(1):33–50.
58. Specchio N, Curatolo P. Developmental and epileptic encephalopathies: what we do and do not know. Brain 2021;144(1):32–43.
59. Hrdlicka M. EEG Abnormalities in Autism: What is the Significance? Autism Open Access 2012;02(03).
60. Wirrell EC. Prognostic significance of interictal epileptiform discharges in newly diagnosed seizure disorders. J Clin Neurophysiol 2010;27(4):239–48.
61. Hughes R, Poon WY, Harvey AS. Limited role for routine EEG in the assessment of staring in children with autism spectrum disorder. Arch Dis Child 2015;100(1):30–3.
62. Myers SM, Challman TC. Autism spectrum disorder. In: Voigt RG, Macias MM, Myers SM, et al, editors. *Developmental-behavioral pediatrics*. 2nd edition. Itasca, IL: American Academy of Pediatrics; 2018. p. 407–75.
63. Pacheva I, Ivanov I, Yordanova R, et al. Epilepsy in Children with Autistic Spectrum Disorder. Children 2019. https://doi.org/10.3390/CHILDREN6020015.
64. Tuchman R. CSWS-related autistic regression versus autistic regression without CSWS. Epilepsia 2009;50(s7):18–20.
65. Barger BD, Campbell J, Simmons C. The relationship between regression in autism spectrum disorder, epilepsy, and atypical epileptiform EEGs: A meta-analytic review. J Intellect Dev Disabil 2017;42(1):45–60.
66. Kwon CS, Wirrell EC, Jetté N. Autism Spectrum Disorder and Epilepsy. Neurol Clin 2022;40(4):831–47.
67. Duan YM, Zhao WD, Luo C, et al. Identifying and Predicting Autism Spectrum Disorder Based on Multi-Site Structural MRI With Machine Learning. Front Hum Neurosci 2022;15.
68. Bahathiq RA, Banjar H, Bamaga AK, et al. Machine learning for autism spectrum disorder diagnosis using structural magnetic resonance imaging: Promising but challenging. Front Neuroinform 2022;16.

Evidence-Based Interventions in Autism

Julia S. Anixt, MD[a,b,*], Jennifer Ehrhardt, MD, MPH[a,b],
Amie Duncan, PhD[a,c]

KEYWORDS

- Autism spectrum disorder • Evidence-based practice • Early intervention
- Behavior intervention

KEY POINTS

- Refer children with suspected autism for diagnostic evaluations and early intervention services as soon as possible.
- Participation in evidence-based interventions for autism improves outcomes across multiple domains: core autism symptoms, communication, cognition, behavior, and adaptive and social skills.
- There is no "one size fits all" approach to autism treatment—consider each child's strengths and challenges and families' priorities and goals.

INTRODUCTION

Primary care pediatricians have a crucial role in screening for autism and other intellectual and developmental disabilities[1] and providing longitudinal care to children with autism spectrum disorder (ASD) and their families. This review provides an overview of evidence-based treatments to support optimal developmental-behavioral outcomes and independent living skills for children with ASD. The review is organized by treatment domains (ie, early intervention, communication, adaptive skills, and so forth) and within those domains information is presented by general age groups (ie, toddlers, preschoolers, adolescents).

Autism is a heterogeneous diagnosis including individuals with a wide range of intellectual abilities, communication skills, and associated behaviors. Every child with ASD has a unique set of strengths and challenges and there is no "one size fits all" model for treatment. Intervention recommendations should be customized to best

[a] Department of Pediatrics, University of Cincinnati College of Medicine, Cincinnati, OH, USA;
[b] Division of Developmental and Behavioral Pediatrics, Cincinnati Children's Hospital Medical Center, 3333 Burnet Avenue, MLC-4002, Cincinnati, OH 45229, USA; [c] Division of Behavioral Medicine and Clinical Psychology, Cincinnati Children's Hospital Medical Center, 3333 Burnet Avenue, MLC-4002, Cincinnati, OH 45229, USA
* Corresponding author. Division of Developmental and Behavioral Pediatrics, Cincinnati Children's Hospital Medical Center, 3333 Burnet Avenue, MLC-4002, Cincinnati, OH 45229, USA
E-mail address: julia.anixt@cchmc.org

Pediatr Clin N Am 71 (2024) 199–221
https://doi.org/10.1016/j.pcl.2024.01.001
0031-3955/24/© 2024 Elsevier Inc. All rights reserved.
pediatric.theclinics.com

meet the needs of each child, align with a family's goals and priorities, and be feasible for the child and family in terms of time and cost. Families seeking care for autistic children may be inundated with information about therapy options of varying levels of evidence. Pediatricians play an important role in advising families that they are likely to hear about interventions for autism that are both evidence-based and non-evidence based. Conversations between pediatricians and families about ASD treatment choices can be enhanced using a shared decision-making approach. This allows the clinician to provide evidence-supported information and to identify a family's goals, priorities, and values to ensure that the treatment plan is a good fit for the child and family. When making decisions about their child's treatment, families should understand which practices have clear evidence of positive outcomes based on multiple research studies. To address the need for evidence-based practice guidelines for ASD based on systematic review of the literature, the National Autism Center published the National Standards Project (NSP2, published in 2015)[2] and the University of North Carolina National Clearinghouse on Autism Evidence and Practice (NCAEP) Review Team published an Evidence-Based Practices report in 2020.[3] Both reports provide comprehensive and detailed information about ASD evidence-based interventions and associated outcomes. The findings from these reports are reflected in this review article.

Pediatricians play an important role in encouraging early diagnosis and intervention, advising families about evidence-based treatments for ASD, and supporting family's emotional health as they care for a child with a developmental disability.[4] The purpose of this article is to provide pediatricians with information about evidence-based autism treatments.

DISCUSSION
Importance of Early Intervention

Autism can be diagnosed with accuracy in children less than 2 years of age[5] and when possible, the goal is to diagnose children before 3 years of age.[6] The rationale for encouraging early identification and diagnosis of ASD is that interventions started before age 3, at a time when the brain is still developing and has more plasticity, are more likely to be effective long-term.[7] The use of evidence-based early intervention (EI) services that promote building developmental skills sequentially and positive parent-child interactions improves outcomes.[8–10] Unfortunately, common misconceptions such as giving it more time with a "wait and see" approach or that young children with developmental delays will "catch up," can lead to delays in referrals to services[11] and lost opportunities for intervention during critical windows for development. Several EI treatment models offer clear benefits to autistic children less than 3 years of age.[5]

Goals of Intervention Across the Lifespan

Younger age at enrollment into EI services has been associated with achieving greater gains in social communication, cognitive abilities, adaptive skills, and reduction of ASD symptom severity.[12] There is a greater positive impact from interventions started before age 3 years compared to those started after age 5 years.[5,13,14] However, intervention services are beneficial for children with ASD at any age and can be started as soon as an ASD diagnosis is suspected or diagnosed. Treatment goals for children with ASD include (1) minimizing impact of challenges associated with core ASD symptoms (social communication difficulty, restricted interests/repetitive behaviors); (2) maximizing functional independence/adaptive skills; and (3) preventing, reducing, or minimizing the impact of behaviors that interfere with acquisition of functional skills.[15] Intervention services need to be individualized to the specific child's strengths and areas of difficulty and aligned with families' goals and priorities. Shared decision-making between clinicians and families can be used to determine the best fit for a child's participation in therapy services. Clinicians should provide information about evidence-based treatment options and consideration should be given to families' sociocultural beliefs, family dynamics and support system, health insurance coverage for treatments, and the family's economic situation, all of which can impact the feasibility of participation in therapy.[5,15]

Determining a treatment plan for a child with autism requires an understanding of evidence-based interventions, the family's goals and priorities, and the unique strengths and needs of the child. Goals and needs may change over time and vary based on the child's developmental stage. **Table 1** provides information about potential evidence-based therapy options.

Federally Mandated Interventions and Services in the United States

Note: this section describes EI and educational services that are federally mandated in the United States and, therefore, may not be applicable in other countries. In 2012, guiding principles were published to support the international community to develop or refine EI programs to yield optimal outcomes for children with developmental delays/disabilities consistent with 2 United Nations international human rights treaties: the Convention on the Rights of the Child and the Convention on the Rights of Persons with Disabilities.[16]

The **Individuals with Disabilities Education Act** (IDEA) authorizes federal funding to states to support EI services for infants and toddlers from birth up to 3 years (part C) and special education services for preschool and school-aged children of 3 to 21 years (part B).[17] This is also discussed in the article Autism Spectrum Disorder at Home and in School.

Early intervention (part C): birth to age 3 years

Participation in EI services for infants and toddlers with developmental delays is associated with positive long-term outcomes in language, cognition, academics, and behavior.[8] An Individual Family Service Plan (IFSP) is developed by the EI professionals with family input documenting the child's goals and services. Best practices for EI services include creating opportunities for "learning in the natural environment" and using a family "coaching" model.[8] The contact information for every state's EI program can be found on the Centers for Disease Control and Prevention (CDC) website: https://www.cdc.gov/ncbddd/actearly/parents/state-text.html. The CDC's "Learn the Signs. Act Early." Program[18] provides resources to parents to track developmental milestones and learn more about EI services.

Part B services: preschool-aged and school-aged services

Preschool-aged children (3–5 years old) with ASD can be referred to their public school district for evaluation for eligibility for special education preschool services (part B). For children less than 3 years receiving EI services, the IFSP team will orient families and facilitate the transition of supports to part B special educations services.[17] Preschool-aged (3–5 years) and school-aged children (6–21 years) referred to the school district will undergo multidisciplinary team evaluations to determine eligibility for Individualized Education Program (IEP) services. Eligibility for an IEP is based on the child meeting criteria for a categorical determination of a disability as defined by IDEA (such as autism, intellectual disability, speech or language impairment, other

Table 1
Intervention services for children with autism

Service/Therapy	Developmental Domains Targeted	Age Range	Funding Source(s)	Intervention Approach & Additional Information
State Early Intervention Services (IDEA part B)	Cognitive Communication Motor Adaptive Social-emotional	0–3 ys	Public Public or private health insurance (for some programs)	• IFSP based on child's needs which then determines goals and services • Parent training model • Professionals: developmental specialist, speech-language pathology, PT, OT
Public school education services (IDEA part C)	Academic Cognitive Communication Social Motor Adaptive Behavior	3–21 ys	Public	• Eligibility for IEP based on multi-disciplinary evaluation determining if child meets criteria for disability category with impairment impacting education. • IEP based on child's needs which then determines goals and services • Professionals: special education (intervention specialist), speech-language pathology, PT, OT, behavior support, school psychologist
Comprehensive treatment models (CTMs) based on principles of ABA (ie, EIBI, ESDM)	Behavior Cognitive Communication Social Adaptive Academic	0–9 ys	Public or private health insurance-Private pay	• Center-based or home-based programming • Follows manualized procedures • Goals determined based on skill acquisition • Frequency: substantial number of hours/week • Longevity: treatment for 1 y or longer

Outpatient therapies (domain-specific)

Intervention	Domains	Ages	Payment	Notes
Speech-language therapy	Communication- receptive, expressive, pragmatic language, social skills	All ages	Public or private health insurance Private pay	• Evidence-based strategies include augmentative and alternative communication (AAC), functional communication training, language training, modeling, scripting • Emerging evidence for virtual or augmented reality (VAR) interventions
Behavioral—mental health treatment	Behavior Emotions (eg, anxiety) Adaptive Social Executive functioning	All ages	Public or private health insurance	• Parent-management training to address behaviors • Cognitive-behavioral therapy for school-aged and adolescent children with adequate communication and cognitive skills • Professionals: psychology, licensed clinical social worker, counselor, behavior therapist
Occupational therapy	Fine motor skills Gross motor skills Sensory processing Adaptive	All ages	Private pay	• Ayres Sensory Integration® approach is evidence-based to improve sensory integration • Treatment may address adaptive behaviors such as feeding and toileting
Social skills intervention	Social	Adolescents	Public or private health insurance	• PEERS—evidence-based, manualized social skills intervention • Professionals: speech-language therapist, psychologist, licensed clinical social worker

Abbreviations: ABA, applied behavioral analysis; EIBI, early intensive behavioral intervention; ESDM; early start Denver model; IDEA, individuals with disabilities education act; IEP, individualized education program; IFSP, individual family service plan; OT, occupational therapist; PT, physical therapist.

health impairment, and so forth) and this condition affecting school performance and learning.[17] If eligible, children can begin to receive services once an IEP is developed. The IEP documents goals and services and is developed with family input. Parents can choose to share independent diagnostic evaluation or therapy reports with the school district to support the development of IEP goals.

EVIDENCE-BASED INTERVENTIONS
Core Autism Spectrum Disorder Symptoms

For children less than 3 year old with ASD, best practice involves participation in interventions starting as early as possible that include a combination of developmental and behavioral approaches, meaning therapies that are evidence-based and are adjusted to the child's developmental level and use behaviorally based strategies and teaching methods.[5] Evidence-based interventions for autism treatment are described in 2 categories: (1) comprehensive treatment models (CTMs) and (2) evidence-based practices (EBPs) or focused intervention practices.[3,19–21] Both CTMs and EBPs are effective across a range of ages and developmental levels, although CTM programs target building essential skills for younger children (0–9 years of age).[2] Additionally, participation in outpatient therapies (described in following paragraph #3) such as speech-language therapy, occupational therapy (OT), and behavior therapy can support skill development to address common symptoms of autism (ie, communication difficulty) and co-occurring developmental delays/disabilities or behavioral challenges.

Comprehensive treatment models: target age range 0 to 9 years

CTMs include intensive EIs that address skills important for early childhood development including communication, social, and adaptive skills. CTMs are based on a conceptual framework that supports broad learning and skill development to impact core features of ASD.[20] Additionally, CTMs are characterized by the use of manualized procedures, intensity (substantial number of hours per week), longevity (treatment occurs for 1 year or longer), and a focus on broad outcomes (ie, communication, behavior, social).[3] CTM programs may use approaches of applied behavioral analysis (ABA) and/or naturalistic approaches (strategies provided in the context of typical social activities in community settings).[15] Examples of CTM programs include Early Intensive Behavioral Intervention (EIBI), Treatment and Education of Autistic and Related Communication-Handicapped Children, the Early Start Denver Model, or similar behavioral inclusive programs.[2,15] **Table 2** describes characteristics of several CTMs. These programs use similar evidence-based strategies such as using a visual schedule to communicate the activities that the child will be doing and providing reinforcement when a child is learning a new skill. In addition to building developmental skills such as self-feeding using utensils or toilet training, CTM programs integrate behavioral approaches to increase or decrease target behaviors. There is no evidence to support which specific CTM approach is the best fit for each child. There are also regional differences in the availability of programs. However, pediatricians can confidently recommend these evidence-supported CTMs (see **Table 2**) and should encourage families to choose a program based on their goals, preferences, and factors such as availability and cost.

Evidence-based practices (also called focused intervention practices): all ages

EBPs are strategies designed to teach an individual skill or to address a specific goal.[19,21] EBPs are the basic units or building blocks that are combined to form educational programs for children with ASD including CTMs, public school special education interventions, and outpatient therapies.[20,21] Some examples of EBPs are discrete trial training (an instruction is given, child responds, a planned consequence is provided,

Table 2
Examples of comprehensive treatment models including evidence-based practices

Model/Intervention	Domains Addressed	Setting	Approach/Program Characteristics
Comprehensive treatment models (CTMs)			
Early Intensive Behavioral Intervention (EIBI)	Addresses core autism spectrum disorder (ASD) symptoms (social-communication, restricted interests, play, imitation)	Structured, predictable setting, low student-to-teacher ratio	• Program supports acquisition, generalization, and maintenance of developmentally appropriate skills • Monitors progress over time • Uses Discrete Trial Training (DTT) (ie, an instruction is given, child responds, a planned consequence is provided, and a pause before presenting next instruction) • Promotes family involvement • Implements functional approach to challenging behaviors
Treatment and Education of Autistic and Related Communication-Handicapped Children (TEACCH)	Targets activities of daily living, communication, social skills, executive functioning, attention, engagement. Skill acquisition in these domains supports intellectual functioning.	Structured setting, environment organized to meet child's needs (ie, minimize distraction), predictable setting	• Individualized curriculum developed based on individual's abilities and needs as measured by standardized assessments • Makes use of structured teaching experiences • Organize tasks/materials to promote independence from prompts, including use of visual supports (ie, visual schedules, video modeling) • Encourages close working relationship between practitioners and parents

(continued on next page)

Table 2
(continued)

Model/Intervention	Domains Addressed	Setting	Approach/Program Characteristics
Naturalistic developmental behavioral interventions (NBIs)— These use strategies involving naturally occurring environments and activities			
Early Start Denver Model (ESDM)	Designed for young children (12–48 mos); addresses core autism spectrum disorder (ASD) symptoms; supports social, communication, cognitive skills	Multiple settings—home, school, clinic; as a group or one-on- one	• Parents and therapists use play to build positive, fun relationships while targeting developmentally appropriate skills • Based on understanding of toddler development and learning • Teaching occurs in natural, everyday settings/activities
Pivotal response treatment	Addresses "pivotal" areas of development: motivation, response to cues, self-management, and initiation of social interaction	Multiple settings- particularly natural environments (school, community)/inclusive settings with typically developing peers	• Parents taught to implement motivational procedures including: following child's lead, offering choices, gaining child's attention, providing opportunities to respond/ take turns, varying tasks, using natural reinforcement, reinforcing attempts at target skills • Family involvement is emphasized
Joint Attention, Symbolic Play, Engagement, and Regulation (JASPER)	Play-based intervention, teaches social communication skills to young children (12 months- 8 ys)	Multiple settings—inclusion/ special education classrooms, home, community	Interventions focused on 4 core domains: 1. Joint attention—teach and model coordination of attention between objects and people for purpose of sharing 2. Symbolic play—model appropriate play, increase flexibility in play, support joint attention in play 3. Engagement—joint engagement with others 4. Regulation—of emotions/behavior

and a pause before presenting next instruction), prompting (verbal or gesture assistance given to learner to support acquiring a skill), video modeling (video-recorded demonstration of a target skill is shown to learner), and visual supports (visual display to support learner engage in behavior without additional prompts).[21] These focused interventions can be used for short periods of time, until a specific goal is achieved, and may address skills in the areas of behavior, development, or education.

Outpatient therapies: all ages

Children with ASD benefit from participation in outpatient therapies delivered by licensed professionals to support skill development across multiple domains. Examples of outpatient therapies include speech-language therapy, OT, and behavior therapy. Children receiving part C or part B services (EI or school-based services) can supplement these interventions with outpatient therapies to provide increased frequency and intensity of intervention and address goals impacting the child outside of the educational setting (ie, difficulty getting haircuts, tantrums when transitioning from activity to another). Caregiver involvement and practicing specific skills at home and within the community are critical components for the success of outpatient therapies. For example, if a child is learning to use 1 to 2 word phrases to request or make choices in speech therapy, the caregiver should work on practicing this skill at home (eg, choosing what snack the child wants, choosing what toy the child wants to play with) and within the community (eg, choosing a book to check out at the library, choosing a cereal to buy at the grocery store). The role of outpatient therapies will be described in each developmental domain section in the following paragraphs (ie, social communication, adaptive, behavior). Of note, for some children, outpatient therapies are not a feasible option due to challenges such as lack of access to pediatric therapists, long wait times, and financial barriers (limited insurance coverage, high co-payment fees).

Applied Behavioral Analysis and Early Intensive Behavioral Intervention

Principles of ABA are the foundation for most evidence-based treatment models for autism. ABA is a general behavioral learning theory, not a specific set of interventions.[22] ABA has been defined as the process of applying learning theory principles to improve socially meaningful behaviors and evaluating if changes in behavior are due to the interventions.[23] ABA methods can include reinforcing social, communication, and other skills and are effective at reducing challenging behaviors that may interfere with a child's progress toward educational or independent living goals.[15,22] The goal of ABA is to promote meaningful growth in skill development (eg, adaptive skills, functional communication, emotional regulation) and generalize skills across environments (eg, community, home, school, different caregivers). EIBI programs, which are CTMs using ABA principles, have demonstrated positive outcomes, including 20% to 50% of children participating in EIBI programs achieving average intelligence quotient and placement in general education settings upon completion of treatment and 20% to 40% achieving moderate gains, but still requiring supports.[13,22]

ABA therapy can be delivered in a variety of settings including 1:1 or group settings, center-based, or in more natural environments (home, school). An individualized treatment plan should be developed collaboratively between the family and the professional supervising the child's ABA therapy program, typically a board-certified behavior analyst, to address identified priorities.

Naturalistic Developmental Behavioral Interventions

Naturalistic developmental behavioral intervention (NDBI) approaches foster back-and-forth engagement between the child and the intervention provider.[12] The intervention provider responds to the child's interests, play, and communication approaches in an intentional way (eg, reading the child a book after a child points and requests it). Cues are provided to the child to promote behaviors with consequences naturally found in the environment providing reinforcement.[2,12] Naturalistic interventions can be incorporated into typical activities and routines to support and encourage learners to build and promote skills in natural and contextually relevant environments, such as home, school, and the community.[2,3,12]

Parent-Mediated Intervention

Parent-mediated intervention, also called parent training, describes a variety of approaches in which parents receive training to implement strategies to promote building their child's social communication skills or reducing challenging behaviors.[2,3,15] Parent training can occur individually or in group settings and can provide strategies to target core ASD symptoms (eg, building expressive language and joint attention skills) to teach new skills to a child (eg, engaging in play with other peers) or to reduce disruptive behaviors.

SOCIAL COMMUNICATION

Building communication and social skills is a key focus of interventions for children with ASD from the toddler/preschool years through adolescence. Interventions supporting communication are generally delivered by speech-language pathologists and those supporting social skills can be delivered by professionals in multiple disciplines, including speech-language pathology, psychology, special education, and OT.

Toddlers and Preschool-Aged Children

When toddlers and preschoolers are diagnosed with ASD, they may have no or limited verbal language and no or limited means of functionally communicating their needs and wants (eg, requesting items, asking for help). Developing both areas is critical at this age, especially the latter. Evidence-based strategies that target communication skills include behavioral interventions, naturalistic teaching strategies, functional communication training, language training (production), modeling, scripting, and augmentative and alternative communication (AAC).[2,3]

Communication goals can be incorporated into treatment programs utilizing behavioral interventions or naturalistic teaching strategies. Functional communication training, as a circumscribed intervention, is complementary to these strategies. It seeks to identify problematic behaviors in a child that serve a communication purpose and replace them with more appropriate means of communication, for example, verbal language or AAC. Language training (production) centers on helping autistic children use their spoken words functionally. Modeling and scripting are ways a desired behavior or response to social situation can be modeled for children with ASD. With scripting, a verbal script for a specific social situation is modeled for and practiced with the child. Given the range of evidence-based strategies available, it is beneficial for children with ASD to have a speech-language pathologist with competencies in ASD as part of their larger treatment team.

AAC focuses on the use of communication systems that do not rely on verbal language, including sign language, Picture Exchange Communication System (PECS), and speech-generating devices (SGDs). Across these approaches, the use of PECS and SGDs, compared to sign language, has been found to be more effective in building fundamental communication skills, like requesting.[24] Effectiveness of AAC is enhanced when it is used to teach communication skills in specific routines (eg, mealtimes).[25]

Many parents express concern that using AAC will prevent their child from developing verbal language. Contrary to this belief, studies have shown that AAC does not impede verbal language and may increase it modestly. More research is needed on child and treatment (frequency and intensity of intervention) factors that influence outcomes with AAC.[26]

The evidence-based strategies described earlier are also effective for building social and play skills (eg, imitative play, make-believe play, turn taking with peers and adults) in toddlers and preschoolers with ASD. Additionally, parent training, peer-mediated interventions, and social narratives are effective in building these skills.[2,3] Social narratives have similarities with modeling and scripting. They utilize visuals and/or written words to describe to the child what they can expect of a specific social situation and how to respond to it. There is emerging evidence for interventions centered on specific social communication skills like imitation, eye contact, gestures, joint attention, and play.[27,28] THe effect sizes for this intervention are moderate and enhanced for children of younger ages with higher dosage of treatment.

School-Aged Children

For school-aged autistic children, the same evidence-based strategies utilized to promote communication and social skills in toddlers and preschoolers with ASD are applicable. Peer-mediated interventions in home or school settings may be more impactful. Peers are trained in how to respond during social interactions with the child who has ASD (eg, engaging in back-and-forth conversation, taking turns playing a game). These interventions have been shown to increase frequency and duration of social interactions, as well as help build the use of AAC.[29] It is unclear if they have impact on verbal language.

Adolescents

In adolescents with ASD, the following evidence-based strategies remain effective for promoting communication and social skills—modeling, scripting, AAC, parent training, and peer-mediated interventions. Additionally, social skills packages are an effective, evidence-based strategy for this age group.[2,3,30] This intervention centers on helping a teenager with ASD build skills needed to participate in social experiences across settings, namely, home, school, and in the community. The Program for the Education and Enrichment of Relational Skills (PEERS) is a manualized social skills intervention package for autistic adolescents and young adults that has been designated as evidence-based in increasing specific social skills[31,32] (eg, reciprocal conversations, interactions with same-aged peers, etc.) both immediately after treatment and at follow-up. PEERS for adolescents consists of 14 weekly and concurrent sessions for both adolescents and their parent/caregiver. In the adolescent group, evidence-based strategies such as direct instruction, modeling, video modeling, and reinforcement are used to teach concepts such as having a back-and-forth conversation, dealing with teasing and bullying, and hosting a get-together for a friend. In the caregiver group, caregivers receive instruction on what the adolescents are learning and also receive coaching on how to provide feedback to adolescents during weekly homework assignments (eg, joining a club or activity, having a friend over, and so forth).Research has shown that many social skills packages have a positive impact on their social knowledge, but it is unclear how much it improves their participation in social activities.[30]

Lastly, there is growing research on extended reality interventions, for example, virtual or augmented reality (VAR) environments, for child and adolescents with ASD. In studies of VAR interventions, the effectiveness of this intervention ranges from weak to strong for promoting social skills.[33,34] Older age was found to contribute to larger improvements, while the presence of comorbid conditions was found to contribute to smaller improvements.

It is important to note that, sometimes, families seek interventions that are not evidence-based. Currently, facilitated communication and rapid prompting method do not have an evidence base for building communication and social skills in children with ASD. They are also not supported by the American Speech-Language-Hearing Association.[35]

ADAPTIVE BEHAVIOR

Adaptive behavior is defined as the ability of an individual to be independent and self-sufficient in the areas of communication, socialization, and daily living skills.[36] The authors will focus on daily living skills in this section since communication and socialization are covered in other sections of this review. Daily living skills are the everyday tasks and behaviors an individual does to take care of themselves at home, school, work, and in the community and are categorized into personal/self-care (eg, getting dressed, brushing teeth, showering, taking medications), domestic (eg, picking up belongings, cleaning one's room, cooking meals, doing laundry), and community (eg, telling time, buying items at the store, getting around the community, and managing and budgeting money).[37] Interventions supporting adaptive skills can be delivered by professionals in multiple disciplines, including OT, psychology, and special education.

Toddlers and Preschool-Aged Children

Daily living skills that are critical for toddlers and preschoolers include getting dressed, eating and drinking, basic personal hygiene (eg, washing hands, brushing teeth), toileting, and simple household chores (eg, picking up toys). Increased age, higher cognitive abilities, few behavior problems, and less severe ASD symptoms are associated with better daily living skills in this age group.[38] Preschool children with autism demonstrate a significant gap between their chronologic age and daily living skills, which suggests these skills need to be prioritized in intervention to increase the likelihood of attaining positive outcomes in adulthood.[38,39] Evidence-based interventions for this age range are typically behavioral (eg, discrete trial training, extinction, reinforcement, prompting), and may also include video modeling, visual supports, social narratives, or the use of technology.[3] It can be highly beneficial for caregivers to work with psychologists or occupational therapists to develop goals and implement evidence-based strategies when targeting the acquisition and mastery of these skills.

School-Aged Children

Daily living skills that are critical for autistic school-aged children include hygiene (eg, taking a bath or shower), cooking snacks and simple meals, helping with their laundry, cleaning their room, understanding the concept of time, and developing an understanding of spending and saving money. The gap between chronologic age and actual daily living skills continues to widen as children start school, which makes it critical to intervene.[39,40] While many evidence-based strategies to address age-appropriate daily living skills continue to be behavioral (eg, reinforcement, prompting), additional strategies such as task analysis and cognitive behavioral intervention strategies may be useful. For example, if a school-aged child is struggling to complete their morning hygiene routine before school, this skill could be explicitly broken down into its component steps (eg, wake up with alarm, get dressed, put pajamas in hamper, brush teeth, comb hair, and so forth) using a task analysis and then used as a checklist to help them consistently and independently complete this routine (**Fig. 1**). The child could then be rewarded (eg, verbal praise, 10 minutes of screen time before school) for completing the routine independently or with minimal prompts from a caregiver.

Adolescents

Daily living skills that are essential for continuing to build independence and autonomy prior to the transition to adulthood include personal care and hygiene (eg, wearing deodorant, taking medications, beginning to manage health care appointments), cooking meals, cleaning the home (eg, vacuum/mop, taking trash out), household maintenance (eg, cutting the grass), managing money (eg, budgeting for expenses), and navigating the community (eg, biking, walking, driving). The gap between daily living skills and chronologic age is often very apparent in adolescence such that a teen's skills may be 6 to 8 years behind their peers,[41,42] which then directly affects their ability to achieve positive adult outcomes in college, employment, independent living, and quality of life.[42] Evidence-based strategies such as prompting, reinforcement, visual supports, and task analysis continue to be effective for teaching these skills. However, additional strategies such as self-monitoring and technology-aided instruction may be particularly effective in adolescence. For example, surviving and thriving in the real world is a manualized intervention that has shown promise in increasing age-appropriate daily living skills in autistic adolescents in the areas of hygiene, laundry, cleaning, cooking, and managing money.[43] An essential intervention component is the use of a contract to define specific daily living skills goals and

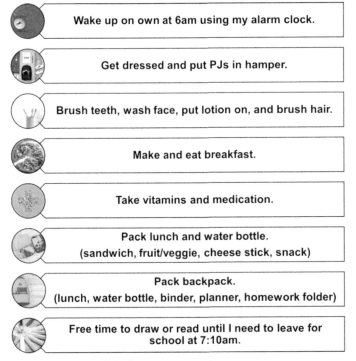

Fig. 1. Example of visual schedule for morning routine.

expectations, monitor daily/weekly progress, and specify the reward or privilege that will be earned. Technology strategies such as alarms (eg, to switch laundry from the washer to the dryer) or reminders (eg, setting a smart speaker to remind the teen to take medication at 7:45 AM everyday) are often incorporated to build autonomy.

BEHAVIOR AND MENTAL HEALTH

While disruptive behaviors are not a core feature of ASD, it is common for children with ASD to experience challenging behaviors such as inattention, hyperactivity, impulsivity, anxiety, irritability, tantrums, refusal behaviors, aggression, and self-injury.[44] In a population of about 600 children with ASD from 13 sites across North America participating in an autism learning health network, 93% of parents of children of ages 6 to 12 years reported problematic behaviors in the past month, with 85% indicating these behaviors were of moderate or worse intensity (moderate [47%], severe [28%], or extremely severe [10%]).[44] Co-occurring psychiatric conditions occur in up to 70% of children with ASD.[45] Attention-deficit/hyperactivity disorder (ADHD), anxiety, and oppositional defiant disorder are among the most commonly reported conditions[45] and 41% to 61% of children with ASD have 2 or more psychiatric conditions.[46]

Identifying Triggers and Patterns of Challenging Behavior

Conducting a functional behavioral assessment (FBA) is the first step to developing an effective intervention plan to address challenging behavior. The FBA involves observation and data collection to identify the "ABCs" of a behavior—the antecedent (what happens before the behavior), the behavior of concern, and the consequence (what happens after the behavior). These data are then used to determine the function of a maladaptive behavior (why is the child engaging in the behavior?) to determine how to respond to the behavior to make a change and disrupt the persistence of the behavior. Common functions of behavior include wanting to get something, such as attention or a tangible object, or wanting to escape something. Sometimes it can be difficult to identify the function of a behavior. If disruptive behavior seems to occur "out of the blue," without an identifiable trigger, it is important to evaluate for possible underlying medical reasons for the behavior such as pain, dental problems, sleep disorders, or constipation, for which children with ASD are at increased risk.[47,48] Additionally, clinicians may want to consider evaluation for a possible co-occurring mood disorder. The FBA approach can be used in therapy and school/classroom settings to develop effective behavior plans.

Behavior and Mental Health Interventions

Parent training
Parent training models are an evidence-based intervention for the treatment of disruptive behaviors including ADHD in **typically developing** children. These include programs such as Incredible Years, Positive Parenting Program, and Parent-Child Interaction therapy.[49–51] Through participation in these programs, parents gain an understanding of the child's behavior and skills to respond to the child and reinforce desired behaviors. However, less is known about the effectiveness of parent-mediated interventions in children with developmental disabilities including autism.[52] While parent training was found to be superior to parent education in reducing disruptive behavior in a randomized control trial,[53] a 2020 systematic review and meta-analysis of parent training for children with ASD concluded that methodological limitations make it difficult to draw conclusions about effectiveness and generalizability of specific parent training programs at this time.[54]

Cognitive behavioral therapy

Cognitive behavioral therapy (CBT) is an effective treatment for pediatric anxiety disorders in the typically developing population, with approximately 60% of children rated as much improved or very much improved on the Clinician Global Impression-Improvement Scale after 14 sessions of CBT.[55] Systematic reviews have found moderate efficacy of CBT for the treatment of anxiety in autistic youth without an intellectual disability.[56,57] Manualized CBT intervention programs have been adapted to meet the needs of individuals with ASD, including adjustments to materials to provide visual cues and role-playing.[2] CBT interventions teach participants to evaluate their thoughts and emotions and then use step-by-step strategies to change their thinking and behavior.[3] These interventions can be helpful at addressing challenging behaviors related to emotions such as anger and anxiety.[3]

Facing your fears

Facing Your Fears (FYF) is a cognitive behavioral intervention for autistic school-aged children (ages 8–14) that uses evidence strategies to increase recognition of anxiety symptoms (eg, thoughts, feelings, physical reactions) and then teaches a range of age-appropriate coping strategies (eg, worry bugs, exposure strategies). FYF sessions are attended by both children and their caregiver, and they then break into separate groups to allow for additional instruction, practice, and coaching. In particular, caregivers are coached to provide supportive feedback and support as their child learns how cope with their anxiety and generalize these skills to other settings (eg, school, social interactions with peers).[58]

Additional evidence-based strategies

For children who do not have the cognitive or communication skills to participate in CBT, other evidence-based strategies and tools can be helpful for reducing stress and anxiety such as use of visual supports. Visual supports provide information in a visual format, which can include photographs, pictures, or checklists that may or may not be paired with words (eg, listing the steps for calming down when feeling frustrated or anxious). Visual schedules are a type of visual support that prepares children to participate in an activity or routine by providing information about what to expect, including what they need to do, what will happen as a result, and when the activity will be done.[3]

Executive Functioning

School-aged and adolescents

It is estimated that between 35% to 70% of autistic children and adolescents have significant challenges in the area of executive functioning, which includes skills such as organization, planning, prioritizing, time management, initiating tasks, persevering on tasks, completing tasks, multitasking, and working memory.[59] Executive functioning impairments have been shown to impact performance at both home (eg, completing homework assignments, getting household chores done) and school (eg, writing down assignments in a planner, taking notes, bringing materials to class) and are also predictors of poor outcomes in adulthood.[60] The profile of executive functioning in autistic individuals appears to be similar to those with a diagnosis of ADHD[61] and they may benefit from similar treatments. For example, several evidence-based supports and strategies (eg, task analysis, graphic organizers, technology such as alarms and reminders) and interventions (eg, Unstuck and On Target, Achieving Independence and Mastery in School) have been identified to be implemented at both home and school to address specific executive functioning difficulties in autistic individuals.[3,62] Children and adolescents may benefit from attending group or individual treatment to learn compensatory strategies (eg, using a binder to organize classroom materials, creating flash cards to study) to address executive functioning challenges. Caregivers are often an integral component of treatment so that they can assist their child in implementing specific strategies (eg, writing down and prioritizing assignments in a planner) at home and school.

Sensory processing

Many children with ASD have difficulty with sensory processing. Hyperactivity or hyporeactivity to sensory input or unusual sensory interests in aspects of the environment is one of the restrictive, repetitive patterns of behavior symptoms included in the Diagnostic and Statistical Manual of Mental Disorders, Fifth Edition, diagnostic criteria for ASD.[63] In children with ASD, sensory processing difficulty can present with a range of behaviors such as food selectivity and restricted eating habits, sensitivity to loud or unexpected noises (covering ears, becoming upset), visual examination (looking at objects out the side of the eye, visual fixation on spinning objects or lights), or tactile sensitivity (not liking how it feels to wear clothes or shoes). Sensory sensitivities can negatively interfere with day-to-day functioning and participation in therapies and educational activities. Occupational therapists can work with a child and their family to gradually expose the child to sensory challenges and support them in learning strategies to cope with it.[22] The evidence-based Ayres Sensory Integration[64] approach uses individually customized activities to support sensory processing, motor planning, movement, and organization in space, and "just right" challenges to help children process and tolerate sensory information from their body and the environment (visual, auditory, tactile, proprioceptive, and vestibular).[3]

Case presentation #1: preschool-aged child with autism, delays in communication and adaptive skills, and behavior challenges. Henry is a 4-year-old boy who was diagnosed with ASD and global developmental delay at the age of 2 years. He has minimal verbal language and only uses a few single words for requesting. He is not toilet trained. He has sensory aversions, especially related to toothbrushing and feeding. He has 10 foods that he eats consistently. Henry also has difficulty with transitions which often cause him to have a meltdown (eg, dropping to the floor, screaming, and throwing things). He was enrolled in EI services when he was 18 month old. After his diagnosis of autism, he also received outpatient speech therapy and OT. His parents tried to enroll him in ABA therapy but were not successful due to long waitlists for ABA programs in their community. Since turning 3 years old, he has been enrolled in an EIBI preschool program. In the classroom, he is using PECS and more single words to communicate. Initially he handled transitions well in the classroom, although transitions continued to be a challenge at home. However, recently he has been having more meltdowns at school. His teachers describe him as seeming more irritable. Henry and his parents are currently concerned that his behavioral meltdowns have become more frequent both at home and at school.

Clinical question. What additional questions would you ask Henry's parents about his behavior? What guidance would you offer them?

Case discussion. This case illustrates some of the challenges that parents of preschool-aged children with ASD face in navigating behavior. The history shared by Henry's parents indicates that he had frequent meltdowns, but they have acutely worsened and are now occurring more frequently at his preschool. It is helpful to think about antecedents or triggers for these meltdowns and it may even be helpful for school personnel to conduct a FBA. For example, in preschool, was there a change in classroom staffing, structure, or routine? Was there recently an extended school holiday (ie, winter break)? Henry's parents responded "no" to these questions and also noted that his daily routine at home is unchanged. Medical factors like dental cavities or constipation can cause discomfort and pain, which, in turn, can result in behavior changes in a child with limited verbal language. Henry's parents explain that he has always been a picky eater. They worry about his nutrition and fiber intake. Usually, he has bowel movements about 2 to 3 times a week, but it has been less frequent in the last month (1–2 times a week). You determine he has constipation and recommend a bowel clean out and use of a daily stool softener. You also discuss the use of visual supports to help with understanding the structure of his day and upcoming transitions. For example, a "first, then" board could help Henry transition to a non-preferred task (eg, get shoes on and get in the car to drive to school) and then be rewarded with a preferred activity (eg, looking at a book about vehicles).

Treatment recommendations

- Continue use of daily stool softener for constipation and monitor symptoms.
- Consider referral for feeding therapy with OT or psychology to work on expanding Henry's food repertoire.
- Continue participation in EIBI program. Discuss Henry's behavior concerns at home with EIBI team for suggestions of strategies that have been helpful at school and could be generalized to the home setting.
- Continue use of visual support strategies, such as "first, then" board and visual schedule to help Henry prepare for transitions and increase his communication skills.
- Consider referral for speech therapy to assist parents with understanding how to build communication skills at home.

Case presentation #2: *school-aged child with autism and executive functioning difficulty.* Leo is a 10-year-old male in the fourth grade who was diagnosed with autism at 4 years of age. He also has a diagnosis of ADHD-combined type and takes a stimulant medication. Leo has an IEP at school and receives speech-language therapy to address social communication difficulties (eg, asking for help, initiating interactions with peers) and OT (eg, coping with changes in his schedule, managing his emotions by taking a break). His cognitive abilities are in the low average range and he struggles with reading comprehension, which is impacting his ability to do well in school and complete homework on his own. He currently struggles with having back-and-forth conversations with peers and adults and wants to have friends, but he struggles to interact with peers at school and at baseball. Leo is very interested in video games, prefers to talk about this topic with others, and wants to play video games whenever he has free time at home. Leo has executive functioning difficulties (eg, organizing materials, planning, and prioritizing tasks). His daily living skills are below average for his age in that he still needs a lot of assistance and prompting to do simple chores (eg, clean his room, put belongings away) and personal hygiene tasks (eg, shower, brush teeth). Leo struggles to cope with his emotions at home and school such that he yells and cries when he is feeling overwhelmed, or when he does not get what he wants.

Clinical question. What types of interventions would be helpful for optimizing Leo's academic success, emotional functioning, and independent living skills?

Case discussion. This case illustrates that children with autism benefit from a multidisciplinary intervention approach. This child in the case is receiving school-based services through an IEP. With an IEP, children with autism can receive educational supports for learning difficulties, in this case with reading comprehension, and related services such as speech-language therapy and OT services. An IEP for a student with Leo's ADHD and executive functioning difficulties could also include accommodations to support slower processing time (ie, extended time on tests) and organizational difficulty (ie, use of a planner to be signed daily by his teacher). In addition to impacting his functioning in an educational setting, Leo's autism-related challenges also affect his social and daily skills functioning at home and in the community. Therefore, Leo would also benefit from receiving outpatient therapies such as social skills training and OT or psychology treatment to support independence with daily living skills and strategies to improve executive functioning.

Treatment recommendations

After meeting with his developmental pediatrician and reviewing his current presentation and caregiver concerns, the following recommendations were made:

- Continue to receive services at school through his IEP and inquire about specific intervention to help with reading comprehension.
- Social communication—(1) enroll in a social skills group to receive instruction on specific skills, (2) set up play dates with peers he is interested in having a relationship with, to practice social skills and provide him with feedback on what he did well and what he can improve upon, (3) continue involvement in extracurricular activities.
- Executive functioning—(1) work with occupational therapist or psychologist to develop strategies that may increase his organization and planning/prioritizing skills (eg, setting up a homework routine that includes a quiet space, creating a "to-do" list of assignments in his planner, working for 20 minutes, and then taking a 5-minute break).
- Daily living skills—work with an occupational therapist or psychologist to develop a plan for building his skills by utilizing evidence-based strategies such as a task analysis (eg, break down the steps for cleaning his room and then teach him how to do each step until he is independent).
- Emotion management—work with a psychologist to develop a plan by utilizing cognitive behavioral–based strategies to increase his ability to identify and then cope with emotions (eg, take a break by going to his room and playing Legos for 5 minutes when he is overwhelmed with homework).

SUMMARY

Developmental outcomes for autistic children are optimized when a diagnosis is made at a young age (<3 years) and with prompt connection to intervention services as early as possible when a diagnosis of ASD is suspected or confirmed. Children less than 3 years of age with suspected ASD or other developmental delays should be referred to their state's EI (part C) services, or if age 3 years or older, to their public school district (part B) for eligibility evaluation and to start services as soon as a concern is identified, even if a child has not yet completed medical diagnostic evaluations. Goals of treatment for ASD include (1) minimizing the impact of core ASD symptom–associated challenges, (2) maximizing adaptive skills and independence, and (3) reducing the impact of behaviors that negatively affect achievement of functional skills.[15]

Evidence-based interventions that address core ASD symptoms are categorized as either CTMs or focused intervention practices. Participation in CTMs, which generally use an ABA approach and focused intervention practices, is associated with optimal outcomes for the child. Younger age at enrollment in CTM intervention is associated with greater gains in social communication, cognitive abilities, adaptive skills, and reduction of ASD symptom severity.[6] Children and adolescents with ASD benefit from connection to multidisciplinary professionals including speech-language pathologists, occupational therapists, and psychologists, behavior therapists, and other mental health professionals. Participation in speech-language therapy supports the development of functional communication skills through strategies such as AAC, modeling, and scripting. PEERS social skills intervention package improves adolescent social knowledge.

Challenging behavior and mental health concerns are common in autistic children and adolescents. Collaboration with psychologists and the use of FBAs can support the development of effective behavior plans to address disruptive behaviors. CBT is an effective treatment for anxiety in autistic youth without intellectual disability. Interventions that address adaptive behaviors and executive functioning promote independent living skills and success in school and work environments. **Table 1** provides a summary of intervention services and therapies that may be considered to support optimal outcomes for children and adolescents with ASD.

CLINICS CARE POINTS

- Children with suspected autism should be referred for diagnostic evaluations and EI services as soon as possible.
- Starting evidence-based EI at a young age (<3 years) is associated with greater positive impact on outcomes.
- CTM interventions are associated with improvement in core autism symptoms, cognitive abilities, communication skills, adaptive skills, and behavior.
- Consider referral for evidence-based therapies to support communication, social skills, adaptive skills, sensory processing, behavior, and mental health in children with autism, depending on each child's strengths and challenges.
- Pediatricians play an important role in advising families about evidence-based versus non-evidence–based treatments for autism.

DISCLOSURE

None of the authors has any commercial or financial conflicts of interest.

Funding sources for all authors. 1) Eunice Kennedy Shriver National Institute of Child Health and Human Development (NICHD): K23HD094855. Surviving and Thriving in the Real World: A Daily Living Skills Intervention for Adolescents with Autism Spectrum Disorder (PI: Amie Duncan), 2) Autism Speaks which supports the Autism Care Netowrk (ACNet) and ECHO Autism at Cincinnati Children's Hospital (PI: Julia Anixt). J.S. Anixt: Autism Speaks: ECHO Autism at Cincinnati Children's Hospital for Primary Care and Allied Health Professionals. Autism Speaks: Improvement Advisor, Autism Care Network (ACNet). Autism Speaks: Cincinnati Children's Hospital Autism Learning Health Network Leadership Site / Autism Care Network (ACNet). NIH: R33 HD100934 (NICHD) Evaluating Assessment and Medication Treatment of ADHD in Children with Down Syndrome (TEAM-DS) (PI: Anna Esbensen, PhD, Tanya Froehlich, MD; my role-co-investigator)HRSA Maternal & Child Health Developmental-Behavioral Pediatrics training Program Award, T7749098 (PI: Tanya Froehlich, MD; my role- faculty member). J. Ehrhardt: N/A. A. Duncan: Eunice Kennedy Shriver National Institute of Child Health and Human Development (NICHD): K23HD094855. Surviving and Thriving in the Real World: A Daily Living Skills Intervention for Adolescents with Autism Spectrum Disorder (PI: Duncan).

REFERENCES

1. Lipkin PH, Macias MM, COUNCIL ON CHILDREN WITH DISABILITIES, SECTION ON DEVELOPMENTAL AND BEHAVIORAL PEDIATRICS. Council on children with disabilities section on developmental behavioral pediatrics. promoting optimal development: identifying infants and young children with developmental disorders through developmental surveillance and screening. Pediatrics 2020; 145(1):e20193449.
2. National Autism Center. Findings and conclusions: National standards project, phase 2. MA: Author Randolph; 2015.
3. Steinbrenner JR, Hume K, Odom SL, et al. Evidence-based practices for children, youth, and young adults with Autism, 2020, The University of North Carolina at Chapel Hill, Frank Porter Graham Child Development Institute, National Clearinghouse on Autism Evidence and Practice Review Team, Chapel Hill; NC.
4. The Roadmap Project. roadmapforemotionalhealth.org Accessed 03/31/2023.
5. Zwaigenbaum L, Bauman ML, Choueiri R, et al. Early Intervention for Children With Autism Spectrum Disorder Under 3 Years of Age: Recommendations for Practice and Research. Pediatrics 2015;136(Suppl 1):S60–81.
6. Lord C, Risi S, DiLavore PS, et al. Autism from 2 to 9 years of age. Arch Gen Psychiatr 2006;63(6):694–701.
7. Dawson G. Early behavioral intervention, brain plasticity, and the prevention of autism spectrum disorder. Dev Psychopathol 2008;20(3):775–803.
8. Adams RC, Tapia C, Council on children with disabilities. Council on children with disabilities. Early intervention, IDEA Part C services, and the medical home: collaboration for best practice and best outcomes. Pediatrics 2013;132(4):e1073–88.
9. Center on the Developing Child. The science of early childhood development (In-Brief). Cambridge, MA: Center on the Developing Child, Harvard University; 2007. Available at: www.developingchild.harvard.edu.
10. Majnemer A. Benefits of early intervention for children with developmental disabilities. Semin Pediatr Neurol 1998;5(1):62–9.
11. Singleton NC. Late talkers: Why the wait-and-see approach is outdated. Pediatric Clinics 2018;65(1):13–29.
12. Landa RJ. Efficacy of early interventions for infants and young children with, and at risk for, autism spectrum disorders. Int Rev Psychiatr 2018;30(1):25–39.
13. Eldevik S, Hastings RP, Hughes JC, et al. Using participant data to extend the evidence base for intensive behavioral intervention for children with autism. Am J Intellect Dev Disabil 2010;115(5):381–405.
14. Kasari C, Gulsrud A, Freeman S, et al. Longitudinal follow-up of children with autism receiving targeted interventions on joint attention and play. J Am Acad Child Adolesc Psychiatry 2012;51(5):487–95.
15. Hyman SL, Levy SE, Myers SM, et al. Council on children with disabilities section on developmental behavioral pediatrics. identification, evaluation, and management of children with autism spectrum disorder. Pediatrics 2020;145(1).
16. Brown SE, Guralnick MJ. International human rights to early intervention for infants and young children with disabilities: tools for global advocacy. Infants Young Child 2012;25(4):270–85.

17. Lipkin PH, Okamoto J, Council on Children with Disabilities, et al. Council on children with disabilities and council on school health. the individuals with disabilities education act (idea) for children with special educational needs. Pediatrics 2015; 136(6):e1650–62.

18. Centers for Disease Control and Prevention (CDC). Learn the Signs. Act Early. https://www.cdc.gov/ncbddd/actearly/index.html. Accessed 04, 01, 2023.

19. Odom SL, Collet-Klingenberg L, Rogers SJ, et al. Evidence-based practices in interventions for children and youth with autism spectrum disorders. Prev Sch Fail: Alternative Education for Children and Youth 2010;54(4):275–82.

20. Wong C, Odom SL, Hume KA, et al. Evidence-based practices for children, youth, and young adults with autism spectrum disorder: a comprehensive review. J Autism Dev Disord 2015;45(7):1951–66.

21. Hume K, Steinbrenner JR, Odom SL, et al. Evidence-based practices for children, youth, and young adults with autism: Third generation review. J Autism Dev Disord 2021;51(11):4013–32.

22. Will MN, Currans K, Smith J, et al. Evidenced-based interventions for children with autism spectrum disorder. Curr Probl Pediatr Adolesc Health Care 2018; 48(10):234–49.

23. Baer DM, Wolf MM, Risley TR. Some current dimensions of applied behavior analysis. J Appl Behav Anal 1968;1(1):91–7.

24. Aydin O, Diken IH. Studies Comparing augmentative and alternative communication systems (AAC) applications for individuals with autism spectrum disorder. Education and Training in Autism and Developmental Disabilities 2020;55(2): 119–41.

25. Logan K, Iacono T, Trembath D. A systematic search and appraisal of intervention characteristics used to develop varied communication functions in children with autism who use aided AAC. Research in Autism Spectrum Disorders 2022;90: 101896.

26. White EN, Ayres KM, Snyder SK, et al. Augmentative and alternative communication and speech production for individuals with ASD: A systematic review. J Autism Dev Disord 2021;51(11):4199–212.

27. Bejarano-Martin A, Canal-Bedia R, Magan-Maganto M, et al. Efficacy of focused social and communication intervention practices for young children with autism spectrum disorder: A meta-analysis. Early Child Res Q 2020;51:430–45.

28. Fuller EA, Kaiser AP. The effects of early intervention on social communication outcomes for children with autism spectrum disorder: A meta-analysis. J Autism Dev Disord 2020;50:1683–700.

29. O'Donoghue M, O'Dea A, O'Leary N, et al. Systematic review of peer-mediated intervention for children with autism who are minimally verbal. Review Journal of Autism and Developmental Disorders 2021;8:51–66.

30. Gilmore R, Ziviani J, Chatfield MD, et al. Social skills group training in adolescents with disabilities: A systematic review. Res Dev Disabil 2022;125:104218.

31. Laugeson EA, Frankel F, Gantman A, et al. Evidence-based social skills training for adolescents with autism spectrum disorders: The UCLA PEERS program. J Autism Dev Disord 2012;42:1025–36.

32. Mandelberg J, Laugeson EA, Cunningham TD, et al. Long-term treatment outcomes for parent-assisted social skills training for adolescents with autism spectrum disorders: The UCLA PEERS program. Journal of Mental Health Research in Intellectual Disabilities 2014;7(1):45–73.

33. Chen Y, Zhou Z, Cao M, et al. Extended Reality (XR) and telehealth interventions for children or adolescents with autism spectrum disorder: Systematic review of qualitative and quantitative studies. Neurosci Biobehav Rev 2022;138:104683.

34. Karami B, Koushki R, Arabgol F, et al. Effectiveness of virtual/augmented reality-based therapeutic interventions on individuals with autism spectrum disorder: a comprehensive meta-analysis. Front Psychiatr 2021;12:665326.

35. American Speech-Language-Hearing Association. Facilitated communication Position Statement. Retrieved from www.asha.org/policy/2018.

36. Sparrow SS, Cicchetti DV, Balla DA. Vineland adaptive behavior scales Vineland-II: survey forms manual. MN: Pearson Minneapolis; 2005.

37. Saulnier CA, Klaiman C. Assessment of adaptive behavior in autism spectrum disorder. Psychol Sch 2022;59(7):1419–29.

38. Di Rezze B, Duku E, Szatmari P, et al. Examining trajectories of daily living skills over the preschool years for children with autism spectrum disorder. J Autism Dev Disord 2019;49:4390–9.

39. Pathak M, Bennett A, Shui AM. Correlates of adaptive behavior profiles in a large cohort of children with autism: The autism speaks Autism Treatment Network registry data. Autism 2019;23(1):87–99.

40. Kanne SM, Gerber AJ, Quirmbach LM, et al. The role of adaptive behavior in autism spectrum disorders: Implications for functional outcome. J Autism Dev Disord 2011;41:1007–18.

41. Glover M, Liddle M, Fassler C, et al. Microanalysis of daily living skills in adolescents with autism spectrum disorder without an intellectual disability. J Autism Dev Disord 2023;53(7):2600–12.

42. Clarke EB, McCauley JB, Lord C. Post–high school daily living skills in autism spectrum disorder. J Am Acad Child Adolesc Psychiatr 2021;60(8):978–85.

43. Duncan A, Liddle M, Stark LJ. Iterative development of a daily living skills intervention for adolescents with autism without an intellectual disability. Clin Child Fam Psychol Rev 2021;24(4):744–64.

44. Anixt JS, Murray DS, Coury DL, et al. Improving behavior challenges and quality of life in the autism learning health network. Pediatrics 2020;145(Supplement_1):S20–9.

45. Simonoff E, Pickles A, Charman T, et al. Psychiatric disorders in children with autism spectrum disorders: prevalence, comorbidity, and associated factors in a population-derived sample. J Am Acad Child Adolesc Psychiatr 2008;47(8):921–9.

46. Lecavalier L, McCracken CE, Aman MG, et al. An exploration of concomitant psychiatric disorders in children with autism spectrum disorder. Compr Psychiatr 2019;88:57–64.

47. Da Silva SN, Gimenez T, Souza RC, et al. Oral health status of children and young adults with autism spectrum disorders: systematic review and meta-analysis. Int J Paediatr Dent 2017;27(5):388–98.

48. Neumeyer AM, Anixt J, Chan J, et al. Identifying associations among co-occurring medical conditions in children with autism spectrum disorders. Academic Pediatrics 2019;19(3):300–6.

49. Kazdin AE. Parent management training: treatment for oppositional, aggressive, and antisocial behavior in children and adolescents. New York, NY: Oxford University Press; 2008.

50. McNeil CB, Hembree-Kigin TL, Anhalt K. Parent-child interaction therapy. 2010.

51. Murray DW, Lawrence JR, LaForett DR. The Incredible years® programs for ADHD in young children: a critical review of the evidence. J Emot Behav Disord 2018;26(4):195–208.
52. Bearss K, Burrell TL, Stewart L, et al. Parent training in autism spectrum disorder: What's in a name? Clin Child Fam Psychol Rev 2015;18:170–82.
53. Bearss K, Johnson C, Smith T, et al. Effect of parent training vs parent education on behavioral problems in children with autism spectrum disorder: a randomized clinical trial. JAMA 2015;313(15):1524–33.
54. Deb S, Retzer A, Roy M, et al. The effectiveness of parent training for children with autism spectrum disorder: a systematic review and meta-analyses. BMC Psychiatr 2020;20:1–24.
55. Walkup JT, Albano AM, Piacentini J, et al. Cognitive behavioral therapy, sertraline, or a combination in childhood anxiety. N Engl J Med 2008;359(26):2753–66.
56. Ung D, Selles R, Small BJ, et al. A systematic review and meta-analysis of cognitive-behavioral therapy for anxiety in youth with high-functioning autism spectrum disorders. Child Psychiatr Hum Dev 2015;46:533–47.
57. Vasa RA, Carroll LM, Nozzolillo AA, et al. A systematic review of treatments for anxiety in youth with autism spectrum disorders. J Autism Dev Disord 2014;44:3215–29.
58. Reaven J, Blakeley-Smith A, Culhane-Shelburne K, et al. Group cognitive behavior therapy for children with high-functioning autism spectrum disorders and anxiety: a randomized trial. JCPP (J Child Psychol Psychiatry) 2012;53(4):410–9.
59. Pennington BF, Ozonoff S. Executive functions and developmental psychopathology. JCPP (J Child Psychol Psychiatry) 1996;37(1):51–87.
60. Kenny L, Cribb SJ, Pellicano E. Childhood executive function predicts later autistic features and adaptive behavior in young autistic people: A 12-year prospective study. J Abnorm Child Psychol 2019;47:1089–99.
61. Elias R, White SW. Autism goes to college: Understanding the needs of a student population on the rise. J Autism Dev Disord 2018;48:732–46.
62. Tamm L, Zoromski AK, Kneeskern EE, et al. Achieving independence and mastery in school: an open trial in the outpatient setting. J Autism Dev Disord 2021;51:1705–18.
63. American Psychiatric Association. Diagnostic and statistical manual of mental disorders (5th ed.). 2013.
64. Ayres AJ, Robbins J. Sensory integration and the child: understanding hidden sensory challenges. Los Angeles, CA: Western psychological services; 2005.

Autism Spectrum Disorder at Home and in School

Megan E. Bone, MD[a,b,*], Mary L. O'Connor Leppert, MB, BCH[b,c]

KEYWORDS

- Autism spectrum disorder • Family • Home • School • Services
- Sibling relationships • Peer relationships • Transition

KEY POINTS

- Children with autism spectrum disorder (ASD) have high utilization of school services, but the nature of services change with age.
- School and family considerations change as children with ASD progress across preschool, school age, and adolescence.
- Sibling, peer, and social relationships become more challenging as children with ASD navigate away from school and into adult services.

Autism spectrum disorder (ASD) affects children and families throughout the lifespan and across all different environments. Parents or caregivers are often the first to identify symptoms of ASD in early childhood,[1] typically because of behavior or communication deficits. The suspicion of ASD begins the logistically and emotionally challenging first step of securing an evaluation of concerning symptoms. The confirmation of an ASD diagnosis begins an odyssey which navigates ever evolving family, medical, educational, legal, and social considerations as symptoms change and comorbidities emerge (**Fig. 1**). Throughout childhood and adolescence, the two primary environments are home and school, which both influence and are influenced by the symptoms of children with ASD. These confounding factors affect the child with ASD and their family as they impact ability and quality of life at home, in school, and in the community.

CASE EXAMPLES

Case 1

A 4-year-old boy with ASD lives with his parents and younger sister. Parents report that he has great difficulty settling down for sleep and often wakes up his younger

^a Department of Neurology, Johns Hopkins University School of Medicine; ^b Department of Neurodevelopmental Medicine, Kennedy Krieger Institute, Baltimore, MD, USA; ^c Department of Pediatrics, Johns Hopkins University School of Medicine
* Corresponding author. 707 North Broadway, Baltimore, MD 21205.
E-mail address: Bone@kennedykrieger.org

Pediatr Clin N Am 71 (2024) 223–239
https://doi.org/10.1016/j.pcl.2024.01.008
0031-3955/24/© 2024 Elsevier Inc. All rights reserved.

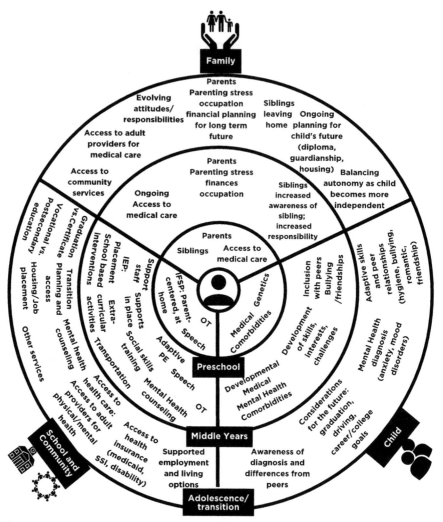

Fig. 1. Considerations in caring for children with autism spectrum.

sister at bedtime with his tantrums. His preferred activity is playing games and watching videos on his tablet. Parents allow him to have his tablet after dinner to keep him occupied while they bathe and put his younger sister to bed. It is difficult to transition him away from the tablet once it is his bedtime, and he will often tantrum with yelling, kicking, and slamming the door. Once parents do get him to bed, it can take 90 minutes for him to fall asleep, and there are multiple attempts to leave his room and find his tablet. Parents brought this up at his 4-year well-child visit, as they are at their wits' end and not getting good sleep.

The pediatrician recommended the following.

1. Eliminate the use of tablet after dinner and at least 2 hours before bedtime and replace with one-on-one time with one parent as the other prepares the baby for bed. Activities during that time should be quiet and devoid of all electronic stimuli.
2. Low-dose melatonin is recommended with or just following dinner.

3. Actual bedtime should consist of the child being prepared for bed, followed by a few minutes of reading, after which the parent should tuck him into bed in a cool, dark, quiet room, and leave the room while he is sleepy but not fully asleep.
4. Once sleep routines are well established, the parents may be able to wean off the melatonin.
5. Behavioral therapy may be pursued if the routine is unsuccessful after consistent practice for 2 to 3 weeks.

Case 2

An 8-year-old boy is in third grade at a public school. He has an individualized education program (IEP) and has been diagnosed with ASD and developmental delay. He receives speech therapy three times per week, occupational therapy (OT) once per week, and spends mornings in a special education classroom that he shares with six classmates, one teacher, and two assistant teachers. He does well in the special education classroom in the morning. In the afternoons, he attends specials with the mainstream third-grade class, including art, physical education, and music class. He consistently elopes from the classroom in the afternoon, sometimes leaving the building entirely out to the parking lot. This elopement behavior only happens at school and only in the afternoons. Parents are concerned that the school may decide to stop mainstreaming him and keep him in the special education classroom the entire day due to this behavior, and it is important to them for him to have time with typically developing peer models. After discussing this with their pediatrician, the following recommendations were made.

1. Pediatrician suggested requesting an IEP meeting to explore a functional behavioral analysis and behavior intervention plan.
2. Suggestion was made for the classroom to implement a peer buddy system, where another child is designated to notify the teacher if the child leaves the group.
3. The child should be supported with a teacher-supervised peer group at lunch time to help facilitate the development of social skills using peer modeling.
4. Resources on safety tracking devices were supplied to the parents for use while working on this behavior.
5. If the suggested strategies prove ineffective even after implementation of the behavior intervention plan, full IEP reassessment for placement may be necessary.

Identification of Autism Spectrum Disorder

The average age of caregiver concern in children who are diagnosed with ASDs is 25 months,[2] yet the average age of diagnosis of ASD worldwide is 60 months, and in the US ranges from 38 to 64 months.[2–4] There is good evidence that the gap between concern and diagnosis is narrowing, as the age at which autism is identified is becoming earlier, perhaps due to early screening.[4,5] One study found that 73% of primary care practices screened for ASD at the American Academy of Pediatrics (AAP) recommended ages and that for those children with positive screens, the age of diagnosis was 10 months earlier than those not screened.[4]

Developmental delays are identified in early childhood in several ways; surveillance of a child identified with a condition associated with a high risk of developmental delay, screening at routine health supervision visits, or by caregiver appraisal of a child's development. Children with conditions associated with higher risk of neurodevelopmental or behavioral disorders may be identified prenatally or soon after birth and automatically placed in early intervention programs. These conditions include but are not limited to congenital malformations, genetic disorders, known intrauterine exposure to infection, medication or substances, preterm birth, or pre-, peri- or neonatal complications. Other high-risk conditions such as vision or hearing impairment may be identified either clinically or through screenings in the weeks or months after birth.

Children without an identified condition that places them at high risk for developmental or behavioral disorders are identified through caregiver concerns or through screening. The AAP recommends surveillance for developmental and behavioral concerns at all health supervision visits, and periodic developmental screening using a validated instrument at the 9-, 18-, and 30-month visits. Autism screenings are recommended at the 18- and 24-month visits.[6] When a caregiver voices concern about development or behavior at non-screening health supervision visits, the AAP recommends performing developmental screening. Validated screening instruments provide objective data to augment clinical assessment. When screening results indicate a concern in any area of development, referral for medical and developmental evaluation is indicated.[6] Medical evaluation may be conducted in the primary care setting or by a specialist. The evaluation includes a thorough history to assess etiologic risks, and a physical examination focused on neurologic or genetic etiologies of delays. The developmental assessment may be conducted by early intervention programs or by specialists and should evaluate all areas of development to determine the nature and degree of delays and to observe behavior, attachment, and interactions. Specialists will provide developmental diagnoses, and early intervention programs will determine eligibility and frequency of developmental services. A referral to the local early intervention program should always be made independent of the medical and developmental specialist evaluation. Early intervention programs do not require formal diagnosis, but rather determine eligibility for services based on risk, atypical development or areas of delayed developmental rather than on diagnoses, and early intervention (EI) programs often provide services before children receive formal diagnoses at diagnostic centers.[7] The initiation of services through early intervention addresses the urgency of the child's needs and the parent's concerns, whereas they also wait for medical or developmental evaluation.

Educational Considerations

Early childhood

Early intervention programs assess the child's risk for developmental or behavioral conditions and the child's developmental levels in all five areas of development to determine eligibility for services. In the United States, children who qualify for services receive an Individualized Family Service Plan (IFSP) which defines necessary services, family resources and priorities, and goals, expectations and timelines of services provided under Part C of the Individuals with Disabilities Education Act (IDEA).[8] IFSP services are generally provided for children until their 3rd birthday, then children transition to IEP services that are facilitated by public school districts. Some states allow continuation of IFSP services or extension of Part C up to kindergarten entry in special circumstances.[9] As the IFSP transitions to IEP services, the natural environment becomes the least restrictive appropriate classroom with peers, where interventions may be offered in a typical classroom setting ("push in services"), as individual or small group sessions away from the typical classroom ("pull out services"), or in special education settings. Among children receiving early intervention services before age 5 years, the most common intervention is speech therapy, followed by occupational therapy, and the vast majority of young children receive their speech and OT services only through school. Behavioral therapy such as applied behavioral analysis is far less frequently provided in the preschool population, and most of the behavioral services are delivered outside the school setting.[10]

Transitioning to school

Ideally, developmental delays are identified in early childhood, but an estimated 50% of children with developmental disorders, including some with ASD, are not identified before kindergarten entry.[11] In addition, some developmental disorders, such as learning disabilities, do not become evident until classroom demands exceed a child's capabilities. School-age children for whom concerns arise regarding developmental or behavioral disorders require referral to the school system. Such a referral may be made by the child's caregiver(s), medical provider, or by childcare or school personnel. The school determines if there is sufficient cause to warrant evaluation, and if so, is required to notify and obtain the consent of the caregiver(s) for the evaluation and to conduct appropriate assessments and determine eligibility for services within 60 days of caregiver consent. Once student eligibility is established, school teams have 30 days to develop the IEP and determine the nature, goals, and frequency of service provision as well as the environment in which services will be delivered.[8]

School-based services for children with identified delays or eligible conditions start at age 3 years, unless there is a circumstance in which a child qualifies for Part C extension services. The Education for All Handicapped Children Act of 1975, renamed as the IDEA, ensures that all children aged 3 to 21 years with disabilities are entitled to a free and appropriate public education in the least restrictive environment that meets their educational needs. Children that meet eligibility criteria under one or more of the 13 disability categories are entitled to an IEP which defines their special education services.[8] In the 2020 to 2021 academic year, 7.2 million students between 3 and 21 years of age received special education services under IDEA (15% of all school children). Among those receiving special education services, 12% were eligible under the ASD category.[12]

Some children with ASD and other disabilities also receive services under Section 504 of the Rehabilitation Act of 1973, which prohibits discrimination of individuals with a disability in any federally funded program including all public schools or private schools which accept federal funding. Under section 504, individuals with disabilities are entitled to reasonable accommodations that optimize their successful participation. All children who qualify for services under IDEA also qualify under Section 504, but not all children with a 504 plan are eligible for IEP services.[8] For example, a child diagnosed with attention deficit hyperactivity disorder (ADHD) may receive accommodations such as preferential seating, extended test time, or a quiet space to complete a test or examination. Unlike IEP requirements, 504 plans are optimally reassessed annually, but there is no requirement to do so. Some children who have a medical diagnosis of ASD do not meet school criteria to qualify for IEP service under autism but may receive services under a different qualifying condition such as speech impairment or other health impairment or may only receive 504 services.

Type of school placement and the services provided vary greatly due to the wide-ranging needs of children with ASD and the variability of symptoms severity. Comorbid conditions such as ADHD, intellectual disability, learning disabilities, motor disabilities, and behavioral disorders can also impact placement. One of the primary considerations for school placement is the cognitive ability of the child. Current CDC data estimate that 38% of 8-year-old children with ASD also have intellectual disability,[13] indicating significant disability of cognitive and adaptive skills in addition to the primary deficits associated with ASD diagnosis. The frequencies of ADHD (28%–35%), learning disabilities (16%–23%), anxiety (5%–20%), motor disabilities (19%–26%), and behavior disorders (4%–25%) in children with ASD vary tremendously based on the age of the child and the method of reporting.[14–16] The goal of placement is for children to learn in the least restrictive environment, but depending on symptom severity and comorbid conditions, the mainstream classroom with same-age peers may or may not be sufficient to meet the child's educational needs. Recent data from the US Department of Education show that 40% of children with ASD spend the majority (>80%) of their day in a typical classroom setting, 18% spend 40% to 80% of their day in a typical classroom, and 33% spend a majority (>60%) of their day outside of a typical classroom with same-age peers[17] (**Fig. 2**).

Services for autism spectrum disorder

In preschoolers, speech therapy is the most common service provided to students with ASD, followed by occupational therapy, behavioral management, learning support, and case management. By middle or early high school, speech service remains the most commonly used service, followed by transportation, adaptive PE, case management, behavioral services, and assistive technology.[18] Additional school-based or school-related services that may be included in IEP or 504 plans include mental health counseling, nursing/personal care needs, resource room access, school aides, extended school year services, and vocational planning services. For all students with an IEP, there is annual reevaluation of needs and services.

The nature and number of services provided for children with ASD change over time and vary with the severity of autism symptoms and comorbidities. In 2010 to 2021, 12% of children received IDEA services under the eligibility category of autism.[12] Children with ASD who also have intellectual disability or more severe core symptoms or communication deficits are more likely to receive special education services.[19] Preschoolers and primary school students with ASD are far more likely to receive speech, occupational therapy, and behavioral management services, whereas secondary school students are more likely to receive mental health services, adaptive physical education, and assistive technology services (**Fig. 3**). Overall, the number of services peaks in third to fourth grade, and children with more significant deficits in using or understanding communication are more likely to receive more types and a greater number of services.[18]

Speech therapy is the most frequently provided service to students with ASD as part of their IEP services, with 85% of preschool and school-age children receiving this service.[18] Speech sound disorders and language disorders are common in children with ASD. Speech sound disorders occur in about 3.6% of 4-year-old children but may occur as much as eight times more frequently in children with autism.[20,21] Language disorders occur in 11% to 18% of children in early childhood and about

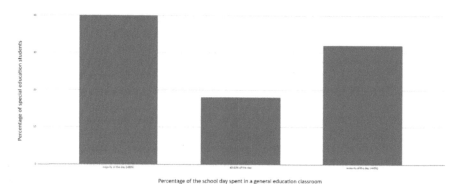

Fig. 2. School placement in General Education. (*Adapted from* US Department of Ed. Ref.[16])

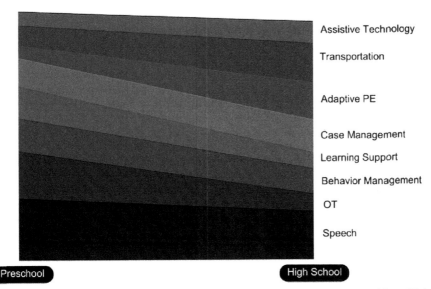

Assistive Technology

Transportation

Adaptive PE

Case Management

Learning Support

Behavior Management

OT

Speech

Preschool   High School

Fig. 3. IEP service provision for children with autism spectrum disorder. (*Adapted from* Wei et al, 2014.)

7% of school-age children.[22] The frequency of language disorder including speech sound disorder, expressive, receptive of mixed receptive and expressive disorders, in children with ASD is much higher, occurring in 50% of preschoolers and 27% of school-age children.[23,24] Although older children with ASD are likely to have standard language measures similar to typically developing peers, there is evidence that the quality and complexity of their language are less sophisticated.[25]

Approximately 30% of children with ASD are minimally verbal,[26] and those with low or no verbalization may benefit from augmentative or alternative communication (AAC). Speech language pathologists are instrumental in the assessment of children's capacity for using AAC devices and matching them with the correct modes or devices. AAC may include no technology (sign language or gesture), low technology (picture exchange systems [PECSs]), or high technology (speech-generating devices). Preschool AAC often uses low-tech PECSs that use pictures to facilitate communication.

Speech-generating communication devices provide mobile, high-tech options for children with limited or no verbal communication and are both an effective and preferred AAC modality, especially in school-age and adolescent children.[27] A recent review of AAC measures indicates that when using evidence-based practice measures (reinforcement, prompting, time delay, discrete trial training, task analysis), high-tech AAC scored slightly better than low tech and was the most preferred AAC mode. Sign language (no tech) did not score well on intervention performance or preference.[27] The use of AAC technology services increases over time, with approximately 20% of preschool and early school-age students accessing AAC, and 30% of older students.[18]

Children with ASD are at relatively high risk for motor impairment, with axial hypotonia and developmental coordination disorder (DCD) commonly diagnosed in children with ASD.[28] DCD is characterized by impairments in gross and fine motor coordination that may significantly impact a child's academic achievement and daily functioning. Children with DCD appear more clumsy and less coordinated than same-age peers in both gross and fine motor function. Difficulty with manual dexterity may be the most lasting and consequential impact of DCD, as it has significant impact on coordination required for activities of daily living including snapping, buttoning, scissor use, and handwriting skills.[29]

OT is the second most common service provided to children with ASD in preschool and early school-age settings, but the frequency of OT services wanes as children get older. An estimated 65% of preschoolers, 50% of school age, and 24% of older students receive OT services.[18] Like speech therapy, OT services in preschoolers are almost entirely received within the IEP/IFSP setting.[10] OT services may be directed toward adaptive skills (snapping, buttoning, dressing), toward skills that impact academics (graphomotor/handwriting) or may focus on training for and use of accommodations for handwriting such as typing programs or specialized keyboards.

Motor impairment, including DCD, may require physical therapy to address coordination, core strength, and physical endurance and to enhance participation in school physical activity, including physical education class, recess, and other activities like field day. Despite the frequency of motor impairments, only about a third of school-age children receive physical therapy services.[28] Unlike speech and OT services, which decrease in frequency across time, adaptive physical education services increase as children age within the school system.[18] The value of physical activity for children is well-documented, but the language and physical demands of general physical education, in addition to the often stimulating environment and competitive nature of general physical education (PE) can be exceedingly challenging for children on the spectrum. Adaptive PE instructors express a need for additional training in behavior management, communication skills, and curriculum development to meet the needs of their ASD students.[30]

Social competency and skills should be discussed and included at IFSP/IEP meetings and included as goals in the educational program.[26] Social skill training aims to improve successful social interaction and navigation with peers, family, teachers, and others. Social skills training may be conducted in individual or group settings and may include direct instruction, practicing in small groups with feedback, and role playing with feedback. Basic instruction in social dynamics may include simple conventions of communication such as eye contact, reciprocal communication, and appropriate initiation of social opportunities. Social skills also target the nuances of communication, like tolerating non-preferred topics of conversation, reading body language, facial expression, and inference such as sarcasm, idioms, and jokes. Social skill services are provided to 49% of children with autism, but far more likely in children with severe ASD,[31] and in children who did not also have intellectual disability.[19]

In addition to the services detailed above, which can be effective for children with a range of different neurodevelopmental disorders, the education of children with ASD may include additional autism-specific approaches. These autism-specific curricula may include comprehensive treatment models such as treatment and education of autistic and communication handicapped children (TEACCH) and learning experiences and alternate programs for preschoolers and their parents (LEAP).[32]

Behavioral health at school

Disruptive behaviors, including aggression, self-injurious behavior (SIB), and tantrums, are a common concern at school and in other settings, with 25% of children with ASD having SIBs.[33] In the school setting, difficult behaviors require a functional behavioral analysis to determine the purpose, antecedents, and reinforcers of behaviors such as aggression and self-injury, as simple interventions or a behavioral intervention plan (BIP) may substantially modify behavior. Children with ASD and ID were more likely to show SIB.[34] In children with ASD, aggressive behavior directed toward self or others may be also due to avoiding demands, may occur impulsively in the context of a tantrum, or may be intended.[34]

The BIP is an individualized plan that uses known triggers and ameliorating factors to help teachers and school staff de-escalate behaviors and help children get back to participating in the learning environment. Addition of the BIP to IEP is most common in preschool settings for children with ASD (45%) and less common in settings for adolescents (35%).[18] In addition to classroom management strategies such as the BIP, many children with ASD benefit from behavioral therapy to address disruptive and externalizing behaviors. Some children ultimately require medication management as well as behavioral therapy due to behaviors that are causing safety concerns or are limiting the child's ability to participate in the classroom or in therapies. Behavioral intervention services are provided to 39% of children with autism but are more likely to be provided to children with severe ASD.[31]

Hyperreactivity and hyporeactivity to sensory stimuli are so common in ASD that they are included in the criteria for diagnosis in the diagnostic and statistical manual of mental disorders, 5th edition (DSM-5).[35] Sensitivities may be oral, auditory, tactile, visual, or olfactory. Sensory therapy aims to reduce sensitivity to triggering stimuli that interfere with participation or function and may be provided by behavioral or occupational therapists. Sensory integration therapies are generally clinic-based rather than school-based and provided as individualized therapy with discrete goals, which have some evidence of improving behaviors associated with sensory sensitivity.[36] Conversely, sensory-based interventions are more often classroom-based interventions to reduce unwanted behavior such as weighted vests, which have little evidence of efficacy but are widely used.[36,37]

Family Considerations

Behavioral disorders, sleep, and feeding

Behavioral disturbance is one of the primary stressors for children with ASD and their caregivers, at home, school, and in the community. Aggression and self-injury are reported in about 35% of children with ASD, may be elevated in children with lower language and cognitive levels, and may worsen if the child is prevented from engaging in repetitive behaviors.[34,38] Parenting-related stress is higher for parents of children with ASD as compared with parents of typically developing children or children with other developmental diagnoses, particularly when externalizing behaviors such as tantrums or self-injury are present.[39,40] Parents of children who have fewer communication skills and higher ASD symptom burden also have increased levels of parenting-related stress.[41] Parent and guardian stress may be compounded by the fact that younger siblings of children with ASD are more likely to be diagnosed with ASD themselves.[41]

Elopement is a particularly frequent behavior, with up to half of children with ASD engaging in wandering or elopement behavior at some point in childhood.[42] Parents report significant worry about elopement and wandering risk: 58.7% worry about their child wandering from home or when out in public, 73.3% limit their child staying with friends or family in their absence due to wandering concerns, and 55% request IEP changes to address elopement safety.[43] Difficulty during car transport including elopement and distracting behaviors is another safety hazard, and families report that fear of driving due to behavioral concerns limits their participation in the community.[33] Issues like elopement and car safety contribute to family feelings of isolation from the community.

Sleep disruption is common in children with ASD, and insufficient sleep may impact function at home and in the classroom, as it exacerbates many of the core symptoms of autism. Parents report that sleep disruption is very common: 44% to 80% of children with ASD have at least some sleep-related symptoms.[44,45] In younger children and toddlers, this manifests primarily as bedtime resistance, nighttime awakenings and parasomnias such as sleepwalking and nightmares. In older children and adolescents, frequent symptoms include delayed sleep onset, shorter sleep duration, and increased daytime sleepiness.[44]

Medical and mental health comorbidities that are common in children with ASD may contribute to sleep disruption, particularly in children with co-occurring ADHD or anxiety. The current guidelines for sleep disruption in children and adolescents with ASD include behavioral and medication approaches. Medical conditions such as obstructive sleep apnea, gastro-esophageal reflux, seizures, ADHD, mental health disorders or medications used for medical conditions that interrupt or disrupt sleep should be managed first.[45] Sleep disruption in all children requires first an assessment of sleep hygiene. In early childhood, a frequent sleep complaint is sleep-onset association type insomnia, in which the conditions a child requires to fall asleep (parent in room, ambient noise, bottle, pacifier) will also be required when the child has normal nighttime arousals. If the same conditions are not present during a night arousal, the child will awaken more fully and demand attention until sleep conditions are met. In older children, sleep hygiene is influenced more commonly by technology devices, especially television, cell phone, or tablet use, which demand attention and delay sleep onset. If children do not respond to sleep hygiene optimization, behavioral strategies such as fading or extinction are helpful in early childhood. Cognitive behavioral therapy is used in older children and adolescents.[45] After appropriate counseling regarding the dose, adverse effects, and lack of long-term data on the use of melatonin, it may be recommended in conjunction with behavioral strategies in children who continue to have sleep disruption.[45]

Feeding behaviors including selective eating are extremely common in children with ASD and can lead to significant stress and disruption around family mealtimes. Up to 75% of children with ASD have selective eating, with many eating less than 20 different foods and requiring separate meals from the rest of the family.[26,46] Food selectivity leads to frequent meltdowns, disrupts family meal routines, and can also cause decreased intake of vitamin D, calcium, and fiber and gastrointestinal disorders, most commonly constipation.[26] There have been rare cases of severe vitamin A, C, and D deficiencies leading to significant medical complications as a result of food selective behaviors in children with ASD.[26] Consultation with a registered dietitian can be helpful for families to help children eat more balanced diets.[26] In more difficult cases, feeding therapy and parent training programs have been shown to increase the variety of foods consumed and decrease disruptive mealtime behaviors.[47] When disrupted feeding behaviors are so severe that there is significant weight loss, growth failure, severe nutrient deficiency, dependence on oral nutritional supplements, or need for enteral feeding, this should lead to consideration of avoidant/restrictive food intake disorder diagnosis and more intensive treatments.[48]

Please see other chapters in this volume for additional information and details on sleep problems, mental health, and evidence-based interventions in this volume.

Emerging mental health concerns
Psychiatric disorders such as anxiety, OCD, and mood disorders occur in children with ASD with a frequency as high as 70% to 90%.[26] The diagnosis of co-occurring mental health disorders can be challenging for families and clinicians, particularly in nonverbal or low-verbal individuals where behavioral changes may be the only manifestation. Behaviors may manifest as increase in core features of autism, with escalation of

repetitive behavior, obsessive compulsive disorder (OCD) or aggression, SIB or as narrowing of behavior such as social withdrawal or further retraction of circumscribed interests. Changes in sleep patterns, appetite, school performance, or participation in extracurricular activity may also be presenting features of emerging mental health concerns.

Although the management of mental health disorders in children with ASD is similar to typically developing children in terms of counseling and psychopharmacology, the diagnosis and mental health counseling may require specialists with an expertise in ASD, particularly when the concern arises in children with intellectual disability or nonverbal or low-verbal ability. Mental health services may be provided in school or clinic-based settings. Mental health service provision increases fourfold between preschool and adolescence.[18] However, mental health or behavioral health services are more difficult to find for children with ASD. Across the United States, only 43% of mental health treatment facilities provide services to children with ASD, and only 12.7% report having clinical specialists with training in ASD.[49] Mothers of children with autism, who experience difficulty locating mental health care, report that the burden also influences their mental health.[50]

Family and peer dynamics

Siblings of children with ASD report higher levels of stress than siblings of children with Down syndrome and more sibling-related stress than children with neurotypical siblings.[51] Studies of impact on neurotypical siblings show higher rates of internalizing behaviors such as worry, anxiety, and withdrawal, greater impairment in social functioning, and more negative sibling relationships.[41] Sibling conflict is common, but tends to emerge at home rather than out in the community.[52] Generally, siblings of children with ASD report feelings of "anxiety, guilt, frustration, love, pride, and protection," but in adolescence, typically developing siblings of children with ASD tend to have more feelings of annoyance, embarrassment, and anger toward their sibling.[41,52]

As children with ASD grow into adolescence, the confluence of many changes begins a new set of challenges for parents and caregivers. The behavioral changes of puberty may be exaggerated, and the increasing academic and social demands of middle and early high school may exacerbate behavior. In addition, the onset of mental illness occurs at increased rates in adolescents with ASD, including depression and anxiety. These changes impact children with ASD both in and out of school. Families also begin to grapple with future planning for postsecondary education, vocational training, independent or supported living, and decision-making.

Friendships and socializing with peers become increasingly important for all children throughout childhood and into adolescence, and for children with ASD, navigating adolescent relationships becomes especially precarious. Adolescents with ASD spend less time with peers and more time with adults and professionals compared with neurotypical same-age peers.[53] Parents report that friendships between teens with ASD and their friends often lack reciprocity, so teens tend to perceive themselves as having more friends than their parents believe them to have.[53] These friendships that lack reciprocity can sometimes lead to bullying situations. Children with ASD are more frequently victims than perpetrators of bullying behavior, which can be a major stressor at school and at home.[54]

As children with ASD get older, parents often wonder at what point they should discuss the child's diagnosis with them, and how to do so. A recent study found that 80% of youth in the study group had been informed of their ASD diagnosis, and that of those who had been informed, 80% first received this information from a parent or guardian, most commonly between the ages of 6 to 12 years.[55] Diagnosis disclosure rates were lower for children who also had co-occurring ID.[55] Parents report that children who are informed of their ASD diagnosis have improved self-awareness of strengths and weaknesses, as well as greater capacity to self-advocate and deal with challenges and setbacks.[55] Parents found it helpful to use informational resources to help with diagnosis disclosure, including books, videos, social stories, Web sites, and support groups.[55]

Transitioning to young adulthood

About 70% of students with disabilities graduate from high school, but 24 states have alternate certificates that are not diploma equivalents. Determination of diploma or certificate path is determined and discussed in IEP meetings, particularly at transition meetings. The pathway, certificate, or diploma have implications for transition plans, so parents need to be aware of which pathway has been suggested or determined for their child.[56] The 2020 data show that 72% of students with ASD graduated from high school, 18% received an alternate certificate, and 6% dropped out, with students with ASD less likely to drop out than students with other disabilities.[17] Plans for graduation or alternative certificate, further education or vocational training, and employment readiness should be discussed in IEP meetings starting in early adolescence.

Young adults with ASD have low rates of participation in the workforce, and by 4 years post-high school completion, as few as 11% of autistic young adults are employed.[57] Vocational support programs include options like supported employment, which can include formal training for employment readiness, strength and support need-based job matching, and ongoing support in the workplace with graduated independence over time.[57] Sheltered workshops are a form of segregated employment where workers with disabilities are paid at less than market wages, including below minimum wage, and are a less favorable option.

Students with ASD are going to college in increasing numbers, and 36% of young adults with ASD attempt at least some college.[58] There are currently more than 30 programs designed to support students with ASD at US universities. These support programs can help mitigate some of the challenges that students with ASD face in college, including difficulty with academic demands, as well as executive functioning, social challenges, and emerging or persisting mental health issues.[58,59] Parents report that college students with ASD have challenges with self-advocacy, regulating emotions, and navigating interpersonal skills during this period.[60]

Decision-making is a frequent concern for parents and families as young adults with ASD come of age. Legislation varies state to state, and options range from guardianship or conservatorship, which entirely transfer decision-making to a court appointed guardian to supported decision-making arrangements, which are less restrictive and involve cooperative decision-making between the disabled adult and one or more trusted advisors. Shared decision-making agreements and other less restrictive legal arrangements have support from organizations including the American Bar Association, The Arc, and the Autistic Self Advocacy Network.[61]

Determining readiness or appropriateness of pursuing a driving license is yet another concern that arises for families in the transition to adulthood. Young adults with ASD have difficulty with several different cognitive skills required for driving, including time estimation[62] and driving hazard detection,[63] and have increased difficulty compared with peers as complexity increases, suggesting that they may benefit from slow and gradual driver's training programs.[64] The use of appropriate driver education may allow many teens and young adults with ASD to gain the skills required for driving: in 2017, one in three adolescents with ASD without co-occurring ID acquired a driver's license, compared with 83.5% of teens without ASD.[65]

Social connectedness is important for quality of life, and once children with ASD graduate from school, the opportunities for them to find community and social connections are reduced. Loneliness and social isolation are more common for autistic adults,[66] and adults with ASD are less likely to participate in community activities compared with neurotypical peers as well as peers with other developmental disabilities.[67] Adults with ASD are more likely to participate in solitary leisure activities and hobbies[67]; however, these interests can sometimes be turned into social opportunities, by connecting them to interest groups. Some autistic adults find meaningful social connection in the workplace, whether paid work or volunteering.[68] Social media networks such as Facebook groups are also an important place for social connection for many autistic adults.[68]

SUMMARY

ASD has an impact throughout the lifespan and across all different environments, especially the home and school. Special education services and therapies in school require continual reassessment to ensure that they are meeting the ever-changing needs of children with ASD (see **Fig. 1**). Families face a unique range of challenges when raising children with ASD, including frequently co-occurring behavioral, sleep, and feeding disturbances, mental health disorders, challenging sibling dynamics, difficulties with socialization, and increased parental stress. As adolescents approach adulthood, weighty decisions are introduced in both the school and home setting and have bearing on the successful transition to adult life. The orchestration of personal, family, educational, medical, and community considerations, needs, and supports of children with ASD is complex, but of inestimable value. Primary care clinicians are at the center of this network of support, providing screening, referrals to appropriate specialists and services, support for families, ongoing surveillance of educational and developmental progress, and for emerging new concerns and co-occurring disorders. Primary care partnership with the child, family, educators, and service providers ensures ongoing support and guidance as the child develops, navigates adolescence, and transitions to adult services and care.

CLINICS CARE POINTS

- The nature and intensity of services needed by children with autism spectrum disorder at home and in the school vary by age and by core and associated symptoms of ASD.
- Children with ASD have high utilization rates of school services.
- There is an evolution of the impacts and considerations of families with children with ASD over time with regard to the child's and family's changing needs.
- As social demands increase with advancing age, peer and sibling relationships become more challenging for children with ASD.
- Children with ASD and their families face challenges of transitioning from entitlement to school services to eligibility for adult service programs.

ACKNOWLEDGMENTS

The authors are grateful for the expertise of Hillary Goldthwait-Fowles, PhD, for her assistance with designing the figures for this article.

DISCLOSURE

M.L. O'Connor Leppert receives funding from Maryland Behavioral Health Administration BH588TEC-1 and from the Henry M. Jackson Foundation for the Advancement of Military Medicine, United States. Uniformed Services University of the Health Services (USU) (HU00012120084).

REFERENCES

1. Goin-Kochel R, Myers B. Parental report of early autistic symptoms: differences in ages of detection and frequencies of characteristics among three autism spectrum disorders. J Dev Disabil 2004;11:21–40.
2. Zuckerman KE, Lindly OJ, Sinche BK. Parental concerns, provider response and timeliness of autism spectrum disorder diagnosis. J Pediatr 2015;166(6):1431–9.
3. van't Hof M, Tisseur C, van Berckelear-Onnes I, et al. Age at autism spectrum diagnosis: A systematic review and meta-analysis from 2012-2019. Autism 2021;25(4):862–73.
4. Carbone PS, Campbell K, Wilkes J, et al. Primary care autism screening and later autism diagnosis. Pediatrics 2020;146(7):e20192314.
5. Shaw KA, Maenner MJ, Bakian AV, et al. Early identification of autism spectrum disorder among children aged 4 years– autism and developmental disabilities monitoring network, 11 Sites, United States 2018. MMWR Surveill Summ 2021; 70(SS-10):1–14.
6. Lipkin PH, Macias MM, Council on Children with Disabilities, Section on Developmental and Behavioral Pediatrics. Council on children with disabilities, section on developmental and behavioral pediatrics. promoting optimal development: identifying infants and young children with developmental disorders through developmental surveillance and screening. Pediatrics 2020;145(1):e20193449.
7. Monteiro SA, Dempse J, Broton S, et al. Early intervention before autism diagnosis in children referred to a regional autism clinic. Journal of Developmental & Behavioral Pediatrics 2016;37(1):15–9.
8. Lipkin PH, Okamoto J, Council on Children with Disabilities, et al. Council on children with disabilities and council on school health. the individuals with disabilities education Act (IDEA) for children with special education needs. Pediatrics 2015; 136(6):e1650–62.
9. Early Childhood Technical Assistance Center. Part C Extension Option. Accessed March 25, 2023. https://ectacenter.org/partc/partc_option.asp.
10. Bilaver LA, Cushing LS, Cutler AT. Prevalence and correlates of educational intervention utilization among children with autism spectrum disorder. J Autism Dev Disord 2016;46:561–71.
11. Glascoe FP, Marks KP. Detecting children with developmental-behavioral problems: The value of collaborating with parents. Psychological Test and Assessment Modeling 2011;52(2):258–79.
12. National Center for Education Statistics. Students with disabilities. condition of education. U.S. Department of Education, Institute of Education Sciences; 2020. https://nces.ed.gov/programs/coe/indicator/cgg. Accessed February 10, 2023.
13. Maenner MJ, Warren Z, Williams AR, et al. Prevalence and characteristics of autism spectrum disorder among children aged 8 years- autism and developmental disabilities monitoring network, 11 Sites, United States. 2020. MMWR Surveill Summ 2023;72(SS-2):1–14.

14. Lai MC, Kassee C, Besney R, et al. Prevalence of co-occurring mental health diagnoses in the autism population: a systematic review and meta-analysis. Lancet Psychiatr 2019 Oct;6(10):819–29.
15. Soke GN, Maenner MJ, Christensen D, et al. Prevalence of co-occurring medical and behavioral conditions/symptoms among 4- and 8-year-old children with autism spectrum disorder in selected areas of the United States in 2010. J Autism Dev Disord 2018;48(8):2663–76.
16. Khachadourian V, Mahjani B, Sandin S, et al. Comorbidities in autism spectrum disorder and their etiologies. Transl Psychiatry 2023;13:71.
17. United States Department of Education, Office of Special Education Programs: OSEP Fast Facts: Children Identified with Autism. Last updated 2020. Accessed March 12, 2023. https://sites.ed.gov/idea/osep-fast-facts-children-with-autism-20//.
18. Wei X, Wagner M, Christiano ERA, et al. Special education services received by students with autism spectrum disorders from preschool through high school. J Spec Educ 2014;48(3):167–279.
19. White SW, Scahill L, Klin A, et al. Educational placements and service use patterns of individuals with autism spectrum disorders. J Autism Dev Disord 2007; 37:1403–12.
20. Wren YE, Miller LL, Peters T, et al. Prevalence and predictors of persistent speech sound disorders at age 8 years old: findings from a population cohort study. J Speech Lang Hear Res 2016;59:647–73.
21. Shrilberg LD, Strand EA, Jakielski KJ, Mabie HL, et al. Estimates of the prevalence of speech and motor speech disorders in persons with complex neurodevelopmental disorders. Clin Linguist Phon 2019;33(8):707–36.
22. Feldman HM. How young children learn language and speech. Pediatr Rev 2019; 40(8):398–411.
23. Marrus N, Hall LP, Paterson SJ, et al. Language delay aggregates in toddler siblings of children with autism spectrum disorder. J Neurodev Disord 2018;10:29.
24. Neumeyer AM, Anixt J, Chan J, et al. Identifying associations among co-occurring medical conditions in children with autism spectrum disorders. Academic Pediatrics 2019;19(3):300–6.
25. Boo C, Alpers-Leon N, McIntyre N, et al. Conversation during a virtual reality task reveals new structural language profiles of children with ASD, ADHD and comorbid symptoms of both. J Autism Dev Disord 2022;52:2970–83.
26. Hyman SL, Levy SE, Meyers SM, et al. Identification, evaluation, and management of children with autism spectrum disorder. Pediatrics 2020;145(1):e20193447.
27. Lorah ER, Holyfield C, Miller J, et al. A systematic review of research comparing mobile technology speech-generating devices to other AAC modes with individuals with autism spectrum disorder. J Dev Phys Disabil 2022;34:187–210.
28. Bhat AN. Is motor impairment in autism spectrum disorder distinct from developmental coordination disorder? a report from the spark study. Phys Ther 2020; 100(4):633–44.
29. Bolk J, Farooqi A, Hafstrom M, et al. Developmental coordination disorder and its association with developmental comorbidities at 6.5 years in apparently healthy children born extremely preterm. JAMA Pediatr 2018;172(8):765–74.
30. Healy S, Judge JP, Block ME, et al. Preparing adapted physical educators to teach students with autism: current practices and future directions. Phys Educat 2016;73:97–109.
31. Zuckerman K, Friedman NDB, Chavez AE, et al. Parent-reported severity and health/educational services use among U.S. children with autism: results from a national survey. J Dev Behav Pediatr 2017;38(4):260–8.

32. Boyd BA, Hume K, McBee MT, et al. Comparative efficacy of LEAP, TEACCH and non-model-specific special education programs for preschoolers with autism spectrum disorders. J Autism Dev Disord 2014;44(2):366–80.

33. Plummer T, Bryan M, Dullaghan K, et al. Parent experiences and perceptions of safety when transporting children with autism spectrum disorder. Am J Occup Ther 2021;7(5):7505205010.

34. Carroll D, Hallett V, McDougle CJ, et al. Examination of aggression and self-injury in children with autism spectrum disorder and serious behavioral problems. Child and Adolescent Psychiatric Clinics of North America 2014;23(1):57–72.

35. American Psychiatric Association. Diagnostic and statistical manual of mental disorders. 5th edition. Arlington, VA: American Psychiatric Association; 2013.

36. Case-Smith J, Weaver LL, Fristad MA. A systematic review of sensory processing interventions for children with autism spectrum disorders. Autism 2015;199(2):133–48.

37. Barton EE, Reichow B, Schnitz A, et al. A systematic review of sensory-based treatments for children with disabilities. Res Dev Disabil 2015;37:64–80.

38. Fitzpatrick SE, Srivorakiat L, Wink LK, et al. Aggression in autism spectrum disorder: presentation and treatment options. Neuropsychiatric Dis Treat 2016;12:1525–38.

39. Olson L, Chen B, Ibarra C, et al. Externalizing behaviors are associated with increased parenting stress in caregivers of young children with autism. J Autism Dev Disord 2022;52(3):975–86.

40. Estes A, Olson E, Sullivan K, et al. Parenting-related stress and psychological distress in mothers of toddlers with autism spectrum disorders. Brain Dev 2013;35(2):133–8.

41. Shivers CM, Jackson JB, McGregor CM. Functioning among typically developing siblings of individuals with autism spectrum disorder: a meta-analysis. Clin Child Fam Psychol Rev 2019a;22(2):172–96.

42. Anderson C, Law JK, Daniels A, et al. Occurrence and family impact of elopement in children with autism spectrum disorders. Pediatrics 2012;130(5):870–7.

43. McLaughlin L, Keim SA, Adesman A. Wandering by children with autism spectrum disorder: key clinical factors and the role of schools and pediatricians. J Dev Behav Pediatr 2018;39(7):538–46.

44. Goldman SE, Richdale AL, Clemons T, et al. Parental sleep concerns in autism spectrum disorders: variations from childhood to adolescence. J Autism Dev Disord 2012;42(4):531–8.

45. Buckley AW, Hirtz D, Oskoui M, et al. Practice guidelines: treatment for insomnia and disrupted sleep behavior in children and adolescents with autism spectrum disorder. Neurology 2020;94(9):392–404.

46. Nadon G, Feldman DE, Dunn W, et al. Mealtime problems in children with autism spectrum disorder and their typically developing siblings: a comparison study. Autism 2011;15(1):98–113.

47. Johnson CR, Brown K, Hyman SL, et al. Parent training for feeding problems in children with autism spectrum disorder: initial randomized trial. J Pediatr Psychol 2019;44(2):164–75.

48. Bourne L, Mandy W, Bryant-Waugh R. Avoidant/restrictive food intake disorder and severe food selectivity in children and young people with autism: A scoping review. Dev Med Child Neurol 2022;64(6):691–700.

49. Cantor J, McBain RK, Kofner A, et al. Fewer than half of us mental health treatment facilities provide services for children with autism spectrum disorder. Health Aff 2020;39(6). https://doi.org/10.1377/hlthaff.2019.01557.

50. Jackson L, Keville S, Ludlow AK. Mothers' experiences of accessing mental health care for their child with an autism spectrum disorder. J Child Fam Stud 2020;29:534–45.
51. Shivers CM, McGregor C, Hough A. Self-reported stress among adolescent siblings of individuals with autism spectrum disorder and Down syndrome. Autism 2019b;23(1):112–22.
52. Guidotti L, Musetti A, Barbieri GL, et al. Conflicting and harmonious sibling relationships of children and adolescent siblings of children with autism spectrum disorder. Child Care Health Dev 2021;47(2):163–73.
53. Kuo MH, Orsmond GI, Cohn ES, et al. Friendship characteristics and activity patterns of adolescents with an autism spectrum disorder. Autism 2013;17(4):481–500.
54. Maïano C, Normand CL, Salvas MC, et al. Prevalence of school bullying among youth with autism spectrum disorders: a systematic review and meta-analysis. Autism Res 2016;9(6):601–15.
55. Kiely B, Adesman A, Rapoport E, et al. Patterns and outcomes of diagnosis disclosure to youth with autism spectrum disorder. J Dev Behav Pediatr 2020;41(6):443–51.
56. Klein, R. These students are finishing high school, but their degrees don't help them go to college. The Hechinger Report. December 2, 2017. Accessed January 20, 2023. https://hechingerreport.org/students-finishing-high-school-degrees-dont-help-go-college.
57. Nicholas DB, Attridge M, Zwaigenbaum L, et al. Vocational support approaches in autism spectrum disorder: A synthesis review of the literature. Autism 2015;19(2):235–45.
58. Anderson C, Butt C. Young adults on the autism spectrum at college: successes and stumbling blocks. J Autism Dev Disord 2017;47(10):3029–39.
59. Hillier A, Ryan J, Buckingham A, et al. Prospective college students with autism spectrum disorder: parent perspectives. Psychol Rep 2021;124(1):88–107.
60. Elias R, White SW. Autism goes to college: understanding the needs of a student population on the rise. J Autism Dev Disord 2018;48(3):732–46.
61. Autistic Self Advocacy Newtork. Available at: https://autisticadvocacy.org/. Accessed March, 31, 2023.
62. Svancara AM, Kana R, Bednarz H, et al. Time-to-collision estimations in in young drivers with autism spectrum disorder and attention-defcit/hyperactivity disorder. J Autism Dev Disord 2022;52:3933–48.
63. Bednarz HM, Kana RK, Svancara AM, et al. Neuropsychological predictors of driving hazard detection in autism spectrum disorder and ADHD. Child Neuropsychol 2021;27(7):857–87.
64. Patrick KE, Hurewitz F, McCurdy MD, et al. Driving comparisons between young adults with autism spectrum disorder and typical development. J Dev Behav Pediatr 2018;39(6):451–60.
65. Curry AE, Yerys BE, Huang P, et al. Longitudinal study of driver licensing rates among adolescents and young adults with autism spectrum disorder. Autism 2018;22(4):479–88.
66. Pellicano E, Fatima U, Hall G, et al. A capabilities approach to understanding and supporting autistic adulthood. Nat Rev Psychol 2022;1(11):624–39.
67. Cameron LA, Borland RL, Tonge BJ, et al. Community participation in adults with autism: A systematic review. J Appl Res Intellect Disabil 2022;35(2):421–47.
68. Chan DV, Doran JD, Galobardi OD. Beyond friendship: the spectrum of social participation of autistic adults. J Autism Dev Disord 2023;53(1):424–37.

Autism and Epilepsy

Jamie K. Capal, MD[a],*, Shafali S. Jeste, MD[b]

KEYWORDS

- Autism spectrum disorder • Epilepsy • Genetics

KEY POINTS

- Epilepsy is one of the most common comorbidities in individuals with autism spectrum disorders (ASDs).
- Risk factors include the presence of developmental delay/intellectual disability, female sex, age, and an underlying genetic condition.
- Due to higher prevalence of epilepsy in ASD, it is important to have a high index of suspicion for seizures and refer to a neurologist if there are concerns.
- Genetic testing is recommended for all children with ASD but it becomes more high yield in children with epilepsy and ASD.

INTRODUCTION

Epilepsy is one of the most common comorbidities in autism spectrum disorder (ASD). This clinical association has been well described during the past 30 years, and during the last decade, advances in genetics have led to insights into the underlying cause of this co-occurrence. Individuals with ASD and epilepsy have higher rates of intellectual disability (ID) and overall, more neurodevelopmental impairment (in language, adaptive skills, and psychiatric conditions) compared with individuals with ASD without epilepsy, thus motivating the need for effective detection and management of seizures.[1–4] In addition, assessing epileptic versus nonepileptic events in this population can sometimes be more complex. Pharmacologic, surgical, and dietary interventions are informed by seizure type, and these approaches still reflect the first-line treatment of epilepsy in ASD. However, as genetic causes are identified, clinical trials have progressed to precision health strategies that target the underlying mechanisms of disease, with the ultimate goal of epilepsy and ASD prevention.

Epidemiology

The prevalence of epilepsy in ASD is estimated between 2% and 46%.[1,3,5–10] Due to the heterogeneous nature of ASD, both in clinical features and in underlying cause,

[a] Department of Neurology, University of North Carolina at Chapel Hill, 170 Manning Drive, CB 7025, Chapel Hill, NC 27599, USA; [b] Children's Hospital of Los Angeles, 4650 Sunset Boulevard, Los Angeles, CA 90027, USA
* Corresponding author.
E-mail address: jamie.capal@cidd.unc.edu

Pediatr Clin N Am 71 (2024) 241–252
https://doi.org/10.1016/j.pcl.2024.01.004
0031-3955/24/© 2024 Elsevier Inc. All rights reserved.

rates differ widely, with rates of epilepsy in nongenetic forms of ASD being lower than rates seen in genetic forms of ASD.[11,12] Conversely, rates of ASD in epilepsy have been reported between 15% and 74%.[7,8,13] Presence of developmental delay, ID, female sex, and overall more severe autism symptoms are associated with increased rates of epilepsy in individuals with ASD.[8,14]

CLINICAL CHARACTERISTICS OF AUTISM SPECTRUM DISORDER/EPILEPSY
Age

Epilepsy in ASD can occur at any developmental stage but the prevalence increases with age.[3,15–18] A systematic review and meta-analysis evaluating 66 studies, ranging from clinic samples to population samples, reported a pooled prevalence rate of epilepsy in 7% of children and 19% of adults with ASD.[19] In a sample of 5185 of individuals with ASD, the prevalence of epilepsy was 12% in children and reached 26% by adolescence, and the odds of being diagnosed with epilepsy in children aged older than 10 years was 2.35 times higher than in children aged younger than 10 years with ASD.[14] Another study evaluating the prevalence of epilepsy in adults aged older than 21 years with ASD reported a mean age of epilepsy onset at 13.3 years with a lifetime prevalence of 22%[15] compared with a prevalence of 1.1% in US adults.[20]

Sex

Both men and women with ASD are at an increased risk for developing epilepsy. Whether or not rates of epilepsy are higher in women is debated.[1,7,10] A meta-analysis evaluating epilepsy rates in children with ASD aged younger than 12 years reported higher rates in women compared with men (34.5% vs 18.5%, respectively).[8] However, another study reported that sex was not an independent risk factor for epilepsy development in ASD.[14] One study prospectively evaluating 130 children and young adults with ASD found that rates of treatment-resistant epilepsy were higher in women compared with men (46.4% vs 23.7%, respectively).[21] As will be discussed later, the association with female sex is likely driven by the causative genetic mutations and variants that do not show the same sex bias as does polygenic risk, those that have been historically considered "idiopathic."

Intellectual Functioning and Overall Neurodevelopmental Disability Severity

The estimated prevalence rate of epilepsy in individuals with ID is approximately 22%.[22] Similarly, higher rates of ID are seen in individuals with epilepsy and ASD.[8,10,18,23] Several studies evaluating rates of epilepsy in ASD reported that rates of epilepsy were higher in individuals with co-occurring ID.[8,15,24,25] A meta-analysis of children with ASD aged younger than 12 years reported rates of epilepsy at 21% in those with co-occurring ID versus those without ID (8%) with the highest rates of epilepsy reported in children with more severe ID (intellectual quotient [IQ] < 40).[8] Other studies support this association, noting that higher IQ was associated with lower odds of developing epilepsy.[14] In a study of 6975 children with ASD, ID was the most important factor to the relative risk for epilepsy in this cohort when controlling for age and sex.[26] ID was also found to be an independent risk marker for both ASD and epilepsy. In contrast, in the previously mentioned cross-sectional analysis of 5815 children with ASD, both age and cognitive ability were independently associated with epilepsy.[14]

Children with ASD and co-occurring epilepsy are also reported to have greater motor atypicalities, greater autism severity as noted by more impaired social awareness and social communication, and more challenging behaviors.[27–30] A study using the

Diagnostic Interview for Social and Communication Disorders found higher rates of developmental delays, motor difficulties, and challenging behavior in public spaces in children with ASD with epilepsy compared with those with ASD without epilepsy.[27] Another study found that children with ASD and co-occurring epilepsy scored higher on an objective ASD measure (Childhood Autism Rating Scale) compared with those without epilepsy, indicating a more severe ASD phenotype.[28]

It is possible that changes in the brain in individuals with ASD are present before the development of epilepsy, and there is interest in determining if these changes can be measured in an attempt to predict the development of epilepsy in individuals with ASD. A prospective analysis of 472 children with ASD through the Autism Treatment Network found that children with epilepsy had lower adaptive functioning and greater hyperactivity even before the onset of seizures, and lower adaptive functioning before seizure onset was predictive of subsequent seizure development.[31] As will be discussed later in this review, in certain genetic syndromes in which both epilepsy and ASD are highly prevalent, such as tuberous sclerosis complex (TSC), there also have been studies asking whether early epilepsy prevention can improve neurodevelopmental outcomes and possibly prevent the development of ASD.

Regression

Approximately one-third of children with ASD experience a developmental regression, most commonly between the ages of 18 and 24 months.[32] It is not known whether regression is more prevalent in certain ASD cohorts, such as those with co-occurring epilepsy, and studies have found conflicting results. Although a few studies have found higher rates of epilepsy in children with ASD and a history of regression,[14,33] several others have not found this association.[5,34–37] Autistic regression usually occurs in the second year of life, as a plateauing or decline in social communication skills, such as eye contact, gesturing, pointing, intentional use of babbling or words, and it may also include the emergence of repetitive behaviors, rigidity, and sensory sensitivities. In other words, autistic regression is characterized by the clear emergence of core autism symptoms.

An epileptic aphasia, by distinction, usually remains isolated to language, and it usually occurs in a school age or older child who at baseline has typical development. The classic syndrome that is associated with this acquired epileptic aphasia is Landau Kleffner syndrome, a rare condition in which a typically developing child undergoes an expressive language regression during a short period (over days to weeks).[38] These children may also display social withdrawal, which is thought to be caused by frustration due to language regression. Most have a history of at least one convulsive seizure. In these children, an electroencephalogram (EEG) shows a pattern of status epilepticus of sleep (ESES) that is treatable with high-dose benzodiazepines or sometimes immunosuppression, and with treatment and normalization of EEG comes a return of expressive language. Autistic regressions are not secondary to ESES and do not warrant treatment with antiseizure medications. Of note, and not in the scope of this review, there is a large clinical spectrum of ESES that is not associated with regression but is associated with global developmental delays and cognitive impairment. There are several options for treatment of ESES more broadly, depending on the clinical and electrophysiological features of the case. Treatment of ESES is aimed to improve cognition and overall behavior and can include traditional antiseizure medications, high-dose benzodiazepines, steroids, and surgical interventions (For review, see van den Munckhof and colleagues, Epilepsia 2015).[39]

Epilepsy Features

There is no predominant seizure type in ASD. Epilepsy severity varies and is affected by co-occurring conditions, such as presence of a brain injury or underlying genetic condition. Similarly, EEG findings largely depend on type of epilepsy, and there is no specific EEG pattern. However, a few studies have reported the presence of focal epileptiform discharges in frontal or temporal/centrotemporal head regions.[5,36,37,40–42]

Several studies also have reported higher rates of interictal epileptiform discharges (IEDs) and other abnormal EEG features in individuals with ASD, even without the presence of clinical seizures. These abnormalities on EEG are reported with rates ranging from 8% to 60%, depending on the study design such as inclusion of individuals with epilepsy or length of EEG recording.[34,36,37,40,41,43–45] For example, studies using overnight EEG monitoring in children with ASD without epilepsy reported higher rates of IEDs in sleep.[7,37,40,41,43] The effects of these abnormalities are largely unknown, with relevant questions asked about whether "spikes can cause autism."[46–49] It is possible that these EEG abnormalities not only serve as biomarkers of atypical brain development and function but also may directly contribute to ongoing behavioral and cognitive impairments.[4,36,37,46–52] It is not clear whether these EEG abnormalities increase the risk for or predict the development of epilepsy because most studies to date are cross-sectional, provide insufficient longitudinal EEG data, involve small sample sizes, or suffer from selection bias based on the indication for obtaining the clinical EEG. Furthermore, although small pilot studies and case reports have described treatment of epileptiform abnormalities in individuals with ASD without epilepsy, there have been no randomized controlled clinical trials to date,[53–57] and these rigorous studies would be needed before antiseizure medications can be recommended for children with ASD without epilepsy. Only with prospective early intervention trials with medications that aim to modify these EEG features will it be able to be determine if these spikes actually "cause" ASD. In the absence of these trials, there is no clinical indication to treat a child with ASD with an antiseizure medication in the absence of clinical seizures. Sometimes, an unexpected electrographic seizure may be seen on an EEG, and in this setting, a decision may be made to treat with an antiseizure medication, most likely after conducting more extensive EEG monitoring to determine the full extent and type of subclinical seizures.

CAUSE

Rates of epilepsy are higher in genetic disorders with many identified genes resulting in a shared phenotype of ASD, ID, and epilepsy. The heritability of ASD ranges from 15% to 90% based on the types of cohorts being studied.[58] Common variation, usually due to common single nucleotide polymorphisms (SNPs), most often explains familial ASD (such as ASD in siblings) and results in smaller effect sizes and often milder phenotypes. A large population-based cohort study of more than 1.5 million children born in Denmark showed that siblings of children with epilepsy have an increased risk of ASD and siblings of children with ASD have an increased risk of epilepsy.[59] Younger siblings had a 70% higher risk of developing epilepsy if their older sibling had ASD (compared with siblings where the older sibling did not have ASD) and a 54% higher risk of ASD if their older sibling had epilepsy.

Rare variants, either copy number variants or SNPs, are usually de novo and lead to more severe impairment across developmental domains. These de novo variants and mutations often cause syndromes that are highly prevalent for epilepsy as well. Several studies have examined overlaps between epilepsy and ASD associated genes, with considerable overlap in genes such as ANK2, CACNA1E, CACNA2D3, GRIA2, and DLG4, to name a few.[60] Many single gene and copy number variant syndromes diagnosed in the setting of developmental delay, ID, or ASD, such as TSC,[61] Dup15q syndrome (caused by 15q11.3–13.1 duplication),[62] Angelman syndrome (AS; caused by maternal UBE3A deletion),[63] and Phelan McDermid syndrome (caused by Shank3 mutation)[64] cause intractable epilepsy.

Preclinical models (from induced pluripotent stem cells [iPSCs] to animal models) of these genetic variations and mutations provide insight into underlying mechanisms of disease, including disruptions in transcription, cellular growth, and proliferation, along with synaptic development, stability, and function,[65] all of which converge on neural circuit structure and function. In fact, these studies have led to the coining of terms such as "synaptopathies" and "developmental disconnections" when describing the ASD and epilepsy risk genes. In clinical practice, genetic testing is the only routinely recommended medical workup for children with ASD, first with chromosomal microarray (CMA), Fragile X testing for boys and MECP2 sequencing for girls. Whole exome sequencing (WES) often is pursued next if CMA does not yield results,[66–69] although WES still is not easily covered by most insurance companies and, as a result, is often performed through commercial panels or through research protocols. However, a recent meta-analysis showed that the yield for combined WES and CMA in children with neurodevelopmental disorders can be as high as 53% especially when the child has multiple neurologic or other medical comorbidities.[69]

Overall, the clinical recommendation for genetic testing in ASD has motivated more widespread genetic testing of children after an ASD diagnosis is made, with a resulting increase in the proportion of children identified with specific genetic causes, such as the ones described earlier. Sometimes, genetic diagnoses may precede clinical diagnoses of ASD or epilepsy, thus opening the door for early precision therapies to be tested that may mitigate or even prevent the onset of epilepsy or neurodevelopmental disorders. Clinical practice still needs to catch up with testing guidelines. A recent study that interviewed caregivers of children with neurodevelopmental disorders to understand the diagnostic journey found that average wait from first parental concerns to getting a genetic diagnosis was 40 months, with on average at least 3 months from the time of diagnosis to consulting with a specialist about the implications of the testing for the clinical care of their child.[70]

Updated practice parameters are warranted for genetic testing in both ASD and epilepsy (either co-occurring or occurring independently). A recent meta-analysis of genetic testing yield for epilepsy found that whole genome sequencing had the highest yield (48%), followed by exome sequencing, targeted gene panels, and then CMA testing. Yield for genetic testing was highest in those with epileptic encephalopathy and/or the presence of a neurodevelopmental disorder (such as ASD). Overall, genetic testing for ASD is still recommended as described in this review but the yield becomes higher in those with co-occurring epilepsy.[71]

RECOMMENDATIONS FOR EVALUATION

Determining seizure is sometimes challenging in this population because children with ASD exhibit behaviors that are rooted in their core deficits, such as staring off and seeming inattentive, not responding to their names, or manifesting stereotyped repetitive movements. However, given the higher prevalence of epilepsy in ASD, it is important to refer to a neurologist if there are concerns for a seizure, which may include behavioral arrest, abnormal paroxysmal movements, cognitive changes or regression, behavioral changes, and disrupted sleep. Anytime possible, it is recommended that the caregiver take a video of the spell because visualizing the behavior is most helpful when risk stratifying. EEGs should not be performed on all children with ASD but only those with a concern for seizure or in a child with a newly diagnosed genetic syndrome that is highly penetrant for epilepsy. A prolonged EEG that can capture sleep is the ideal study because spikes can emerge in sleep, although sometimes this duration of testing is challenging for children with ASD.[72] Imaging with brain MRI is recommended only if there are focal deficits on neurologic examination, abnormalities on EEG (especially if focal), history that is concerning for brain injury, or a genetic syndrome that is associated with structural brain abnormalities. As indicated earlier, genetic testing is the one test that is recommended for all children with ASD, and this testing becomes even higher yield if a child has comorbid epilepsy and/or ID.

TREATMENT: STANDARD EPILEPSY CARE AND PRECISION HEALTH

Similarly, for individuals with epilepsy without ASD, treatment of epilepsy should be based on the seizure type, epilepsy syndrome diagnosis if applicable, and considerations of patient characteristics that may influence therapeutic effectiveness, such as side effect profile, need for safety monitoring, and drug–drug interactions. Ultimately, the principles that guide standard best practices in epilepsy care also should be followed for children with ASD and epilepsy. The identification of specific genetic causes further informs and focuses therapeutic options. At the most basic level, with more natural history and cohort studies of specific genetic syndromes, there is more understanding of the specific seizure types and effective antiepileptic medications within specific genetic subtypes. For example, in TSC, vigabatrin has been shown to be most effective for infantile spasms, and therefore, it is considered the first-line treatment instead of steroids or adrenocorticotropic hormone (ACTH).[73] In Dup15q syndrome, it is known that children often suffer from multiple seizure types that are intractable and require multiple antiepileptics, so clinicians may progress more quickly to polypharmacy in these children. More recently, genetic discoveries have opened the door for precision therapies,[74] with gene-based therapies that include gene replacement, gene addition, gene silencing, gene editing, and gene activation/deactivation. Challenges and unanswered questions remain with these approaches, including timing and duration of treatment, route of administration and mode of delivery to the brain, overall feasibility for patients, and measurable outcomes but ultimately these targeted treatments hold the promise of stopping disease progression and even preventing epilepsy and/or neurodevelopmental disabilities.

Tuberous Sclerosis Complex

TSC is a rare genetic condition resulting from a mutation in either the TSC1 or TSC2 genes, which can affect multiple organ systems. TSC is associated with high rates of ASD, ID, and epilepsy.[61,75,76] ASD is reported in approximately 25% to 50% of individuals with TSC with an increased prevalence seen in those with developmental delay/ID, early onset of epilepsy, and history of infantile spasms.[61,75,77,78] Lifetime prevalence of epilepsy in TSC is approximately 90% of patients, with two-thirds of individuals developing epilepsy in the first year of life.[61,76] Because TSC is often diagnosed early, natural history studies have been able to study the early development of ASD and epilepsy with subsequent attempts to ameliorate or even prevent the onset of both conditions. Nonpharmacological studies using behavioral interventions in infants with TSC at high risk for developing ASD are ongoing (JETS: NCT03422367). Similarly, studies attempting to prevent or delay the onset of seizures in this cohort using vigabatrin, an antiseizure drug FDA approved to treat infantile spasms in TSC (Preventing Epilepsy Using Vigabatrin In Infants With Tuberous Sclerosis Complex, PREVeNT; U01-NS092595) or sirolimus, an mammalian target of rapamycin (mTOR) inhibitor known to modify the disrupted pathway in TSC (Stopping TSC Epilepsy

Prevention Study, TSC STEPS; clinicaltrials.gov NCT05104983), are aiming to improve both seizure and neurodevelopmental outcomes in this condition.

15q Disorders

AS is a rare neurodevelopmental disorder caused by loss of function in the maternally derived copy of the UBE3A gene located on chromosome 15q11.2-q13. Loss of function is most commonly caused by a deletion in the 15q region but can also be caused by a mutation in the maternal allele, paternal uniparental disomy, or an imprinting defect.[79] This loss of function results in the phenotype of AS, which consists of neonatal hypotonia, feeding difficulties, and atypical sleep patterns, followed by global developmental delay, language, and motor impairments.[79–81] Approximately, 42% of AS individuals meet diagnostic criteria for ASD, whereas others exhibit subthreshold autistic behaviors.[82] Epilepsy is commonly reported and is often resistant to treatment.[83] Currently, disease-modifying treatments in the form of antisense oligonucleotides that unsilenced paternal UBE3A expression are being tested,[84,85] and several international clinical trials are underway (NCT04428281, NCT03882918).

Duplications of 15q11.2 to 13.1 (Dup15q syndrome) also result in a neurodevelopmental disorder and epilepsy, with epilepsy occurring in almost 50% of children with this copy number variant. This genetic region contains the Angelman Syndrome/Prader Willi Critical region and also several other genes critical for neural function, including 3 γ-aminobutyric acid type A (GABAa) receptor genes. A recent clinical characterization study in Dup15q syndrome found that children with epilepsy have a more severe developmental phenotype, with lower cognitive function and more delays in adaptive skills than those without epilepsy[86] but it is still unclear why some children develop epilepsy and others do not. A new clinical trial in this syndrome has repurposed a GABA-negative allosteric modulator, with the goal of improving neurodevelopmental outcomes and epilepsy in this condition.

Many families of these rare genetic syndromes have formed patient advocacy groups, with the goal of bringing together families of children with the same syndrome in order to share experiences, engage in advocacy efforts, and promote research, from natural history studies to development of preclinical models, with the ultimate goal of clinical trials and effective treatments. Recently, an umbrella organization called AGENDA (Alliance for Genetic Etiologies of Neurodevelopmental Disorders and Autism) was created that brings together these various patient advocacy groups to talk about common issues and practices and ultimately to accelerate progress in clinical trial readiness and therapeutics.

In summary, epilepsy is a common comorbidity in ASD, particularly in those with more severe neurodevelopmental disabilities, with rare de novo genetic variants and mutations often causing both of these conditions. All children with ASD should undergo genetic testing but an EEG should be ordered only for those children where seizures or epileptic encephalopathy is a concern. Early detection and treatment of seizures is important to potentially improve neurodevelopmental outcomes, and treatments range from traditional seizure management to precision health initiatives that treat the underlying pathophysiological mechanisms of disease.

CLINICS CARE POINTS

- Clinicians should have a high suspicion of seizures in children with ASD, with the highest suspicion in children with ID and/or a genetic syndrome.
- Early referral to a neurologist is recommended if there is suspicion for seizures

- Genetic testing is indicated for all individuals with ASD, particularly those with co-occurring epilepsy, and may result in targeted treatments.
- Treatment of seizures is still based on the epilepsy type and possible side effect profiles but precision health can lead to treatments of the underlying genetic cause in some cases.

DISCLOSURE

J.K. Capal has no financial or commercial conflicts of interest. She receives funding from the Department of Defense, United States and National Institute of Health (NIH), United States for unrelated projects. She receives grant funding from NIH and the Simons Foundation, United States. S.S. Jeste serves on the data safety monitoring board for Ionis Pharmaceuticals. She previously consulted for Roche pharmaceuticals. She receives funding from the NIH, Roche pharmaceuticals, the Saban Research Institute, United States, the Autism Science Foundation, United States, and the Simons Foundation for unrelated projects.

REFERENCES

1. Danielsson S, Gillberg IC, Billstedt E, et al. Epilepsy in young adults with autism: a prospective population-based follow-up study of 120 individuals diagnosed in childhood. Epilepsia 2005;46(6):918–23.
2. Hara H. Autism and epilepsy: a retrospective follow-up study. Brain Dev 2007; 29(8):486–90.
3. Viscidi EW, Johnson AL, Spence SJ, et al. The association between epilepsy and autism symptoms and maladaptive behaviors in children with autism spectrum disorder. Autism 2014;18(8):996–1006.
4. Trauner DA. Behavioral correlates of epileptiform abnormalities in autism. Epilepsy Behav 2015;47:163–6.
5. Rossi PG, Parmeggiani A, Bach V, et al. EEG features and epilepsy in patients with autism. Brain Dev 1995;17(3):169–74.
6. Tuchman R, Rapin I. Epilepsy in autism. Lancet Neurol 2002;1(6):352–8.
7. Hughes JR, Melyn M. EEG and seizures in autistic children and adolescents: further findings with therapeutic implications. Clin EEG Neurosci 2005;36(1): 15–20.
8. Amiet C, Gourfinkel-An I, Bouzamondo A, et al. Epilepsy in autism is associated with intellectual disability and gender: evidence from a meta-analysis. Biol Psychiatr 2008;64(7):577–82.
9. Kohane IS, McMurry A, Weber G, et al. The co-morbidity burden of children and young adults with autism spectrum disorders. PLoS One 2012;7(4):e33224.
10. Jokiranta E, Sourander A, Suominen A, et al. Epilepsy among children and adolescents with autism spectrum disorders: a population-based study. J Autism Dev Disord 2014;44(10):2547–57.
11. Bill BR, Geschwind DH. Genetic advances in autism: heterogeneity and convergence on shared pathways. Curr Opin Genet Dev 2009;19(3):271–8.
12. Betancur C. Etiological heterogeneity in autism spectrum disorders: more than 100 genetic and genomic disorders and still counting. Brain Res 2011;1380: 42–77.
13. Strasser L, Downes M, Kung J, et al. Prevalence and risk factors for autism spectrum disorder in epilepsy: a systematic review and meta-analysis. Dev Med Child Neurol 2018;60(1):19–29.

14. Viscidi EW, Triche EW, Pescosolido MF, et al. Clinical characteristics of children with autism spectrum disorder and co-occurring epilepsy. PLoS One 2013;8(7): e67797.

15. Bolton PF, Carcani-Rathwell I, Hutton J, et al. Epilepsy in autism: features and correlates. Br J Psychiatry 2011;198(4):289–94.

16. Deykin EY, MacMahon B. The incidence of seizures among children with autistic symptoms. Am J Psychiatr 1979;136(10):1310–2.

17. Volkmar FR, Nelson DS. Seizure disorders in autism. J Am Acad Child Adolesc Psychiatry 1990;29(1):127–9.

18. Woolfenden S, Sarkozy V, Ridley G, et al. A systematic review of two outcomes in autism spectrum disorder - epilepsy and mortality. Dev Med Child Neurol 2012; 54(4):306–12.

19. Liu X, Sun X, Sun C, et al. Prevalence of epilepsy in autism spectrum disorders: A systematic review and meta-analysis. Autism 2021. 13623613211045029.

20. Kobau R, Luncheon C, Greenlund K. Active epilepsy prevalence among U.S. adults is 1.1% and differs by educational level-National Health Interview Survey, United States, 2021. Epilepsy Behav 2023;142:109180.

21. Blackmon K, Bluvstein J, MacAllister WS, et al. treatment resistant epilepsy in autism spectrum disorder: increased risk for females. Autism Res 2016;9(2): 311–20.

22. Robertson J, Hatton C, Emerson E, et al. Prevalence of epilepsy among people with intellectual disabilities: a systematic review. Seizure 2015;29:46–62.

23. Tuchman R, Cuccaro M, Alessandri M. Autism and epilepsy: historical perspective. Brain Dev 2010;32(9):709–18.

24. Berg AT, Plioplys S. Epilepsy and autism: is there a special relationship? Epilepsy Behav 2012;23(3):193–8.

25. Tuchman R. What is the relationship between autism spectrum disorders and epilepsy? Semin Pediatr Neurol 2017;24(4):292–300.

26. Ewen JB, Marvin AR, Law K, et al. epilepsy and autism severity: a study of 6,975 children. Autism Res 2019;12(8):1251–9.

27. Turk J, Bax M, Williams C, et al. Autism spectrum disorder in children with and without epilepsy: impact on social functioning and communication. Acta Paediatr 2009;98(4):675–81.

28. Shubrata KS, Sinha S, Seshadri SP, et al. Childhood autism spectrum disorders with and without epilepsy: clinical implications. J Child Neurol 2015;30(4):476–82.

29. Ko C, Kim N, Kim E, et al. The effect of epilepsy on autistic symptom severity assessed by the social responsiveness scale in children with autism spectrum disorder. Behav Brain Funct 2016;12(1):20.

30. Smith KR, Matson JL. Behavior problems: differences among intellectually disabled adults with co-morbid autism spectrum disorders and epilepsy. Res Dev Disabil 2010;31(5):1062–9.

31. Capal JK, Macklin EA, Lu F, et al. Factors Associated With Seizure Onset in Children With Autism Spectrum Disorder. Pediatrics 2020;145(Suppl 1):S117–25.

32. Barger BD, Campbell JM, McDonough JD. Prevalence and onset of regression within autism spectrum disorders: a meta-analytic review. J Autism Dev Disord 2013;43(4):817–28.

33. Kobayashi R, Murata T. Setback phenomenon in autism and long-term prognosis. Acta Psychiatr Scand 1998;98(4):296–303.

34. Tuchman RF, Rapin I. Regression in pervasive developmental disorders: seizures and epileptiform electroencephalogram correlates. Pediatrics 1997;99(4):560–6.

35. Baird G, Robinson RO, Boyd S, et al. Sleep electroencephalograms in young children with autism with and without regression. Dev Med Child Neurol 2006;48(7): 604–8.
36. Mulligan CK, Trauner DA. Incidence and behavioral correlates of epileptiform abnormalities in autism spectrum disorders. J Autism Dev Disord 2014;44(2):452–8.
37. Capal JK, Carosella C, Corbin E, et al. EEG endophenotypes in autism spectrum disorder. Epilepsy Behav 2018;88:341–8.
38. Kleffner FR, Landau WM. The landau-kleffner syndrome. Epilepsia 2009;50 Suppl 7:3.
39. van den Munckhof B, van Dee V, Sagi L, et al. Treatment of electrical status epilepticus in sleep:a pooled analysis of 575 cases. Epilepsia 2015;56(11):1738–46.
40. Chez MG, Chang M, Krasne V, et al. Frequency of epileptiform EEG abnormalities in a sequential screening of autistic patients with no known clinical epilepsy from 1996 to 2005. Epilepsy Behav 2006;8(1):267–71.
41. Parmeggiani A, Barcia G, Posar A, et al. Epilepsy and EEG paroxysmal abnormalities in autism spectrum disorders. Brain Dev 2010;32(9):783–9.
42. Yasuhara A. Correlation between EEG abnormalities and symptoms of autism spectrum disorder (ASD). Brain Dev 2010;32(10):791–8.
43. Kim HL, Donnelly JH, Tournay AE, et al. Absence of seizures despite high prevalence of epileptiform EEG abnormalities in children with autism monitored in a tertiary care center. Epilepsia 2006;47(2):394–8.
44. Kawasaki Y, Yokota K, Shinomiya M, et al. Brief report: electroencephalographic paroxysmal activities in the frontal area emerged in middle childhood and during adolescence in a follow-up study of autism. J Autism Dev Disord 1997;27(5): 605–20.
45. Kanemura H, Sano F, Tando T, et al. Can EEG characteristics predict development of epilepsy in autistic children? Eur J Paediatr Neurol 2013;17(3):232–7.
46. Ballaban-Gil K, Tuchman R. Epilepsy and epileptiform EEG: association with autism and language disorders. Ment Retard Dev Disabil Res Rev 2000;6(4): 300–8.
47. Deonna T, Roulet-Perez E. Early-onset acquired epileptic aphasia (Landau-Kleffner syndrome, LKS) and regressive autistic disorders with epileptic EEG abnormalities: the continuing debate. Brain Dev 2010;32(9):746–52.
48. Spence SJ, Schneider MT. The role of epilepsy and epileptiform EEGs in autism spectrum disorders. Pediatr Res 2009;65(6):599–606.
49. Tuchman R. Treatment of seizure disorders and EEG abnormalities in children with autism spectrum disorders. J Autism Dev Disord 2000;30(5):485–9.
50. Hernan AE, Alexander A, Jenks KR, et al. Focal epileptiform activity in the prefrontal cortex is associated with long-term attention and sociability deficits. Neurobiol Dis 2014;63:25–34.
51. Lado FA, Rubboli G, Capovilla G, et al. Pathophysiology of epileptic encephalopathies. Epilepsia 2013;54(Suppl 8):6–13.
52. Jeste SS, Geschwind DH. Disentangling the heterogeneity of autism spectrum disorder through genetic findings. Nat Rev Neurol 2014;10(2):74–81.
53. Nass R, Petrucha D. Acquired aphasia with convulsive disorder: a pervasive developmental disorder variant. J Child Neurol 1990;5(4):327–8.
54. Plioplys AV. Autism: electroencephalogram abnormalities and clinical improvement with valproic acid. Arch Pediatr Adolesc Med 1994;148(2):220–2.
55. Golla S, Sweeney JA. Corticosteroid therapy in regressive autism: Preliminary findings from a retrospective study. BMC Med 2014;12:79.

56. Rossignol DA, Frye RE. A systematic review and meta-analysis of immunoglobulin g abnormalities and the therapeutic use of intravenous immunoglobulins (IVIG) in autism spectrum disorder. J Personalized Med 2021;11(6).

57. Lewine JD, Andrews R, Chez M, et al. Magnetoencephalographic patterns of epileptiform activity in children with regressive autism spectrum disorders. Pediatrics 1999;104(3 Pt 1):405–18.

58. Rylaarsdam L, Guemez-Gamboa A. genetic causes and modifiers of autism spectrum disorder. Front Cell Neurosci 2019;13:385.

59. Christensen J, Overgaard M, Parner ET, et al. Risk of epilepsy and autism in full and half siblings-A population-based cohort study. Epilepsia 2016;57(12): 2011–8.

60. Peng J, Zhou Y, Wang K. Multiplex gene and phenotype network to characterize shared genetic pathways of epilepsy and autism. Sci Rep 2021;11(1):952.

61. Capal JK, Bernardino-Cuesta B, Horn PS, et al. Influence of seizures on early development in tuberous sclerosis complex. Epilepsy Behav 2017;70(Pt A): 245–52.

62. DiStefano C, Gulsrud A, Huberty S, et al. Identification of a distinct developmental and behavioral profile in children with Dup15q syndrome. J Neurodev Disord 2016;8:19.

63. Thibert RL, Larson AM, Hsieh DT, et al. Neurologic manifestations of Angelman syndrome. Pediatr Neurol 2013;48(4):271–9.

64. de Coo IFM, Jesse S, Le TL, et al, European Phelan-McDermid syndrome consortium. Consensus recommendations on Epilepsy in Phelan-McDermid syndrome. Eur J Med Genet 2023;104746.

65. Lee BH, Smith T, Paciorkowski AR. Autism spectrum disorder and epilepsy: Disorders with a shared biology. Epilepsy Behav 2015;47:191–201.

66. Michelson DJ, Shevell MI, Sherr EH, et al. Evidence report: Genetic and metabolic testing on children with global developmental delay: report of the Quality Standards Subcommittee of the American Academy of Neurology and the Practice Committee of the Child Neurology Society. Neurology 2011;77(17):1629–35.

67. Moeschler JB, Shevell M, Committee on G. Comprehensive evaluation of the child with intellectual disability or global developmental delays. Pediatrics 2014;134(3):e903–18.

68. Schaefer GB, Mendelsohn NJ, Professional Practice and Guidelines Committee. Clinical genetics evaluation in identifying the etiology of autism spectrum disorders: 2013 guideline revisions. Genet Med 2013;15(5):399–407.

69. Srivastava S, Love-Nichols JA, Dies KA, et al. Meta-analysis and multidisciplinary consensus statement: exome sequencing is a first-tier clinical diagnostic test for individuals with neurodevelopmental disorders. Genet Med 2019;21(11): 2413–21.

70. Simon J, Hyde C, Saravanapandian V, et al. The diagnostic journey of genetically defined neurodevelopmental disorders. J Neurodev Disord 2022;14(1):27.

71. Sheidley BR, Malinowski J, Bergner AL, et al. Genetic testing for the epilepsies: A systematic review. Epilepsia 2022;63(2):375–87.

72. Paasch V, Hoosier TM, Accardo J, et al. Technical tips: performing EEGs and polysomnograms on children with neurodevelopmental disabilities. Neurodiagn J 2012;52(4):333–48.

73. Villeneuve N, Soufflet C, Plouin P, et al. Vigabatrin monotherapy as first line in infantile spasms. Traitement des spasmes infantiles par vigabatrin en premiere intention et en monotherapie: A propos de 70 nourrissons 1998;5(7):731–8.

74. Davidson BL, Gao G, Berry-Kravis E, et al. Gene-based therapeutics for rare genetic neurodevelopmental psychiatric disorders. Mol Ther 2022;30(7):2416–28.

75. Jeste SS, Sahin M, Bolton P, et al. Characterization of autism in young children with tuberous sclerosis complex. J Child Neurol 2008;23(5):520–5.

76. Chu-Shore CJ, Major P, Camposano S, et al. The natural history of epilepsy in tuberous sclerosis complex. Epilepsia 2010;51(7):1236–41.

77. Capal JK, Williams ME, Pearson DA, et al. Profile of autism spectrum disorder in tuberous sclerosis complex: results from a longitudinal, prospective, multisite study. Ann Neurol 2021;90(6):874–86.

78. van Eeghen AM, Chu-Shore CJ, Pulsifer MB, et al. Cognitive and adaptive development of patients with tuberous sclerosis complex: a retrospective, longitudinal investigation. Epilepsy Behav: E&B 2012;23(1):10–5.

79. Tan WH, Bacino CA, Skinner SA, et al. Angelman syndrome: Mutations influence features in early childhood. Am J Med Genet 2011;155a(1):81–90.

80. Zori RT, Hendrickson J, Woolven S, et al. Angelman syndrome: clinical profile. J Child Neurol 1992;7(3):270–80.

81. Tietze AL, Blankenburg M, Hechler T, et al. Sleep disturbances in children with multiple disabilities. Sleep Med Rev 2012;16(2):117–27.

82. Peters SU, Beaudet AL, Madduri N, et al. Autism in Angelman syndrome: implications for autism research. Clin Genet 2004;66(6):530–6.

83. Wang TS, Tsai WH, Tsai LP, et al. Clinical characteristics and epilepsy in genomic imprinting disorders: Angelman syndrome and Prader-Willi syndrome. Ci Ji Yi Xue Za Zhi 2019;32(2):137–44.

84. Huang HS, Allen JA, Mabb AM, et al. Topoisomerase inhibitors unsilence the dormant allele of Ube3a in neurons. Nature 2011;481(7380):185–9.

85. Lee HM, Clark EP, Kuijer MB, et al. Characterization and structure-activity relationships of indenoisoquinoline-derived topoisomerase I inhibitors in unsilencing the dormant Ube3a gene associated with Angelman syndrome. Mol Autism 2018; 9:45.

86. DiStefano C, Wilson RB, Hyde C, et al. Behavioral characterization of dup15q syndrome: Toward meaningful endpoints for clinical trials. Am J Med Genet 2020;182(1):71–84.

Sleep Problems in Autism Spectrum Disorder

Navjot Sidhu, MD[a], Zoe Wong, BS[b],
Amanda E. Bennett, MD, MPH[a,b,c,d,*],
Margaret C. Souders, PhD, CRNP[e]

KEYWORDS

- Autism spectrum disorder • Sleep disorders/disturbances • Prevalence • Treatment
- Children • Assessment • Impact

KEY POINTS

- Sleep problems have prevalence estimates ranging from 40% to 80% among pediatric patients with autism spectrum disorder (ASD).
- The types of sleep disorders predominantly seen in patients with ASD include insomnia, parasomnias, and circadian rhythm sleep-wake disorders.
- Sleep problems have a bidirectional relationship with behaviors, developmental skills, and the health of autistic children and can affect the quality of life of both patients and their caregivers.
- All children with autism should be properly and regularly screened for sleep problems and evaluated for co-occurring medical contributors.
- Behavioral interventions coupled with caregiver education remain first-line treatment for sleep problems for both neurotypical and neurodiverse youth; other therapies, including melatonin supplementation, can also be considered.

CASE PRESENTATION

A 3-year-old girl with autism spectrum disorder (ASD), mixed receptive–expressive language disorder, and global developmental delay presents for a follow-up visit with her parent. She is nonverbal and has limited functional communication skills. The mother reports that her daughter "never sleeps." She typically falls asleep

[a] Division of Developmental and Behavioral Pediatrics, The Children's Hospital of Philadelphia, 3550 Market Street, 3rd Floor, Philadelphia, PA 19104, USA; [b] The Children's Hospital of Philadelphia, Center for Autism Research, Sidney Kimmel Medical College, Thomas Jefferson University; [c] Department of Pediatrics, The University of Pennsylvania Perelman School of Medicine; [d] Autism Integrated Care Program, Division of Developmental and Behavioral Pediatrics, The Children's Hospital of Philadelphia, 3550 Market Street, 3rd Floor, Philadelphia, PA 19104, USA; [e] The University of Pennsylvania School of Nursing, The Children's Hospital of Philadelphia
* Corresponding author. 3550 Market Street, 3rd Floor, Philadelphia, PA 19204.
E-mail address: bennettam@chop.edu

Pediatr Clin N Am 71 (2024) 253–268
https://doi.org/10.1016/j.pcl.2024.01.006
pediatric.theclinics.com
0031-3955/24/© 2024 Elsevier Inc. All rights reserved.

between 12 AM and 1 AM in her own bedroom, alongside mom, while watching content on her tablet. She will wake up within 4 hours, walk over to parents' room and insist on playing. The sleep disruption also impacts caregivers' own sleep and daily functioning. The mother seeks insight into the likely causes of her daughter's sleep issues and guidance on next steps for management.

INTRODUCTION

Sleep is a natural, recurring state of rest fundamental to mental, physical, and emotional well-being and healthy development. Individuals with ASD have a greater risk of developing sleep problems compared with neurotypical peers.[1] Insufficient or poor-quality sleep has been linked to increased internalizing and externalizing behaviors and decreased adaptive functioning[2] which is required for learning, emotional regulation, memory consolidation, and neuroplasticity.[3,4] Downstream effects of poor sleep are expansive, impacting school attendance, hospitalizations, family relations, and parental employment.[5-9] Given the potential for significant impact, screening for, assessing, and treating underlying sleep disorders is crucial for the overall health of individuals with ASD and their families.

This review follows the path of a patient in the primary care setting from screening to assessment to interventions and resources, highlighting the most common types of sleep problems and their association with other medical and behavioral health conditions seen among autistic children. Recommendations for management of sleep problems will be presented in alignment with current practice guidelines.

WHY SHOULD CLINICIANS SCREEN FOR SLEEP PROBLEMS IN AUTISTIC YOUTH?

Among the most frequent co-occurring conditions, disrupted sleep can be a burdensome and challenging issue for individuals with ASD and their families. Sleep problems have a prevalence of 40% to 80% among children with ASD in comparison to 25% to 40% among typically developing (TD) children.[10] Sleep problems are commonly reported in children with ASD starting at around 30 months of age.[11]

Current evidence is inconclusive as to whether specific cohorts of autistic individuals have a higher predisposition for sleep disorders. Some studies have suggested that patients with both ASD and intellectual disability may experience more sleep problems or obtain fewer hours of sleep per night.[12,13] The predisposition of sleep problems in ASD at different ages and stages of development is also debatable. Although some studies report no correlation, others have observed either a decline in sleep problems with age or a persistence of problems into adulthood.[4,13]

The etiology of sleep problems in ASD is multifactorial in nature and varies among individuals. Disrupted sleep has been linked to dysfunction in the homeostatic sleep process and/or endogenous circadian rhythm, two key regulators of sleep.[13] A variety of factors including genetics (eg, circadian-relevant CLOCK genes), abnormal melatonin and/or serotonin production, and delayed or atypical brain maturation and development have been hypothesized as predisposing factors for sleep dysfunction.[1-3,13-15]

The core features of ASD (eg, deficits in social communication, difficulty with transitions, sensory hyperreactivity) can interfere with sleep onset and the establishment of sound bedtime behaviors.[4,10,13] Environmental (eg, alteration in nighttime routine), psychological (eg, anxiety, attention deficit hyperactivity disorder [ADHD]), and physical (eg, constipation, epilepsy, gastroesophageal reflux disease, acute illness) stressors can also exacerbate and trigger sleep problems.[12,13,16] Once developed, the persistence of sleep problems may be attributed to psychological factors including learned association and cognitive/physiologic arousal induced by intrusive thoughts, rumination, and anxiety secondary to sleeplessness.

HOW TO EFFECTIVELY IDENTIFY SLEEP PROBLEMS IN AUTISTIC PATIENTS
Screening for Sleep Disturbances

Given the high prevalence of sleep disorders in ASD and their far-reaching impact, screening autistic individuals for sleep problems is crucial. Caregivers of autistic children are often managing multiple behavioral challenges and can perceive poor sleep as an inherent aspect of autism. Therefore, they may not share sleep-related concerns proactively.[2,17] Screening for sleep problems should thus be performed for all autistic youth.

Marvin and colleagues investigated the efficacy of sleep screening and discovered that asking a single, broad question about sleep (eg, "does your child have any sleep problems?", "how satisfied are you with your child's sleep?") would yield vague responses and thus leave a significant number of children with sleep disorders undiagnosed. Using a brief, validated questionnaire or posing more specific questions would aid in identifying children with sleep disorders more accurately.[17]

One such validated screening tool is the Children's Sleep Habits Questionnaire (CSHQ) which has been adapted for use in children with ASD. The extensive, in-depth CSHQ consists of 33 parent-reported items across eight subscales that address behaviors such as bedtime resistance, sleep onset, sleep duration, sleep anxiety, nighttime awakenings, parasomnias, sleep-disordered breathing, and daytime sleepiness.[2,16,18] Parents rate each item on a 3-point Likert-type scale; higher scores signify a more severe sleep disturbance. A total score of 41 has a sensitivity of 80% and a specificity of 70% for sleep disorders.[13] Alternatively, the Composite Sleep Disturbance Index (CSDI) is brief and assesses the frequency and duration of six sleep habits. The overall CSDI score is calculated by summing the total of the six sleep habit questions rated on a 3-point Likert-type scale; a score of greater than 4 indicates a severe sleep disturbance.[17] A compilation of accessible screening questionnaires is presented in **Table 1**.[19,20]

Although several validated screening measures exist, the Autism Speaks Autism Treatment Network (ASATN) Sleep Committee established the following expert-consensus-based screening questions to facilitate Primary Care Providers (PCPs) in efficiently assessing potential sleep disturbances in their clinical practice.[10] The questions are.

1. Does the child fall asleep within 20 minutes after going to bed?
2. Does the child fall asleep in the parent's or sibling's bed?
3. Does the child sleep too little?
4. Does the child awaken at least once during the night?

Children who screen positive based on initial evaluation for sleep issues during their routine well-visits should undergo comprehensive follow-up assessments, including in-depth questioning, to determine the specific type of sleep disorder and evaluate for any potential co-occurring medical contributors. Providers should inquire about their patient's bedtime routine, timing of sleep onset, frequency and duration of any nighttime awakenings, parental response to awakenings, sleep environment, nocturnal disturbances (eg, snoring, body movements), residual daytime symptoms and behaviors, and the familial impact of sleep disruption.[1,13,19,21] In addition, a caregiver-completed sleep diary spanning 1 to 2 weeks can help provide valuable information regarding sleep patterns and behaviors.[21,22]

Table 1 Sleep screening questionnaires		
Screening Questionnaire	**Age**	**Target Sleep Disorder**
Children's Sleep Habits Questionnaire (CSHQ)	2–18 y of age	Bedtime resistance, sleep anxiety, parasomnias, daytime sleepiness
Composite Sleep Disturbance Index (CSDI)	2–18 y of age	Scores frequency and duration of six sleep habits over previous month (settling at bedtime, sleep induction, waking during night, resettling, early wake time and co-sleeping)
Family Inventory of Sleep Habits (FISH)	4–10 y of age	Dysfunctional sleep habits and environments ("sleep hygiene")
Pediatric Sleep Questionnaire (PSQ)	2–18 y of age	Sleep-disordered breathing and periodic limb movements

Types of Sleep Disorders in Autism Spectrum Disorder

The most common sleep disorders in individuals with ASD include insomnia, parasomnias, and circadian rhythm sleep-wake disorders.[2,4,17] These primary sleep disorders can be further subdivided based on the predominant behavioral manifestation.

Insomnia is the most prevalent sleep disorder seen in patients with ASD, occurring at a rate two to three times higher than their TD peers.[13] The condition is characterized by ongoing challenges in sleep initiation, maintenance, duration, or quality. Behaviors commonly associated with insomnia include bedtime resistance, frequent nighttime awakenings, and the inability to sleep independently. Although there are many different subtypes, behavioral insomnia is particularly pertinent to children with ASD, as it arises from learned behaviors and routines and is influenced by environmental factors. Behavioral insomnia can be further classified into two categories: sleep-onset association type (ie, involves the child/adolescent developing a dependence on specific conditions or associations to help initiate sleep and requires identical conditions to fall back asleep) or limit-setting type (ie, involves caregivers struggling with initially setting and then consistently enforcing appropriate bedtime routines and limits, resulting in delayed sleep onset and resistance to bedtime).[13,21]

Circadian rhythm sleep-wake disorders stem from disruptions in the typical sleep-wake cycle that signify a misalignment between the internal circadian rhythm and the external environment.[4] They occur at higher rates in comparison to neurotypical peers. These disorders can manifest in a variety of ways, most commonly delayed sleep phase (ie, difficulty initiating sleep) and irregular sleep-wake rhythm (ie, difficulty maintaining sleep leading to a fragmented sleep pattern).[3,4,22,23] A common clinical picture may be of patients with difficulty falling asleep and waking up at appropriate times due to inconsistent sleep patterns with variable bedtime and wake times. Recall that the circadian rhythm is influenced by genetic factors, fluctuations in melatonin production, and an individual's sensitivity to surrounding environmental cues.

Parasomnias are characterized by experiences or physical behaviors that occur amid sleep or during periods of arousal from sleep. These episodes are often related to the activation of the autonomic nervous system with associated skeletal muscle activity and cognitive confusion.[4,21,22] Parasomnias can be further classified into non-rapid eye movement (NREM) parasomnias and rapid eye movement (REM) parasomnias. NREM parasomnias primarily occur in the first half of the night during deep stages of sleep, whereas REM parasomnias occur in the latter half of the night during REM sleep. The most common NREM parasomnias include night terrors, sleepwalking, and sleep talking; all can be associated with a varying degree of movements, vocalizations, autonomic arousal, amnesia, and level of unresponsiveness.[21] This can present as a child having multiple, weekly episodes of unusual behaviors in the night (wandering from bedroom, talking to self, or screaming/thrashing during sleep) often accompanied by limited consciousness or recollection of the event. The most common REM-associated parasomnia in children is nightmares that often lead to sudden awakenings. Children with appropriate communication skills are typically able to recall details about their nightmares and maintain a degree of responsiveness to their surroundings; episodes may be triggered by stress or anxiety.[4,21,22]

Evaluation for Co-occurring Medical Contributors

Autistic individuals are at an increased risk of co-occurring conditions that may cause or contribute to sleep problems. These include gastrointestinal (GI) disorders (eg, gastroesophageal reflux, constipation), asthma, obstructive sleep apnea, ADHD, epilepsy, restless leg syndrome, depression, and anxiety. The administration of certain medications commonly prescribed for individuals with ASD (eg, antipsychotics, stimulants, selective serotonin reuptake inhibitors) may also interfere with the sleep-wake cycle. Investigating and addressing these medical contributors is, therefore, vital to proper sleep-related screening and treatment. The ASATN Sleep Committee developed a list of questions, as detailed in the 2012 AAP *Pediatrics* article about insomnia management in ASD, which can be used by providers to screen for medical contributors to sleep problems.[10]

If sleep-disordered breathing such as obstructive sleep apnea is suspected, a more thorough sleep investigation is warranted. Suspicious symptoms for this condition include snoring and observed periods of gasping or halted breathing during sleep which can result in sleep fragmentation.[19] Although the overall prevalence of obstructive sleep apnea (OSA) is not elevated in individuals with ASD in comparison to the general pediatric population, certain subgroups within the ASD population, such as those with hypotonia or substantial weight gain induced by atypical antipsychotics, exhibit a greater susceptibility to developing OSA.[19,24] Polysomnography (PSG) is considered the gold standard for objective sleep measurement and for a definitive diagnosis of obstructive sleep apnea. Other clinical uses for PSG studies are discussed as follows.

The interdependent relationship between sleep disorders and epilepsy is well established in the general population. Acute and/or chronic sleep deprivation may have seizure-inducing effects.[15] In addition, patients with epilepsy are more frequently diagnosed with sleep disorders.[19] Overall management of sleep and other comorbidities such as OSA and epilepsy are also interconnected. Research conducted in patients with epilepsy and concurrent OSA has demonstrated enhanced seizure control following treatment.[25–27]

ADVANCED TESTING FOR SLEEP DISORDERS

PSG, the collective process of monitoring and recording physiologic data during sleep, is an objective measurement of sleep. It has been used to investigate the sleep patterns of autistic children for decades,[28,29] and results suggest that children with autism may have differences in brain maturation that affect their sleep. More recent PSG studies have indicated shorter sleep times, longer times to fall asleep, and more frequent night wakings for children with ASD and sleep concerns.[12,30–32]

As mentioned previously, PSG is the gold standard for diagnosing obstructive sleep apnea or other sleep-related breathing disorders and evaluating treatment efficacy for such conditions. PSG studies may also be useful in the setting of suspected restless leg syndrome, narcolepsy, sleep-related epilepsy, and other excessive movements during sleep.[33,34] PCPs should refer patients with these concerns to a sleep center or sleep specialist for further evaluation and PSG testing.

Actigraphy (ACT) has also been used in individuals with ASD as an objective measure of sleep. ACT is a miniaturized wristwatch-like microcomputer that senses physical motion and generates a signal each time it is moved (accelerated) and generally placed on the wrist.[35] The stored movement data can be transferred to a computer for interpretation and estimation of sleep parameters. This technology is used in many wearable fitness trackers, and these devices may have a future role in helping families with ASD improve their sleep.

ACT is useful for determining sleep patterns and circadian rhythms, may be worn for several weeks at a time, and is less expensive and cumbersome than PSG. ACT has been used in estimating the prevalence of insomnia in children with ASD[12,32,35,36] and as an objective sleep measure in intervention studies. Yavuz-Kodat and colleagues used equivalence tests to study the validity of ACT compared with PSG in children with ASD and found the difference between ACT and PSG measures to be clinically acceptable. Agreement analysis revealed a high sensitivity and moderate specificity, suggesting ACT as a valid method to evaluate sleep in ASD.[37]

CASE DISCUSSION FOLLOW-UP

After more detailed questioning about the child's sleep routine, the mother shares that her daughter cannot fall to sleep without the iPad and often insists on having it when she wakes in the middle of the night. Parents have tried changing the bedtime routine by putting her to bed without the iPad, but she still wakes and insists in lying next to her mother on those nights. On nights when mother has tried to have her fall to sleep on her own, she is up for hours crying or leaving her bed repeatedly.

IMPLICATIONS OF NOT TREATING SLEEP PROBLEMS IN CHILDREN WITH AUTISM SPECTRUM DISORDER

Sleep problems have been associated with other medical and behavioral conditions for both TD and autistic children.[38,39] Although sleep difficulties can be easily identified because of some conditions (eg, gastroesophageal reflux or asthma), other associations are likely bidirectional in nature, particularly those between sleep and behavior. For many youth with ASD, sleep problems are also related to core behaviors associated with autism.

Sleep Problems and Daytime Behaviors

Like the TD population, sleep disturbances in children with ASD are associated with challenging daytime behaviors including inattention, hyperactivity, irritability, aggression (including self-injurious behaviors), and heightened sensory sensitivities.[38,40–47] These associations were found across different age groups, adaptive function profiles, and living environments (ie, children in residential placement). Mazurek and Sohl found night-waking behaviors to have the strongest association with these challenges.[44]

Sleep difficulties have also been associated with symptoms of mood disorders like anxiety and depression.[38,43,45] Furthermore, sleep problems have been linked to an increased risk of hospitalization for psychiatric symptoms.[9] Thus, properly addressing sleep concerns can have a profound impact on an individual's mental health.

The direction of these relationships is difficult to predict, and many studies assume that disrupted sleep plays a role in the worsening of daytime behaviors. However, a few studies have found aggressive behavior, anxiety, and sensory under-responsiveness or over-seeking to be predictors of future sleep problems.[48,49] Addressing some of these behavioral challenges early may thus impact the development of future sleep problems.

Sleep Problems and Developmental Skills

Several studies have explored the relationship between poor sleep and certain developmental skills including language and social interaction. Goldman and colleagues found that autistic children with moderate to severe sleep problems had increased challenges with language and social interaction when compared with those with no or mild sleep problems.[41] Sleep problems have also been linked to reduced adaptive skills.[47] Sleep severity, however, did not seem to differentiate adaptive functioning as it did with language skills, social interaction, or daytime behaviors.

Autism symptom severity has sometimes been used as a variable when measuring sleep associations. Core autism features (eg, differences in social-emotional reciprocity and nonverbal communicative behaviors) have been found to be predictive of sleep problems.[48] Improvement in these skills have been linked to improved sleep function, suggesting a relationship between social communication skills and sleep.[42]

Sleep problems and health/quality of life

GI problems (eg, diarrhea, constipation, challenging eating behaviors) have been identified as both a predictor and consequence of sleep difficulties in autistic youth.[48,50] Sleep problems can also have profound impact on the quality of life for both children and their families. Delahaye and colleagues found sleep problems to be associated with lower physical, psycho-social, and total health-related quality of life,[51] whereas Johnson and colleagues noted increased parental stress in autistic youth with sleep concerns.[52] Properly addressing sleep difficulties can thus have a marked impact on both the individual and family unit.

HOW TO ADDRESS SLEEP PROBLEMS IN AUTISM SPECTRUM DISORDER

The ASATN and the American Academy of Neurology have emphasized the importance of delivering competent sleep care to autistic youth by creating evidence-based practice and treatment guidelines.[10,53] These works support behavioral intervention and parent education as first-line treatment for sleep problems and disorders. Pharmacologic therapies may be offered in combination with behavioral intervention or if behavioral strategies have been unsuccessful. Alternative therapies, such as weighted blankets, aromatherapy, and specialized mattress technology, have limited evidence supporting their efficacy or use.

Behavioral and Educational Interventions

Behavioral strategies remain first-line treatment for sleep problems in both neurotypical and neurodiverse children.[53–56] The efficacy of these approaches for autistic youth has been most studied in relation to nighttime or early morning awakenings, sleep-onset difficulties, self-settling practices, and co-sleeping behaviors.[57–59] Effective behavioral interventions incorporate multiple strategies based on an individual's unique sleep concerns. **Table 2** provides examples of behavioral sleep strategies for various sleep problems, including references to protocols to assist in implementing such interventions. These and other strategies have been incorporated into family-based cognitive behavioral therapy with reported success.[53,60–62]

The inclusion of caregiver education and training has been shown to improve sleep outcomes in response to behavioral interventions and be highly valued by caregivers

Table 2
Examples of behavioral sleep principles and strategies

Sleep Problem	Behavioral Sleep Principle	Example of Behavioral Sleep Strategy
Bedtime Resistance Child resists bedtime and/or has difficulties following bedtime routine	*Extinction*: removing reinforcement of undesirable sleeping behaviors	*Graduated planned ignoring*: ignoring behavior (eg, crying or fussing) for a set time interval (eg, 5 min) before allowing a brief check-in, with time intervals progressively lengthened.[63]
	Positive reinforcement: using rewards to promote desired behaviors	*Bedtime pass*: note card given to child at bedtime and exchangeable for one "free" parent visit or trip out of bed after bedtime. If the pass is not used, it can be exchanged for a reward in the morning.[64,65]
	Cueing: using components of modeling, visual supports, sticker charts, and social stories to promote positive bedtime behaviors	*Visual schedule for bedtime routines*: set of pictures depicting bedtime routine to help break down tasks, set expectations, and create consistency.[66]
Insomnia Child has difficulty falling or staying asleep	*Relaxation*: using relaxation techniques to promote sleep	*Relaxation training*: parent teaching child controlled breathing, progressive muscle relaxation, or visual imagery skill to assist in falling asleep.[62]
	Time Restriction: limiting time spent in bed when a child cannot fall asleep	*Restricted time in bed*: Encourage child to leave bed/bedroom and participate in quiet activity (eg, reading) if they cannot fall asleep within 30 min.[62]
Delayed Sleep Phase Child falls asleep and wakes up later than desired	*Bedtime fading*: progressively setting bedtime routine at earlier times until the desired bedtime is achieved.	*Faded bedtime with response cost*: setting initial bedtime near time of average sleep onset (determined with sleep log). Bedtime is progressively moved to an earlier time (eg, by 15–30 min) if child initiates sleep within 15 min. If sleep is not initiated within 15 min, child is encouraged to leave bed and bedtime is reset to a later time.[67-69]
	Light Exposure: timed exposure to bright light to help reset circadian rhythm	*Morning light exposure*: daily bright light exposure (eg, 2500 lux) for 1–3 h in the morning (eg, 7–9 AM) combined with restricted evening light to achieve earlier sleep times and improve morning alertness.[70]

(continued on next page)

Table 2
(continued)

Sleep Problem	Behavioral Sleep Principle	Example of Behavioral Sleep Strategy
Parasomnias Child experiences abnormal or undesired behaviors during sleep or partial arousals from sleep	*Scheduled awakening:* purposeful, brief awakenings 15–30 min before the typical time of night-waking events in hopes of alleviating behaviors that would typically occur after this experience.[71]	
Sleep-Onset Association Disorder Child requires presence of person or object to initiate sleep	*Stimulus fading:* gradual removing of an object or person from the child's space until the child is able to fall asleep without the stimulus.	*Camping out:* parent sits in chair or cot bed next to child's bed until child falls asleep and then gradually moves further away over next few nights. Process is repeated until child can fall asleep alone.[62]
All Sleep Problems	*Sleep hygiene:* implementation of a bedtime routine, creating an environment conducive to sleep, and avoidance of activities before bedtime that may arouse the child	*Positive routines:* parent creating and consistently implementing a ~30 min pre-bedtime routine that includes sleep readiness activities (dressing, washing, story time) and avoids activities that provoke challenging behaviors (eg, screen time) and extensions of routine (eg, one more turn, one more minute).[66,72]

of children with ASD.[73] For example, the ASATN developed a sleep toolkit involving caregiver education on sleep hygiene, bedtime routines, and behavioral modification strategies (eg, graduated extinction, bedtime passes).[66] This toolkit was found effective in improving sleep-onset delay in children with ASD and has since been expanded to include written training materials for parents and caregivers. However, pamphlet materials for caregivers alone were ineffective in providing sufficient education or making a positive impact on sleep.[74]

Pharmacologic Intervention

There are currently no medications approved for pediatric insomnia by the US Food and Drug Administration. Nevertheless, medications and supplements are frequently used to treat sleep disturbances in autistic children.[2] The largest body of evidence exists for the use of exogenous melatonin to improve sleep-onset insomnia and sleep maintenance insomnia in this population.[13,53,58]

Initiation of melatonin should begin at the lower range for a patient's age and be titrated weekly as needed. Over-the-counter preparations have variable concentrations and purities, making melatonin obtained by prescription most representative of literature results.[53] No serious adverse effects have been reported from short- or long-term melatonin use in this population; commonly reported side effects include morning drowsiness, increased enuresis, dizziness, and headaches.[13,53,75,76]

For sleep-onset insomnia, immediate-release (half-life of 40 minutes) forms of melatonin are available and most effective if given 30 minutes before desired sleep onset.[13,53] Most studies support the effectiveness of a 3 to 5 mg dose, although some studies have reported using doses up to 10 mg.[13,53] For sleep maintenance insomnia, a 2 to 5 mg dose of extended-release (mimicking the endogenous release of melatonin for up to 8–10 hours) melatonin has been shown to increase total sleep time and duration of uninterrupted sleep when given 30 to 60 minutes before desired sleep onset[75,77]

Other pharmacologic treatments, including clonidine, risperidone, clonazepam, and secretin supplementation, have limited studies evaluating or supporting their efficacy for sleep in autistic children. These options are also associated with more significant adverse effects than melatonin and non-pharmacologic strategies. Of the non-melatonin pharmacologic interventions, clonidine, a centrally acting α_2-adrenergic agonist, is most commonly prescribed for sleep and has a few studies suggesting possible effectiveness for night waking, sleep latency, and sleep duration.[2,58,78]

Clonidine is typically initiated at 25 to 50 μg at bedtime and slowly titrated up by 25 μg increments as needed.[78] The agent is available in multiple forms, including an extended-release tablet and transdermal patch. Clinically, clonidine is often considered for sleep concerns in autistic children with associated behavioral symptoms, as some evidence exists supporting its effectiveness for addressing agitation, aggression, and other challenging behaviors.[79] Although it is typically well-tolerated, clonidine is associated with more adverse effects than melatonin including daytime drowsiness. Caution should be taken in its use for children on other CNS depressants or who have a history of hemodynamic instability or cardiac pathology. If clonidine is ineffective or produces unwanted side effects, the agent must be tapered slowly over 2 to 7 days to avoid rebound hypertension.

Complementary and Alternative Interventions

Limited studies exist investigating or supporting the use of complementary or alternative interventions for sleep in children with autism. For example, Malow and colleagues found no evidence supporting the use or efficacy of massage therapy and aromatherapy.[10] Williams Buckley and colleagues found only weighted blankets and specialized mattress technology to have sufficient-quality studies for further results analyses.[53] Although neither strategy improved sleep by objective measures, weighted blankets were well-tolerated and favored by children and parents and may serve as a reasonable non-pharmacologic approach for some individuals.[53,80]

Referral to Sleep Specialists

Although the management of medical contributors to sleep disorders typically requires the expertise of subspecialists, the initial management of primary sleep disturbances can be efficiently handled by the PCP, especially considering resource constraints and limited specialist availability in certain communities. Treatment objectives for managing primary sleep disorders should be to optimize the quality of sleep by reducing sleep latency to less than 30 minutes, achieving age-appropriate sleep duration, improving sleep-sensitive behaviors, and enhancing parental/caregiver satisfaction with their child's sleep patterns.[20] When educational/behavioral interventions prove ineffective, pharmacologic management becomes overly complex, or reaching treatment goals proves challenging, the PCP should consider referring the patient to a sleep specialist for a more specialized, targeted approach to sleep management.[10]

CASE DISCUSSION RESOLUTION

Family reports some positive responses to behavioral strategies discussed after the last visit. She is falling to sleep more quickly with 3 mg of melatonin given as part of her bedtime routine, and they have been able to successfully remove the iPad from her bedroom using a visual schedule and gradually dimming the brightness and volume of the iPad over several days. Mother is currently working to remove herself from the bedtime routine by sitting next to the bed rather than lying next to the child. Although night waking still occurs, it is happening less frequently and with quicker return to sleep.

SUMMARY

This review highlights the significant prevalence and multifactorial etiology of sleep problems among children with ASD. Proper understanding and screening by health care providers is crucial for appropriate diagnosis and treatment given the degree of cognitive, emotional, physical, and behavioral impact sleep disorders can have on the patient and caregiver. Health care providers should construct an individualized plan for sleep management and should incorporate behavioral interventions with potential pharmacologic support. Similar to the enigmatic nature of ASD itself, the relationship between ASD and sleep disorders is complex and heterogeneous. Consequently, further research is needed to understand the intricate connection between these two conditions and further optimize evidence-based interventions for this specific population.

CLINICS CARE POINTS

- Given the high prevalence of sleep disorders in pediatric patients with autism spectrum disorder, all autistic youth should be regularly screened for sleep problems.
- Health care providers screening with a single, nonspecific question pertaining to sleep results in a significant number of individuals left with undiagnosed sleep disorders. Providers should instead ask specific, probing questions related to sleep routine/patterns or use a validated screening questionnaire (eg, Children's Sleep Habits Questionnaire or Composite Sleep Disturbance Index) for a more accurate evaluation.
- While evaluating sleep problems, health care providers should investigate any potential co-occurring medical contributors (eg, constipation, gastroesophageal reflux, obstructive sleep apnea).
- Behavioral interventions remain the first-line treatment for sleep disorders in both neurotypical and neurodiverse youth. Inclusion of caregiver education and training has been shown to improve sleep outcomes in response to behavioral intervention and be highly valued by caregivers of children with autism.
- Of the pharmacologic intervention options, the largest body of evidence exists for the use of exogenous melatonin to improve sleep in autistic youth.

DISCLOSURE

A.E. Bennett has received research funding from the following organizations: Autism Speaks, Roche Pharmaceuticals, Acadia Pharmaceuticals, GW Pharmaceuticals, Maplight Pharmaceuticals. M.C. Souders has received research funding from the University Research Fund, University of Pennsylvania.

REFERENCES

1. Hyman SL, Levy SE, Myers SM. Identification, Evaluation, and Management of Children With Autism Spectrum Disorder. Pediatrics 2020;145(1):e20193447.

2. Malow BA, Katz T, Reynolds AM, et al. Sleep Difficulties and Medications in Children With Autism Spectrum Disorders: A Registry Study. Pediatrics 2016; 137(Supplement_2):S98–104. https://doi.org/10.1542/peds.2015-2851H.

3. Carmassi C, Palagini L, Caruso D, et al. Systematic Review of Sleep Disturbances and Circadian Sleep Desynchronization in Autism Spectrum Disorder: Toward an Integrative Model of a Self-Reinforcing Loop. Front Psychiatr 2019;10:366.

4. Cohen S, Conduit R, Lockley SW, et al. The relationship between sleep and behavior in autism spectrum disorder (ASD): a review. J Neurodev Disord 2014;6(1):44.

5. Hysing M, Haugland S, Stormark KM, et al. Sleep and school attendance in adolescence: Results from a large population-based study. Scand J Publ Health 2015;43(1):2–9. https://doi.org/10.1177/1403494814556647.

6. Malow BA, Marvin AR, Coury D, Bennett A, Lipkin PH Law JK. Sleep Problems in Children with ASD: Effects on Parental Employment, 29932, 2019, International Society for Autism Research Annual Meeting (INSAR), Available at: www.autism-insar.org.

7. Martin J, Hiscock H, Hardy P, et al. Adverse Associations of Infant and Child Sleep Problems and Parent Health: An Australian Population Study. Pediatrics 2007;119(5):947–55.

8. Martin CA, Papadopoulos N, Chellew T, et al. Associations between parenting stress, parent mental health and child sleep problems for children with ADHD and ASD: Systematic review. Res Dev Disabil 2019;93:103463. https://doi.org/10.1016/j.ridd.2019.103463.

9. Righi G, Benevides J, Mazefsky C, et al. Predictors of Inpatient Psychiatric Hospitalization for Children and Adolescents with Autism Spectrum Disorder. J Autism Dev Disord 2018;48(11):3647–57. https://doi.org/10.1007/s10803-017-3154-9.

10. Malow BA, Byars K, Johnson K, et al. A Practice Pathway for the Identification, Evaluation, and Management of Insomnia in Children and Adolescents With Autism Spectrum Disorders. Pediatrics 2012;130(Supplement_2):S106–24.

11. Humphreys JS, Gringras P, Blair PS, et al. Sleep patterns in children with autistic spectrum disorders: a prospective cohort study. Arch Dis Child 2014;99(2):114–8.

12. Elrod MG, Hood BS. Sleep Differences Among Children With Autism Spectrum Disorders and Typically Developing Peers: A Meta-analysis. J Dev Behav Pediatr 2015;36(3):166. https://doi.org/10.1097/DBP.0000000000000140.

13. Souders MC, Taylor BJ, Zavodny Jackson S. Sleep Problems in Autism Spectrum Disorder. In: White SW, Maddox BB, Mazefsky CA, editors. The oxford handbook of autism and Co-occurring psychiatric conditions. Oxford University Press; 2020. https://doi.org/10.1093/oxfordhb/9780190910761.013.14.

14. Cortesi F, Giannotti F, Ivanenko A, et al. Sleep in children with autistic spectrum disorder. Sleep Med 2010;11(7):659–64.

15. Malow BA. Sleep disorders, epilepsy, and autism. Ment Retard Dev Disabil Res Rev 2004;10(2):122–5.

16. Reynolds AM, Soke GN, Sabourin KR, et al. Sleep Problems in 2- to 5-Year-Olds With Autism Spectrum Disorder and Other Developmental Delays. Pediatrics 2019;143(3):e20180492. https://doi.org/10.1542/peds.2018-0492.

17. Marvin AR, Coury DL, Malow BA, et al. Brief report: Measures of effectiveness for single-question sleep problem screeners in children with autism spectrum disorder. Research in Autism Spectrum Disorders 2021;80:101699.

18. Mannion A, Leader G, Healy O. An investigation of comorbid psychological disorders, sleep problems, gastrointestinal symptoms and epilepsy in children and adolescents with Autism Spectrum Disorder. Research in Autism Spectrum Disorders 2013;7(1):35–42.
19. Accardo JA, Malow BA. Sleep, epilepsy, and autism. Epilepsy Behav 2015;47: 202–6.
20. Banaschewski T, Bruni O, Fuentes J, et al. Practice Tools for Screening and Monitoring Insomnia in Children and Adolescents with Autism Spectrum Disorder. J Autism Dev Disord 2022;52:3758–68.
21. Becker RE, Owens JA. Sleep and Sleep Disorders in Children. In: Feldman HM, editor. Developmental-behavioral pediatrics. 5th ed. Elsevier; 2022. p. 711–21. https://bookshelf.health.elsevier.com/books/9780323809740.
22. El Shakankiry HM. Sleep physiology and sleep disorders in childhood. Nat Sci Sleep 2011;3:101–14. https://doi.org/10.2147/NSS.S22839.
23. Lee EK. Introduction to Circadian Rhythm Disorders. In: Auger R, editor. Circadian rhythm sleep-wake disorders. Springer; 2020. p. 1–9. https://doi.org/10.1007/978-3-030-43803-6_3.
24. Tomkies A, Johnson RF, Shah G, et al. Obstructive Sleep Apnea in Children With Autism. J Clin Sleep Med 2019;15(10):1469–76.
25. Koh S, Ward SL, Lin M, et al. Sleep apnea treatment improves seizure control in children with neurodevelopmental disorders. Pediatr Neurol 2000;22(1):36–9.
26. Malow BA, Weatherwax KJ, Chervin RD, et al. Identification and treatment of obstructive sleep apnea in adults and children with epilepsy: a prospective pilot study. Sleep Med 2003;4(6):509–15.
27. Tirosh E, Tal Y, Jaffe M. CPAP treatment of obstructive sleep apnoea and neurodevelopmental deficits. Acta paediatrica (Oslo, Norway: 1992) 1995;84(7):791–4.
28. Ornitz EM, Ritvo ER, Brown MB, et al. The EEG and rapid eye movements during REM sleep in normal and autistic children. Electroencephalogr Clin Neurophysiol 1969;26(2):167–75.
29. Tanguay PE, Ornitz EM, Forsythe AB, et al. Rapid eye movement (REM) activity in normal and autistic children during REM sleep. J Autism Child Schizophr 1976; 6(3):275–88.
30. Buckley AW, Rodriguez AJ, Jennison K, et al. Rapid eye movement sleep percentage in children with autism compared with children with developmental delay and typical development. Arch Pediatr Adolesc Med 2010;164(11):1032–7.
31. Malow BA, Marzec ML, McGrew SG, et al. Characterizing sleep in children with autism spectrum disorders: a multidimensional approach. Sleep 2006;29(12): 1563–71.
32. Petruzzelli MG, Matera E, Giambersio D, et al. Subjective and Electroencephalographic Sleep Parameters in Children and Adolescents with Autism Spectrum Disorder: A Systematic Review. J Clin Med 2021;10(17):3893.
33. Aurora RN, Lamm CI, Zak RS, et al. Practice parameters for the non-respiratory indications for polysomnography and multiple sleep latency testing for children. Sleep 2012;35(11):1467–73.
34. Kushida CA, Littner MR, Morgenthaler T, et al. Practice parameters for the indications for polysomnography and related procedures: an update for 2005. Sleep 2005;28(4):499–521.
35. Wiggs L, Stores G. Sleep patterns and sleep disorders in children with autistic spectrum disorders: insights using parent report and actigraphy. Dev Med Child Neurol 2004;46(6):372–80.

36. Souders MC, Mason TB, Valladares O, et al. Sleep behaviors and sleep quality in children with autism spectrum disorders. Sleep 2009;32(12):1566–78.

37. Yavuz-Kodat E, Reynaud E, Geoffray MM, et al. Validity of Actigraphy Compared to Polysomnography for Sleep Assessment in Children With Autism Spectrum Disorder. Front Psychiatr 2019;10:551.

38. Gregory AM, Sadeh A. Sleep, emotional and behavioral difficulties in children and adolescents. Sleep Med Rev 2012;16(2):129–36. https://doi.org/10.1016/j.smrv.2011.03.007.

39. Lewandowski AS, Ward TM, Palermo TM. Sleep problems in children and adolescents with common medical conditions. Pediatr Clin 2011;58(3):699–713.

40. Cohen S, Fulcher BD, Rajaratnam SMW, et al. Sleep patterns predictive of daytime challenging behavior in individuals with low-functioning autism. Autism Res 2018;11(2):391–403.

41. Goldman SE, McGrew S, Johnson KP, et al. Sleep is associated with problem behaviors in children and adolescents with Autism Spectrum Disorders. Research in Autism Spectrum Disorders 2011;5(3):1223–9.

42. May T, Cornish K, Conduit R, et al. Sleep in high-functioning children with autism: longitudinal developmental change and associations with behavior problems. Behav Sleep Med 2015;13(1):2–18. https://doi.org/10.1080/15402002.2013.829064.

43. Mazurek MO, Petroski GF. Sleep problems in children with autism spectrum disorder: Examining the contributions of sensory over-responsivity and anxiety. Sleep Med 2015;16(2):270–9.

44. Mazurek MO, Sohl K. Sleep and Behavioral Problems in Children with Autism Spectrum Disorder. J Autism Dev Disord 2016;46(6):1906–15.

45. Mazurek MO, Dovgan K, Neumeyer AM, et al. Course and Predictors of Sleep and Co-occurring Problems in Children with Autism Spectrum Disorder. J Autism Dev Disord 2019;49:2101–15.

46. Richdale AL, Baker E, Short M, et al. The role of insomnia, pre-sleep arousal and psychopathology symptoms in daytime impairment in adolescents with high-functioning autism spectrum disorder. Sleep Med 2014;15(9):1082–8.

47. Sikora DM, Johnson K, Clemons T, et al. The Relationship Between Sleep Problems and Daytime Behavior in Children of Different Ages With Autism Spectrum Disorders. Pediatrics 2012;130(Supplement_2):S83–90.

48. Hollway JA, Aman MG, Butter E. Correlates and Risk Markers for Sleep Disturbance in Participants of the Autism Treatment Network. J Autism Dev Disord 2013;43(12):2830–43.

49. Shui AM, Katz T, Malow BA, et al. Predicting sleep problems in children with autism spectrum disorders. Res Dev Disabil 2018;83:270–9.

50. Neumeyer AM, Anixt J, Chan J, et al. Identifying Associations Among Co-Occurring Medical Conditions in Children With Autism Spectrum Disorders. Acad Pediatr 2019;19(3):300–6.

51. Delahaye J, Kovacs E, Sikora D, et al. The relationship between Health-Related Quality of Life and sleep problems in children with Autism Spectrum Disorders. Research in Autism Spectrum Disorders 2014;8(3):292–303.

52. Johnson CR, Smith T, DeMand A, et al. Exploring sleep quality of young children with autism spectrum disorder and disruptive behaviors. Sleep Med 2018;44:61–6.

53. Williams Buckley A, Hirtz D, Oskoui M, et al. Practice guideline: Treatment for insomnia and disrupted sleep behavior in children and adolescents with autism spectrum disorder. Neurology 2020;94(9):392–404.

54. Edinger JD, Arnedt JT, Bertisch SM, et al. Behavioral and psychological treatments for chronic insomnia disorder in adults: An American Academy of Sleep Medicine clinical practice guideline. J Clin Sleep Med 2021;17(2):255–62.
55. Mindell JA, Meltzer LJ. Behavioural sleep disorders in children and adolescents. Ann Acad Med Singapore 2008;37(8):722–8.
56. Morgenthaler TI, Owens J, Alessi C, et al. Practice Parameters for Behavioral Treatment of Bedtime Problems and Night Wakings in Infants and Young Children. Sleep 2006. https://doi.org/10.1093/sleep/29.10.1277.
57. Carnett A, Hansen S, McLay L, et al. Quantitative-Analysis of Behavioral Interventions to Treat Sleep Problems in Children with Autism. Dev Neurorehabil 2020; 23(5):271–84.
58. Cuomo BM, Vaz S, Lee EAL, et al. Effectiveness of Sleep-Based Interventions for Children with Autism Spectrum Disorder: A Meta-Synthesis. Pharmacotherapy 2017;37(5):555–78.
59. Keogh S, Bridle C, Siriwardena NA, et al. Effectiveness of non-pharmacological interventions for insomnia in children with Autism Spectrum Disorder: A systematic review and meta-analysis. PLoS One 2019;14(8):e0221428.
60. McCrae CS, Chan WS, Curtis AF, et al. Cognitive behavioral treatment of insomnia in school-aged children with autism spectrum disorder: A pilot feasibility study. Autism Res 2020;13(1):167–76.
61. Nadeau JM, Arnold EB, Keene AC, et al. Frequency and Clinical Correlates of Sleep-Related Problems Among Anxious Youth with Autism Spectrum Disorders. Child Psychiatr Hum Dev 2015;46(4):558–66.
62. Pattison E, Mantilla A, Fuller-Tyszkiewicz M, et al. Acceptability of a behavioural sleep intervention for autistic children: A qualitative evaluation of Sleeping Sound. Sleep Med 2022;100:378–89.
63. Reid MJ, Walter AL, O'Leary SG. Treatment of Young Children's Bedtime Refusal and Nighttime Wakings: A Comparison of "Standard" and Graduated Ignoring Procedures. J Abnorm Child Psychol 1999;27(1):5–16. https://doi.org/10.1023/A:1022606206076.
64. Friman PC, Hoff KE, Schnoes C, et al. The Bedtime Pass: An Approach to Bedtime Crying and Leaving the Room. Arch Pediatr Adolesc Med 1999; 153(10):1027–9. https://doi.org/10.1001/archpedi.153.10.1027.
65. Moore BA, Friman PC, Fruzzetti AE, et al. Brief Report: Evaluating the Bedtime Pass Program for Child Resistance to Bedtime—A Randomized, Controlled Trial. J Pediatr Psychol 2007;32(3):283–7. https://doi.org/10.1093/jpepsy/jsl025.
66. Malow BA, Adkins KW, Reynolds A, et al. Parent-Based Sleep Education for Children with Autism Spectrum Disorders. J Autism Dev Disord 2014;44(1).
67. Cooney MR, Short MA, Gradisar M. An open trial of bedtime fading for sleep disturbances in preschool children: a parent group education approach. Sleep Med 2018;46:98–106.
68. Delemere E, Dounavi K. *Parent-Implemented* Bedtime Fading and Positive Routines for Children with Autism Spectrum Disorders. J Autism Dev Disord 2018; 48(4):1002–19.
69. Piazza CC, Fisher W. A Faded Bedtime with Response Cost Protocol for Treatment of Multiple Sleep Problems in Children. J Appl Behav Anal 1991;24(1): 129–40.
70. Barion A, Zee PC. A clinical approach to circadian rhythm sleep disorders. Sleep Med 2007;8(6):566–77.
71. Owens J, Mohan M. Behavioral Interventions for Parasomnias. Curr Sleep Medicine Rep 2016;2(2):81–6.

72. Mindell JA, Williamson AA. Benefits of a bedtime routine in young children: Sleep, development, and beyond. Sleep Med Rev 2018;40:93–108.

73. Kirkpatrick B, Louw JS, Leader G. Efficacy of parent training incorporated in behavioral sleep interventions for children with autism spectrum disorder and/or intellectual disabilities: A systematic review. Sleep Med 2019;53:141–52.

74. Adkins KW, Molloy C, Weiss SK, et al. Effects of a Standardized Pamphlet on Insomnia in Children With Autism Spectrum Disorders. Pediatrics 2012; 130(Suppl 2):S139–44.

75. Maras A, Schroder CM, Malow BA, et al. Long-Term Efficacy and Safety of Pediatric Prolonged-Release Melatonin for Insomnia in Children with Autism Spectrum Disorder. J Child Adolesc Psychopharmacol 2018;28(10):699–710.

76. Yuge K, Nagamitsu S, Ishikawa Y, et al. Long-term melatonin treatment for the sleep problems and aberrant behaviors of children with neurodevelopmental disorders. BMC Psychiatr 2020;20:445.

77. Gringras P, Nir T, Breddy J, et al. Efficacy and Safety of Pediatric Prolonged-Release Melatonin for Insomnia in Children With Autism Spectrum Disorder. J Am Acad Child Adolesc Psychiatr 2017;56(11):948–57.e4.

78. Blackmer AB, Feinstein JA. Management of Sleep Disorders in Children With Neurodevelopmental Disorders: A Review. Pharmacotherapy 2016;36(1):84–98.

79. Banasm K, Sawchuk B. Clonidine as a Treatment of Behavioural Disturbances in Autism Spectrum Disorder: A Systematic Literature Review. Journal of the Canadian Academy of Child and Adolscent Psychiatry 2020;29(2):110–20.

80. Gringras P, Green D, Wright B, et al. Weighted Blankets and Sleep in Autistic Children—A Randomized Controlled Trial. Pediatrics 2014;134(2):298–306.

Mental Health Crises in Autistic Children

A Framework for Prevention and Intervention in Primary Care

Roma A. Vasa, MD[a],*, Kate Neamsapaya, BA[b],
Elizabeth A. Cross, PhD[a], Luther Kalb, PhD, MHS[a]

KEYWORDS

- Autism spectrum disorder • Psychiatric and behavioral disorders
- Mental health crisis • Mental health crisis assessment scale
- Prevention and intervention

KEY POINTS

- Autistic children are at increased risk for mental health crisis compared to non-autistic peers.
- A mental health crisis has 2 components: behavior that poses immediate danger and resources that are ineffective or insufficient to manage the situation.
- There are 4 stages in the evolution of a mental health crisis: not in crisis, pre-crisis, crisis, post-crisis.
- Implementing prevention and intervention efforts in outpatient settings for those in the early stages of crisis is important to reduce risk of a full-blown crisis.
- Parents can prepare for a mental health crisis using a variety of strategies.

INTRODUCTION

Children with autism are 2 to 4 times more likely to have a psychiatric diagnosis than their neurotypical peers and at greater risk than children with intellectual disabilities and/or special health care needs.[1,2] Approximately 70% of autistic children in community settings have a co-occurring psychiatric diagnosis, and 40% have 2 or more psychiatric diagnoses.[3] The prevalence in psychiatric clinic samples is significantly higher with 95% of children having 3 or more psychiatric disorders and 74% having 5 or more

[a] Center for Autism and Related Disorders, 3901 Greenspring Avenue, Baltimore, MD 21211, USA; [b] Department of International Health, Johns Hopkins Bloomberg School of Public Health, 615 North Wolfe Street, Suite E8527, Baltimore, MD 21205, USA
* Corresponding author. Center for Autism and Related Disorders, 3901 Greenspring Avenue, Baltimore, MD 21211.
E-mail address: vasa@kennedykrieger.org

psychiatric disorders.[4] Further, suicide attempts occur at a rate 3 times higher and 2.8 years earlier in autistic compared to non-autistic adolescents and young adults.[5,6]

In addition to psychiatric disorders, autistic children show higher rates of externalizing behaviors, with about 50% presenting with 1 or more externalizing behaviors, including irritability, physical and verbal aggression, non-compliance, property destruction, hyperactivity/impulsivity, self-injury, and elopement.[7,8] Sometimes these behaviors occur simultaneously and lead to a dysregulated state or meltdown. A meltdown refers to an intense response to an overwhelming situation resulting in a temporary loss of behavioral control that manifests verbally and/or physically.[9] These behaviors often co-occur and have complex underlying root causes including psychiatric disorders, medical conditions, communication difficulties, psychosocial stressors, and operant factors.[10]

Given the high rates of psychiatric and behavioral disorders, autistic children are at increased risk for mental health crisis when these disorders exacerbate and lead to a state of immediate risk for harm. The American Psychiatric Association (APA) defines a psychiatric emergency, which is analogous to a mental health crisis, as an acute psychiatric or behavioral event that poses imminent danger to oneself or others, in which the resources available to manage the event are insufficient to de-escalate the situation.[11,12] Several lines of evidence suggest that autistic children are at higher risk of experiencing a mental health crisis compared to non-autistic children. First, data over the past decade indicate that autistic children have higher rates of emergency department (ED) visits,[13–15] prolonged ED stays,[16] and elevated rates and duration of inpatient psychiatric hospitalizations compared to non-autistic peers.[17,18] Second, in an online survey of an autism research community, 32% of the parents reported that their autistic child had experienced a mental health crisis during the last 3 months.[19] Last, data from 2 specialized autism centers indicate that 1 in 5 autistic children were at risk for mental health crisis.[20] Prevention and treatment of mental health crises are therefore critical to reducing child morbidity, improving quality of life, and diverting more restrictive care.

Primary care providers may be the first-line providers to treat psychiatric and behavioral disorders in autistic children, and therefore can play a key role in preventing and managing crisis in their practice. The goal of this article is therefore to provide primary care clinicians with the tools to address mental health crisis in autistic children. We will first discuss research measurement of crisis, including the development of the Mental Health Crisis Assessment Scale (MCAS), which could be implemented in primary care. Next, the authors provide information on the current state of ED and inpatient visits for crisis in autistic children, to inform clinicians how they can best engage with these acute care systems. They also present an example of a community-based wrap around program (START Program) to reduce crisis risk. Lastly, and the heart of this article, is the presentation of a 4-stage model of crisis that includes assessment and management strategies that clinicians can offer caregivers to help their child manage crisis.

In this article, the terms "autistic children" or "children with autism" will be used interchangeably to reflect the different perspectives of autism advocates.[21] The term "children" refers to children and adolescents, ages 3 to 18 years, and the term "crisis" refers to "mental health crisis." Before launching into the article, the authors first present a fictitious case of an autistic child in crisis to orient the reader to this phenomenology.

Jason is a 14-year-old male with autism and moderate intellectual disability. Jason has a long history of frequent meltdowns at home and at school. The meltdowns have increased in severity and frequency over the last few years and are characterized by aggression toward others (eg, hitting and biting others), self-injurious behaviors (eg, banging his head on hard surfaces), and property destruction (eg, destroying electronics). Sometimes the meltdowns have clear antecedents such as having to transition from a preferred to a non-preferred activity. Other times, the meltdowns occur without a clear trigger. The meltdowns last up to 45 minutes and occur several times per day, and the parents' strategies to calm Jason have been ineffective and resulted in scratches on their arms. He is taking medications, and his parents are working with a psychologist to implement behavioral interventions, though his meltdowns continue to occur. The school has suggested that Jason may need a more restrictive school placement. Jason's parents are concerned about their son's safety, are extremely exhausted, and have modified their work schedules to care for their son. They are worried that Jason's behavior will become unmanageable and do not know what to do.

MEASUREMENT OF MENTAL HEALTH CRISIS

Systematic research on mental health crises in autistic children is a relatively new and evolving field. While various measures have been developed to psychiatric and behavioral symptoms in autistic children, only a few measures assess when these conditions become a crisis. Weiss and colleagues were among the earliest pioneers of crisis research in autistic children.[22] They developed the first crisis scale in autism, the Brief Family Distress Scale, a single-item score that assesses the global state of the family as it relates to crisis.[23] They later conducted qualitative research, which identified 4 features of mental health crisis in autistic children: acute behaviors of the child, impact of the child's behavior on the family, use of psychiatric emergency services, and greater need for parental support.[22]

Building on the findings of Weiss and colleagues and the APA definition of crisis, Kalb and colleagues developed the first crisis scale, the Mental Health Crisis Assessment Scale-Revised (MCAS-R), which is a 23-item informant report scale that takes 5 to 10 minutes to implement.[11,20] The MCAS-R assesses 13 psychiatric and behavioral conditions that can lead to crisis (eg, aggression, self-injury), includes questions about the dangerousness of the behavior, and the caregiver's ability to safely manage the behavior. This scale has demonstrated robust psychometric properties and is freely available by emailing the first or last author of this article.[11]

Suicide screening scales are also being tested in autistic children. The Ask Suicide-Screening Questionnaire (ASQ) was implemented in all medical clinics in a pediatric university-affiliated hospital. Results showed that parents of children with neurodevelopmental disorders found the screening to be acceptable and that children with autism had the highest rate of positive screens.[24] Recent evidence suggests that the Columbia Suicide Severity Rating Scale may be a useful measure to assess suicidal thoughts and behaviors in autistic children who present to the ED setting.[25] Both scales require validation in autistic children; the National Institutes of Mental Health is currently conducting a validation study of the ASQ (https://clinicaltrials.gov/study/NCT04317118).

SYSTEMS OF CARE TO ADDRESS MENTAL HEALTH CRISIS IN AUTISTIC CHILDREN

In the early twentieth century, individuals with developmental disabilities in the United States were housed in public institutions to isolate them from society where they experienced atrocities including use of restraint and seclusion, abuse and trauma, and deprivation of basic life needs.[26] In the wake of these scandals, enormous health care costs, legislation such as the Olmstead Act and Public Law 94 to 142, and other factors, public institutions began closing. This led to the transition of individuals with developmental disabilities into the community at a time when insufficient community mental health services were available to address the needs of this group.

While efforts over the past 50 years have attempted to build mental health programs and services, significant gaps in service provision for autistic individuals persist and are of concern as the prevalence of autism continues to rise.[27] To this day, over 50% of parents of autistic children report difficulty accessing mental health services.[28] Only about a third of mental health care facilities in the United States are accepting new autistic patients, about 1 in 10 have a specialized mental health provider trained to see autistic children, and the next generation of child psychiatrists is not adequately trained to work with this group.[29,30] Autistic Latinx children are the least likely racial/ethnic group to receive mental health treatment in this country.[28] Factors contributing to these disparities include clinician bias, health literacy, structural and language barriers, and systemic racism.[31–33] Autistic children in rural settings also face significant access barriers, largely due to nationwide workforce shortages.[29,34]

Many systems are involved in managing crisis in autistic children including community providers, the ED, inpatient unit, law enforcement, emergency medical providers, and state mental health and developmental disabilities systems, among others. In the following paragraphs, the authors present 3 systems relevant to managing crisis in autistic children.

Emergency Department Care

Prior research has shown that autistic children are 9 times more likely compared to non-autistic children to use the ED for psychiatric purposes,[13] and ED visits for psychiatric reasons in autistic children have substantially increased between 2005 and 2013.[14] Furthermore, autistic children who present to the ED in crisis are also more likely than non-autistic peers to remain in the ED for extended periods of time while waiting for inpatient hospitalization.[16]

Several factors may be contributing to the sustained high levels of ED visits among autistic children including the dire shortage of community professionals, which sometimes means that the ED is the first point of mental health contact for autistic children.[35] Psychiatric disorders also persist and new disorders such as psychosis and bipolar disorder increase with age, thereby leading to crisis.[36,37] Last, home and community-based services for autistic individuals, which are essential to lowering ED visits, are lacking.[38]

While ED visits have remained high, the authors' clinical experiences indicate that some families are hesitant to seek ED care for crisis, possibly because the ED milieu is not well-suited for autistic children and could even be traumatic.[13–15] ED settings are typically loud and unpredictable, and some professionals lack understanding of autism. These stressors can trigger anxiety and resulting externalizing behaviors, which can increase risk of restraint and medication use. Further, the stresses of prolonged boarding with uncertainty about disposition plans can be disruptive to the family.

Efforts are underway to improve the ED experience for autistic children. For example, the ED at the Children's Hospital at TriStar Centennial has created a friendly environment for autistic children, including quiet rooms, dimmers to reduce light, noise canceling headphones, softer gowns, and sensory-friendly toys.[39] Hospitals are also making efforts to gather information about autistic individuals' needs. For example, Boston Children's Hospital has implemented the Autism Support Checklist, a tool that allows caregivers to document their child's needs, which are then added to the patient's electronic medical record for providers to review (see https://healthcity.bmc.org/population-health/hospital-initiative-strives-autism-friendly-experience).

Inpatient Psychiatric Hospitalization

Data over the last 2 decades suggest that autistic children have higher rates of psychiatric hospitalization than non-autistic children.[15,16] In a recent population-wide cohort study in Sweden, autistic females and males were 5.6 and 3.8 times more likely than same-sex individuals without autism to experience a psychiatric hospitalization, respectively.[17] Similarly, a California-based analysis found that the odds of mental health-related hospitalization were 3.8 to 8.2 times greater for autistic children compared to the general population.[18] Like the ED, autistic individuals have longer inpatient stays (ie, 30+ days) compared to those without autism,[40] which may reflect the increased time needed to achieve behavioral stabilization and develop a disposition plan.

Evidence suggests that autistic children who receive treatment in specialized inpatient units demonstrate reductions in maladaptive behaviors both at discharge and 2 months after discharge.[41,42] In 2012, Siegel and colleagues identified 9 specialized inpatient psychiatric units around the country for autistic children, most of which resided in academic settings[43]; these units offered comprehensive and tailored care for autistic children. Since then, the number of these units has expanded across the country although the exact number is unavailable. Specialized units offer a milieu that communicates expectations through both written and visually based modalities, offers sensory-oriented activities, and includes a contingency management system with rewards that are meaningful to the child.

Despite the growth in specialized inpatient units, most autistic children continue to be hospitalized in general child psychiatry inpatient units. These units often do not have the resources to serve autistic children, which increases risk for crisis intervention, seclusion, and restraints.[44] However, several clinical groups around the country have developed best practice guidelines for treating children with autism and co-occurring psychiatric and behavioral challenges in psychiatric inpatient units[45,46] with preliminary evidence indicating positive outcomes including reduced risk for crisis and shorter lengths of stay.[47]

Systemic, Therapeutic, Assessment, Resources, and Treatment Program

One community-based program that has shown promise in reducing mental health crises is the Systemic, Therapeutic, Assessment, Resources, and Treatment (START) program. START is a lifespan model that serves individuals with intellectual disability and co-occurring mental health needs. The goal of START is to enhance local capacity, promote the development of least-restrictive life-enhancing services, and provide education and training to providers and caregivers. START is overseen by the National Center for START Services, which is located at the University of New Hampshire Institute on Disability. START is currently serving individuals across 10 states in the United States.

Several studies have demonstrated improved outcomes associated with START. This includes reductions in psychiatric hospitalizations and ED visits, improvements in mental health symptoms, and increased satisfaction with the mental health system.[48,49] START improves these outcomes through clinical service provision and co-ordination, with the latter requiring certification through the National Center. All START programs have a clinical team comprising at minimum a director, medical director, clinical director, clinical team leader, and START Coordinators. Primary components of START, beyond coordination and team-based care, include cross system crisis planning, 24-h mobile crisis response and intervention, outreach and coaching, service linkages, and family support. For more details on START, see https://iod.unh.edu/national-center-start-services.

CRISIS PREVENTION AND INTERVENTION

The authors' group developed a 4-stage crisis model to help clinicians gauge an autistic child's stage of crisis and provide guidance to families. This 4-stage framework has been adapted from other existing crisis models (eg, Professional Crisis Management)[50] and behavioral escalation cycles (eg, Positive Behavior Intervention Supports).[51] The authors addition to this model is the inclusion of specific crisis management strategies for autistic children at each stage.

Fig. 1 presents the authors crisis model, which illustrates the 4 stages in the evolution of a crisis: not in crisis, pre-crisis, crisis, post-crisis.[52] Children and families can move in and out of these stages, slowly or rapidly, based on treatment and other factors. Thus, a child may be present in a pre-crisis stage during one visit, however, with appropriate interventions, the child may move into the not in crisis stage.

Given the shortage of mental health providers, the authors encourage primary care providers to take an active role in assessing and managing crisis using the authors' crisis framework. Clinicians can choose to present this model to caregivers, keeping in mind that the term "mental health crisis" or "crisis" may trigger fear and uncertainty for some caregivers. Therefore, clinicians are encouraged to use a personalized approach to determine whether using this would be helpful to parents.

Determining a child's stage of crisis is a focused assessment that involves asking the caregiver questions about the nature of the child's externalizing behaviors, the child's safety, and the caregiver's ability to manage these behaviors. Some starting questions for the clinician include the following.

- Is your child demonstrating irritability, aggression, self-injury, or meltdowns?
- How often do these behaviors occur, and how long do they last?
- What do you think triggers these behaviors?
- Are you concerned about your child's or your safety during these episodes?
- Has anyone been injured?
- What strategies do you use to calm your child?
- Are these strategies effective?

Following determination of the stage of crisis, clinicians can offer caregivers strategies to prevent/manage the child's behaviors. The strategies listed under each stage in **Fig. 1** and elaborated on later are tailored to the autistic population, considering learning preferences (eg, use of visual strategies), sensory processing differences, and preference for predictability. These strategies are based on principles of applied behavior analysis and have been drawn from evidence-based treatments for challenging behaviors in autistic children such as the Research Units in Behavioral Interventions (RUBI) Parent Training program.[53] These recommendations are general and by no means comprehensive - they are intended to provide tools to prevent escalation to a crisis and are not designed to lead to long-term behavioral change.

Stage 1: Not in Crisis

Children who are not in crisis have low levels of externalizing behavior. The clinician's goal during this stage is to screen for psychiatric and behavioral disorders and offer parents behavioral strategies to maintain low levels of behavior. These strategies involve changing the environment and the way in which parents interact with their children.

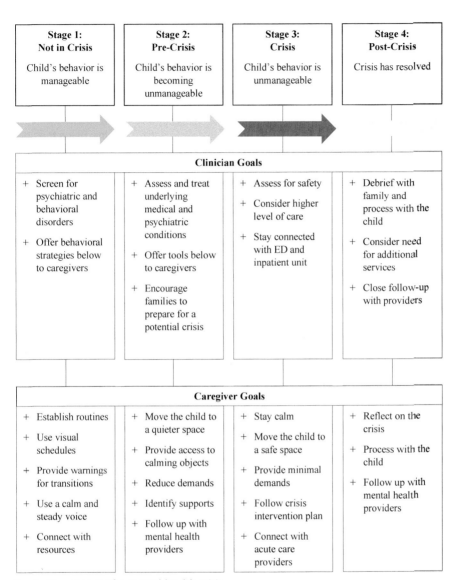

Fig. 1. Four stages of a mental health crisis.

Screening

Tools for assessing challenging behaviors include various parent-report scales including general psychopathology screening measures such as the Child Behavior Checklist, as well as tools to assess more specific behaviors.[54] Some of these tools may not be validated for autistic children and should be interpreted cautiously. Tools for assessing externalizing behaviors are available for clinicians at https://docs. autismspeaks.org/screening-and-assessment/.

The Ask Suicide-Screening Questionnaire shows promise as a screening tool in autistic children, and research in a university-affiliated pediatric hospital setting indicates that it is feasible to implement the measure in outpatient medical clinics.[24]

Nurses can administer this questionnaire during the triage assessment to children who they determine will demonstrate understanding of the questions.[24]

Prevention strategies

Clinicians can offer parents crisis prevention strategies to maintain low levels of behavior and reduce the likelihood of inadvertently reinforcing externalizing behavior. Some of these strategies include.

- Establish consistent and *predictable routines and schedules*; this helps the child understand demands and expectations, and predictability is an effective prevention tool for many autistic children.
- Encourage use of *visual schedules* to inform children of the schedule for the day. The schedule can include upcoming appointments, events, responsibilities, or routines. This increases predictability and supports learning preferences.
- Provide *advanced notice about transitioning* from a preferred to a non-preferred activity to reduce uncertainty and risk of challenging behaviors. This can be done by using visual schedules, countdowns, and/or a timer.
- Use a *calm and steady voice* to prevent escalation of behaviors and to model the behavior we want children to use.
- Keep the environment safe by *removing sharp/dangerous objects.*
- Make specific *positive comments* when the child responds to directions.
- Keep strongly *preferred items out of sight* to minimize conflicts (eg, iPads or preferred foods).
- *Connect* with family and advocacy resources to help navigate the complex world of schools and services.

Stage 2: Pre-crisis

Pre-crisis reflects a state where a child's behavior is escalating and becoming unmanageable. It may feel as if the child may escalate into a full-blown crisis within minutes or hours. During the pre-crisis stage, a child may become agitated, irritable, loud, aggressive, or self-injurious. The clinician's goals when the child is in a pre-crisis are to work collaboratively with parents to implement behavioral strategies and a crisis plan, and to prepare for potential crisis.

Depending on comfort and skill level, the clinician can also evaluate the root cause of the child's externalizing behavior. The etiology of externalizing behaviors is often multifactorial and includes underlying psychiatric disorders, medical conditions, and communication challenges, among other factors. McGuire and colleagues have published guidelines to systematically evaluate the underlying cause of irritability and externalizing behaviors in autistic individuals.[10] One key point that is emphasized in these guidelines is to always consider the possibility of an underlying medical etiology when a child's behaviors intensify. Constipation, respiratory infections, dental problems, and pain can all cause discomfort and trigger externalizing behavior. Treating these medical conditions could immediately reduce externalizing behaviors and prevent escalation to crisis. Clinical practice guidelines have also been developed to evaluate and treat underlying psychiatric disorders that could lead to externalizing behaviors, such as attention-deficit hyperactivity disorder and anxiety.[55,56] Effective treatment of these underlying psychiatric disorders may reduce the risk of pre-crisis and crisis behaviors.

Behavioral strategies that can be offered to parents during the pre-crisis stage include some strategies from the pre-crisis stage as well as new recommendations. These include.

- *Move the child* to a quieter, less stressful, safer space.
- *Identify calming objects* for the child such as a toy or stuffed animal; these items should be available across settings. These are objects that should not cause a conflict (eg, highly preferred electronics) and should be accessible when needed. Consider the child's sensory preferences when selecting these objects.
- *Reduce demands* that may trigger challenging behavior, and only place demands when there is a plan in place to address potential challenging behaviors.
- *Identify someone who can assist* with the child and help calm the situation. Whether it is a friend or family member, this person should feel comfortable with the child. They must also be helpful.
- *Seek or follow up* with mental health providers to assess and treat psychiatric and behavioral causes.
- *Prepare for a potential crisis* by identifying local resources, for example, local ED, urgent care. Crisis toolkits and guidelines can be found at https://www. autismspeaks.org/tool-kit-excerpt/planning-crisis and https://sparkforautism. org/discover_article/when-a-psychiatric-crisis-hits-children-with-autism-in-the-emergency-room/.

Stage 3: In Crisis

When assessing a child in crisis, the clinician's primary goal is to evaluate the child's risk for danger to self and others and create a crisis intervention plan. Part of this evaluation includes asking caregivers if they have the necessary resources to de-escalate the behaviors safely and efficaciously at home, school, and other settings. Based on this assessment, clinicians can develop a crisis plan, which may include calling 911 or going to the ED or a local urgent care center.

Crisis plans are developed with consideration of available resources, treatment options, and caregiver preferences. If the child is sent to the ED, calling in advance to notify the ED of the child's arrival and providing relevant history and strategies to make the visit more comfortable could improve the child and family's experience in the ED. Staying connected with the ED and inpatient teams can facilitate optimal care and plans for close follow-up upon discharge. During a crisis, providers can offer the following strategies to caregivers.

- *Stay calm* and use a neutral tone of voice.
- *Avoid long conversations* with the child.
- *Move the child* to a safe space without access to dangerous items.
- *Provide minimal demands.* Do not ask the child to complete activities during the crisis.
- *Follow the established crisis plan.* If the plan involves calling 911 or going to the ED, inform the providers that the child has autism and share information about effective calming strategies, mode of communication, sensory preferences, past triggers for pre-crisis or crisis behavior, and likes and dislikes.

Stage 4: Post-crisis

After a crisis has occurred, the clinician's goals are to debrief with the caregiver, revisit prevention plans, and encourage caregivers to maintain close follow-up with the primary care clinician and mental health providers. Some points to discuss.

- What *triggers* led to the crisis?
- What *approaches* were helpful, unhelpful, or were not used?
- Does the child *need additional services* to reduce the risk of crisis (eg, wrap around services)?

- *Is the child maintaining close follow-up* with mental health providers and working collaboratively with them to develop a treatment plan?
- Has a *crisis intervention plan* been developed, or does it need to be updated?

Crisis events can be traumatic for the child. Suggestions for caregivers to process the event with the child and restore calm include.

- *Re-connect* with the child (eg, doing a quiet, preferred activity together).
- If the child can participate in the conversation, *review what happened* (eg, gently ask what triggered the crisis, and what the child could do differently next time).
- Caregivers and providers can *actively listen*, acknowledge the child's feelings, and express empathy.

Summary

This article reviews the high rates of mental health crisis in autistic children. The authors provide epidemiologic service data showing that autistic children have high rates of ED and inpatient hospitalization for psychiatric and behavioral reasons. In terms of solutions, they present a novel measure, the MCAS-R, as a reliable, valid, and accurate screening tool for identifying autistic children in crisis. They also discuss efforts to improve the ED and inpatient experience, and highlight a community-based crisis intervention program, START, which has demonstrated promising outcomes. Finally, they present a new 4-stage framework for managing crises in autistic children and offer interventions at each stage. The authors hope these efforts and others will advance the care of autistic children in crisis.

CLINICS CARE POINTS

- Autistic children have high rates of psychiatric and behavioral conditions, which can potentially lead to a mental health crisis.
- Routine follow-up care is important to enable screening and early intervention of mental health conditions, though it can be challenging to access mental health services for autistic youth.
- Given the shortage of mental health providers for autistic children, primary care providers can assess where a child is in the crisis cycle and offer caregivers a set of behavioral strategies to help prevent escalation to a crisis.
- When a child's behavior is escalating, it is important for clinicians to assess and treat underlying causes of crisis, which sometimes can be due to a medical condition.
- When a crisis occurs, the top priority is to develop and implement a plan to ensure the child's safety.

DISCLOSURE

L. Kalb conducts research with and for the National Center for START Services at the Institute on Disability at the University of New Hampshire. He receives compensation for these efforts.

REFERENCES

1. Kerns CM, Rast JE, Shattuck PT. Prevalence and correlates of caregiver-reported mental health conditions in youth with autism spectrum disorder in the United States. J Clin Psychiatry 2021;82(1):11637.

2. Rast J, Roux AM, Anderson KA, et al. National Autism Indicators Report: Health and Health Care. Philadelphia, PA: A.J. Drexel Autism Institute, Drexel University; 2020. Life Course Outcomes Program.

3. Simonoff E, Pickles A, Charman T, et al. Psychiatric disorders in children with autism spectrum disorders: Prevalence, comorbidity, and associated factors in a population-derived sample. J Am Acad Child Adolesc Psychiatry 2008;47(8): 921–9.

4. Joshi G, Petty C, Wozniak J, et al. The heavy burden of psychiatric comorbidity in youth with autism spectrum disorders: A large comparative study of a psychiatrically referred population. J Autism Dev Disord 2010;40(11):1361–70.

5. Chen MH, Pan TL, Lan WH, et al. Risk of suicide attempts among adolescents and young adults with autism spectrum disorder. J Clin Psychiatry 2017;78(9): e1174–9.

6. Kõlves K, Fitzgerald C, Nordentoft M. Assessment of suicidal behaviors among individuals with autism spectrum disorder in Denmark. JAMA Netw Open 2021; 4(1):e2033565.

7. Kanne SM, Mazurek MO. Aggression in children and adolescents with ASD: prevalence and risk factors. J Autism Dev Disord 2011;41(7):926–37.

8. Steenfeldt-Kristensen C, Jones CA, Richards C. The prevalence of self-injurious behaviour in autism: A meta-analytic study. J Autism Dev Disord 2020;50: 3857–73.

9. Lipsky D, Richards W. Introduction. In: Managing meltdowns: using the S.C.A.R.E.D calming technique with children and adults with autism. London: Jessica Kingsley Publishers; 2009. p. 20. https://doi.org/10.1007/s10803-009-0909-y. Cited by: Mazefsky CA. Erratum to: Deborah Lipsky, Will Richards: Managing Meltdowns: Using the S.C.A.R.E.D Calming technique with Children and Adults with Autism. Journal of Autism and Developmental Disorders 2010;40:918.

10. McGuire K, Fung LK, Hagopian L, et al. Irritability and problem behavior in autism spectrum disorder: A practice pathway for pediatric primary care. Pediatrics 2016;137(Suppl 2):S136–48.

11. Kalb IG, Hagopian LP, Gross AL, et al. Psychometric characteristics of the mental health crisis assessment scale in youth with autism spectrum disorder. J Child Psychol Psychiatry 2017;59(1):48–56.

12. Allen M, Forster P, Zealberg J, et al. Report and recommendations regarding psychiatric emergency and crisis services. A review and model program descriptions. American Psychiatric Association; 2002.

13. Kalb LG, Stuart EA, Freedman B, et al. Psychiatric-related emergency department visits among children with an autism spectrum disorder. Pediatr Emerg Care 2012;28(12):1269–76.

14. Liu G, Pearl AM, Kong L, et al. A profile on emergency department utilization in adolescents and young adults with autism spectrum disorders. J Autism Dev Disord 2016;47(2):347–58.

15. Beverly J, Giannouchos T, Callaghan T. Examining frequent emergency department use among children and adolescents with autism spectrum disorder. Autism 2021;25(5):1382–4.

16. Wharff EA, Ginnis KB, Ross AM, et al. Predictors of psychiatric boarding in the pediatric emergency department: Implications for emergency care. Pediatr Emerg Care 2011;27(6):483–9.

17. Martini MI, Kuja-Halkola R, Butwicka A, et al. Sex differences in mental health problems and psychiatric hospitalization in autistic young adults. JAMA Psychiatr 2022;79(12):1188–98.

18. Nayfack AM, Huffman LC, Feldman HM, et al. Hospitalizations of children with autism increased from 1999 to 2009. J Autism Dev Disord 2014;44:1087–94.
19. Vasa RA, Hagopian L, Kalb LG. Investigating mental health crisis in youth with autism spectrum disorder. Autism Res 2019;13(1):112–21.
20. Kalb LG, DiBella F, Jang YS, et al. Mental health crisis screening in youth with autism spectrum disorder. J Clin Child Adolesc Psychol 2022. https://doi.org/10.1080/15374416.2022.2119984.
21. Dwyer P, Ryan JG, Williams ZJ, et al. First do no harm: Suggestions regarding respectful autism language. Pediatrics 2022;149(Supplement 4):e2020049437N.
22. Weiss JA, Wingsiong A, Lunsky Y. Defining crisis in families of individuals with autism spectrum disorders. Autism 2014;18(8):985–95.
23. Weiss JA, Lunsky Y. The Brief Family Distress Scale: A measure of crisis in caregivers of individuals with autism spectrum disorders. J Child Fam Stud 2011;20(4):521–8.
24. Rybczynski S, Taylor RC, Wilcox HC, et al. Suicide risk screening in pediatric outpatient neurodevelopmental disabilities clinics. J Dev Behav Pediatr 2022;43(4):181–7.
25. Schwartzman JM, Muscatello RA, Corbett BA. Assessing suicidal thoughts and behaviors and nonsuicidal self-injury in autistic and non-autistic early adolescents using the Columbia Suicide Severity Rating Scale. Autism 2023. https://doi.org/10.1177/13623613231162154. 13623613231162154.
26. Braddock DL, Parish SL. An Institutional History of Disability. In: Albrecht GL, Seelman KD, Bury M, editors. Handbook of disability studies. Thousand Oaks (CA): Sage Publications; 2001. p. 11–68.
27. Maenner MJ, Warren Z, Williams AR, et al. Prevalence and characteristics of autism spectrum disorder among children aged 8 years - Autism and Developmental Disabilities Monitoring Network, 11 Sites, United States, 2020. MMWR Surveill Summ 2023;72(No. SS-2):1–14.
28. Rast JE, Garfield T, Roux AM, et al. National autism Indicators report: mental health. Philadelphia, PA: A.J. Drexel Autism Institute, Drexel University; 2021. Life Course Outcomes Program.
29. Cantor J, McBain RK, Kofner A, et al. Fewer than half of US mental health treatment facilities provide services for children with autism spectrum disorder. Health Aff 2020;39(6):968–74.
30. Marrus N, Koth KA, Hellings JA, et al. Psychiatry training in autism spectrum disorder and intellectual disability: Ongoing gaps and emerging opportunities. Autism 2023;27(3):679–89.
31. Guerrero MGB, Sobotka SA. Understanding the barriers to receiving autism diagnoses for Hispanic and Latinx families. Pediatr Ann 2022;51(4):e167–71.
32. Suite DH, La Bril R, Primm A, et al. Beyond misdiagnosis, misunderstanding and mistrust: Relevance of the historical perspective in the medical and mental health treatment of people of color. J Natl Med Assoc 2007;99(8):879–85.
33. Mandell DS, Wiggins LD, Carpenter LA, et al. Racial/ethnic disparities in the identification of children with autism spectrum disorders. Am J Public Health 2009;99(3):493–8.
34. McBain RK, Kareddy V, Cantor JH, et al. Systematic review: United States workforce for autism-related child healthcare services. J Am Acad Child Adolesc Psychiatry 2020;59(1):113–39.
35. Brookman-Frazee L, Drahota A, Stadnick N, et al. Therapist perspectives on community mental health services for children with autism spectrum disorders. Adm Policy Ment Health 2012;39(5):365–73.

36. Roestorf A, Howlin P, Bowler DM. Ageing and autism: A longitudinal follow-up study of mental health and quality of life in autistic adults. Front Psychol 2022; 13:741213.

37. Yeh TC, Chen Mu Hong, Bai YM, et al. Longitudinal follow-up of subsequent psychiatric comorbidities among children and adolescents with autism spectrum disorder. J Affect Disord 2023;331:245–50.

38. Liu G, Velott DL, Kong L, et al. The association of the Medicaid 1915(c) home and community-based services waivers with emergency department utilization among youth with autism spectrum disorder. J Autism Dev Disord 2022;52(4): 1587–97.

39. Wood EB, Halverson A, Harrison G, et al. Creating a sensory-friendly pediatric emergency department. J Emerg Nurs 2019;45(4):415–24.

40. Ailey SH, Johnson TJ, Cabrera A. Evaluation of factors related to prolonged lengths of stay for patients with autism with or without intellectual disability. J Psychosoc Nurs Ment Health Serv 2019;57(7):17–22.

41. Siegel M, Milligan B, Chemelski B, et al. Specialized inpatient psychiatry for serious behavioral disturbance in autism and intellectual disability. J Autism Dev Disord 2014;44(12):3026–32.

42. Pedersen KA, Santangelo SL, Gabriels RL, et al. Behavioral outcomes of specialized psychiatric hospitalization in the autism inpatient collection (AIC): A multisite comparison. J Autism Dev Disord 2018;48(11):3658–67.

43. Siegel M, Doyle K, Chemelski B, et al. Specialized inpatient psychiatry units for children with autism and developmental disorders: A United States survey. J Autism Dev Disord 2012;42(9):1863–9.

44. Gabriels RL, Agnew JA, Beresford C, et al. Improving psychiatric hospital care for pediatric patients with autism spectrum disorders and intellectual disabilities. Autism Res Treat 2012;2012:685053.

45. McGuire K, Erickson C, Gabriels RL, et al. Psychiatric hospitalization of children with autism or intellectual disability: Consensus statements on best practices. J Am Acad Child Adolesc Psychiatry 2015;54(12):969–71.

46. Cervantes P, Kuriakose S, Donnelly L, et al. Sustainability of a care pathway for children and adolescents with autism spectrum disorder on an inpatient psychiatric service. J Autism Dev Disord 2019;49(8):3173–80.

47. Kuriakose S, Filton B, Marr M, et al. Does an autism spectrum disorder care pathway improve care for children and adolescents with ASD in inpatient psychiatric units? J Autism Dev Disord 2018;48(12):4082–9.

48. Beasley JB, Kalb L, Klein A. Improving mental health outcomes for individuals with intellectual disability through the Iowa START (I-START) Program. J Ment Health Res Intellect Disabil 2018;11(4):287–300.

49. Kalb LG, Beasley J, Caoili A, et al. Improvement in mental health outcomes and caregiver service experiences associated with the START Program. Am J Intellect Dev Disabil 2019;124(1):25–34.

50. Fleisig N. Professional crisis management: practitioner manual. Sunrise, FL: Professional Crisis Management Association; 2022.

51. Strickland-Cohen MK, Newson A, Meyer K, et al. Strategies for de-escalating student behavior in the classroom. Portland, OR: Center on PBIS, University of Oregon; 2022.

52. Kalb L, Sollins E, Horton J, et al. Autism crisis prevention workbooks. Baltimore, MD: Kennedy Krieger Institute; 2022.

53. Scahill L, Bearss K, Lecavalier L, et al. Effect of parent training on adaptive behavior in children with autism spectrum disorder and disruptive behavior:

Results of a randomized trial. J Am Acad Child Adolesc Psychiatry 2016;55(7): 602–9.e3.

54. Achenbach TM. The Child Behavior Checklist and related instruments. In: Maruish ME, editor. The use of psychological testing for treatment planning and outcomes assessment. 2nd edition. Lawrence Erlbaum Associates Publishers; 1999. p. 429–66.

55. Mahajan R, Bernal MP, Panzer R, et al. Clinical practice pathways for evaluation and medication choice for attention-deficit/hyperactivity disorder symptoms in autism spectrum disorders. Pediatrics 2012;130(Suppl 2):S125–38.

56. Vasa RA, Mazurek MO, Mahajan R, et al. Assessment and treatment of anxiety in youth with autism spectrum disorders. Pediatrics 2016;137(Suppl 2):S115–23.

Psychopharmacology Management in Autism Spectrum Disorder

Jay A. Salpekar, MD[a],*, Lawrence Scahill, MSN, PhD[b]

KEYWORDS

- Autism • Autism spectrum disorder • Psychopharmacology • Treatment
- Clinical trial • Antipsychotic • Behavior • Neuropsychiatry

KEY POINTS

- Autism spectrum disorder (ASD) may include symptoms that are intrinsic to the disorder such as repetitive behavior and symptoms that are not intrinsic such as hyperactivity, disruptive behavior, anxiety, or insomnia but may cause marked distress or impairment.
- Repetitive behavior and these co-occurring problems in ASD may be amenable to medical (pharmacologic) or nonmedical (psychotherapeutic or structural behavioral) treatments.
- Many different classes of medicines including antipsychotics, antiseizure medicines, antidepressants, and stimulant medicines may be effective for symptomatic relief.

INTRODUCTION

Autism spectrum disorder (ASD; autism) is a heterogenous condition that varies in symptom severity and is often accompanied by a range of behavioral problems. The common thread for diagnostic purposes is a persistent pattern of atypical development and characterized by several defining symptoms. Practically, the diagnosis of ASD in children is made through clinical assessment supported by parent-reported rating scales, structured interviews, and direct assessment of the child. As discussed in other articles in this volume, stereotyped behaviors or movements, restricted range of interests, idiosyncratic language patterns, altered social connectedness, or sensory sensitivities are the core elements of ASD.[1] Across these symptom domains, however, there is wide variability and a wide range of functional capacity. Indeed, autism-like phenotypes may be present even in individuals who are functional or even successful by common parlance of society.

Targets for pharmacology treatment focus on symptom clusters that compromise function rather than categorical diagnostic criteria. Some target symptoms reflect

a Neuropsychiatry Center, Kennedy Krieger Institute, Johns Hopkins University School of Medicine, 1741 Ashland Avenue, Baltimore, MD 21205, USA; b Emory University School of Medicine, Marcus Autism Center, 1920 Briarcliff Road, Atlanta, GA 30329, USA
* Corresponding author.
E-mail address: salpekar@kennedykrieger.org

Pediatr Clin N Am 71 (2024) 283–299
https://doi.org/10.1016/j.pcl.2023.12.001
0031-3955/24/© 2023 Elsevier Inc. All rights reserved.

pediatric.theclinics.com

constituent aspects of autism. In many cases, however, the targets focus on co-occurring symptoms such as hyperactivity, irritability, anxiety, or depression. These co-occurring symptoms may add to overall impairment and may warrant intervention. ASD is not protective for psychiatric illness and may in fact increase the likelihood of some psychiatric disorders. In many cases, isolation of symptoms from integral symptoms of ASD can be challenging. As a practical consideration, psychopharmacological approaches for individuals with ASD may be similar to those without ASD. Symptomatic relief may improve function and quality of life whether or not an ASD diagnosis can be confidently established. In this review, available evidence will be discussed but where evidence is lacking, practical considerations will be emphasized.

THEROETICAL UNDERPINNINGS OF AUTISM SPECTRUM DISORDER APPLICABLE TO PSYCHOPHARMACOLOGIC APPROACHES TO TREATMENT

ASD is, by definition, a condition of early onset. Atypical brain development and growth in infancy and in utero is commonly presumed. There is evidence of increased cortical thickness, as well as increased head circumference.[2] Atypical neuronal development may result in anomalous connectivity, which presumably involves cortical connections, as well as subcortical ones.[3] Subcortical structures such as the caudate nucleus may play a role in behavioral inhibition. Dysfunction in that network may result in disinhibition or impulsive behavior, which may be targets for psychopharmacology.[4]

Some theorize that a cortical/subcortical or thalamocortical resonance play a role in anomalous connectivity.[5] Altered regional connectivity is also considered pertinent for seizure pathophysiology. In epilepsy, electrical voltage gradients may be awry and important in seizure propagation. Given that epilepsy is overrepresented in ASD, processes that involve anomalous connectivity may be relevant.[6]

Along those same lines, others have theorized that autism is a disorder of neuronal hyperexcitability.[7] Hyperexcitability is presumed to result from increased signaling of glutamate, which is an excitatory neurotransmitter.[8] This increase is speculated to yield increased synaptic connectivity and may be indirectly related to sensory sensitivities in ASD. In experimental animal models, the excess glutamatergic activity implies atypical processing of sensory input and possibly altered capacity for sensory reception.[8] Many children with autism become overwhelmed in environments with high sensory stimuli, for example, they may overreact to specific smells, sounds, or exhibit extreme responses to tactile stimuli (eg, tags on clothing and seams on socks). These sensory sensitivities may be due to increased neuronal processing of sensory information. Neuronal hyperexcitability, along with anomalous connectivity, may partially explain the overlap between seizure disorders and ASD.[9] The fact that antiseizure medicines (ASMs) often target glutamatergic neurons provides a rationale for using this class of drugs in ASD.

APPROACH TO PSYCHOPHARMACOLOGY

Despite the proven efficacy of some medications in children and adolescents with ASD, nonpharmacological treatments (eg, function-based behavioral intervention) may also be effective for symptom control. A psychopharmacological treatment may target tantrums or aggression. However, careful consideration of the event or situation that precedes tantrums or aggression can provide insight that may inform behavioral intervention as a first-line treatment strategy or in combination with medication.

The field of Applied Behavior Analysis proposes that maladaptive behavior often serves a purpose for the child and that environmental response may reinforce the behavior.

Reactive outbursts may occur in response to routine environmental demands. For example, when a child is engaged in a preferred activity (eg, playing games on a tablet computer), a temper outburst may occur when the child is directed to switch to a nonpreferred activity (eg, getting ready for bed). Understandably, to prevent an outburst, a parent may withdraw the routine demand and let the child continue with the preferred activity. In this scenario, the outburst is not spontaneous. The child may learn that tantrums result in escape from the routine environmental demand. Thus, the tantrum is context dependent, and the purpose (ie, the function) of the behavior is to escape from a routine demand. Behavioral techniques to manage the antecedent (the context) and the reinforcement (not allowing escape) may avert the need for medication. Even so, medication may still be considered in order to decrease the rapidity and severity of reactive outbursts.

In some cases, however, tantrums, aggressive outbursts, or self-injurious behaviors occur with no clear external antecedent, and may be somehow self-reinforcing. In such cases, the behavior may be repetitive in nature or driven by an intrinsic physiologic disturbance. Medication could be useful in addressing impulse control or emotion dysregulation. Note that even if an outburst is spontaneous, it may be mild and medication may not be necessary. A medication decision flow chart is presented in **Fig. 1**.

APPROACH TO IDENTIFYING TARGET SYMPTOMS FOR TREATMENT IN AUTISM SPECTRUM DISORDER

Alleviating targeted symptoms is the goal for pharmacologic treatments. However, in ASD, confidently identifying symptoms amenable to pharmacotherapy may be challenging. Many patients are nonverbal or have limited ways to express emotional states. The decision on whether to use medication or not is tied to the process of identifying a symptom target and then selecting a medication for that target. Although an algorithmic approach

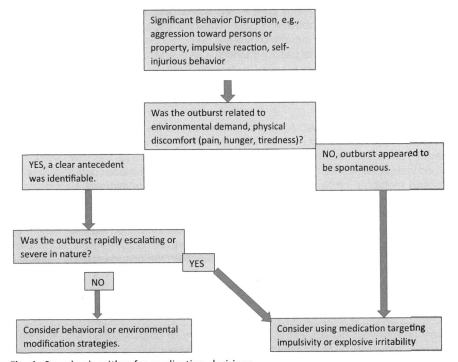

Fig. 1. Sample algorithm for medication decisions.

may be reassuring, many patients present with interwoven problems that elude stepwise decision-making processes. Illustrative examples are presented as follows:

CASE 1: Jimmy

Jimmy is a 14-year-old boy with ASD. He has become increasingly difficult to manage with worsening verbal and physical outbursts during the past year. In the past 3 months, outbursts have occurred several times a day. Minor outbursts include loud protests in response to routine requests, for example, "Turn off the phone and come to dinner." A few times a week, protests escalate to throwing objects and physically pushing parents, although without causing injury. However, as he has grown in physical size and strength, it is more difficult to redirect him physically. His parents sought consultation with their pediatrician due to the increased frequency of outbursts that occur during transitions from one activity to the next. After incomplete response to behavioral approaches, a medication trial was recommended.

Jimmy's parents report that he is not isolating himself or having crying spells, thus his outbursts do not seem to be driven by anxiety. Although not completely ruled out, this information deemphasizes an anxiety or mood problem. Jimmy's parents describe the situation as volatile. He seems generally irritable and unable to manage his emotions. The steady increase in the frequency and the trend toward aggression and property destruction cause parents to be on edge. The target symptom would be the combination of tantrums with aggression.

Aggression

Aggressive outbursts may be the most common reason for use of medication in youth with ASD. The core of aggressive outbursts is a problem of impulse control. Impulsiveness reflects impaired capacity to delay between intention and action and may be due to poor intrinsic inhibitory neural control. Aggressive outbursts may also be described as outwardly directed (to obtain an object of interest, escape a routine demand, or for attention). To be sure, poor impulse control and outbursts that serve a purpose (acquiring a tangible object, escape, or gaining attention) can overlap. Measures of aggression or irritability include the Open Source-Challenging Behavior Scale[10] and the Aberrant Behavior Checklist (ABC).[11] A variety of medications may target impulsiveness and aggression, including mood stabilizers, second-generation antipsychotics, lithium, alpha agonists, and stimulants.[12]

For Jimmy, the pediatrician decided to initiate treatment with risperidone 0.5 mg every morning because he did not seem to have hyperactivity or impulsivity that would suggest use of a stimulant. He asked the caregivers to complete an ABC at baseline. Jimmy had blood tests in the past that showed normal ranges for complete blood count and comprehensive metabolic profile. Some clinicians recommend a pretreatment electrocardiogram to check for prolonged Q-T interval on an electrocardiogram (QTc) and a lipid profile—mindful that in some cases, increases in triglycerides and cholesterol can occur.[13,14] Height and weight should be measured before and during treatment. If no improvement occurs in the first week or two, and there are no dose-limiting adverse effects (sedation and excessive appetite increase), then the dosage may be increased weekly by 0.5 mg increments during the first 4 to 6 weeks of treatment. The usual dose for a teenager is about 2 mg/d in 2 divided doses.

CASE 2: Mary

Mary is a 12-year-old girl with ASD and a history of preoccupation with women's fashion, rereading fashion magazines and excessively talking about topics related to her preoccupation. On occasion, she gets upset if she is interrupted in her rereading or repetitive comments. During the past 6 months, she has increasingly isolated herself, declined to go to public places that she used to enjoy—such as the mall—saying that it made her uneasy. She exclaimed that things were not going well for her and frequently asked for reassurance that things will be ok. The pediatrician faced a dilemma of targeting the long-standing repetitive behavior or the emergence of anxiety and depression.

Repetitive behavior

Repetitive behavior in ASD may include a wide range of motor behavior (stereotyped movements, pacing), or preoccupation with a circumscribed interest (rereading a store catalog, watching the same video repeatedly, and lining up objects). The classic symptoms of obsessive-compulsive disorder (OCD) such as fears of contamination and washing rituals may also be present but are not present in Mary's case. Indeed, the stereotyped movements and circumscribed interests are constituent parts of ASD and phenomenologically separate from OCD. Evidence from pharmacologic studies also suggests that repetitive behavior in ASD and OCD are mechanistically separate. For example, some selective serotonin reuptake inhibitors (SSRIs) have Food and Drug Administration (FDA) approval and are often effective in OCD but the SSRI citalopram was not found to be effective for repetitive behavior in ASD.[15] In a secondary analysis of federally funded risperidone trials, Scahill and colleagues reported that this second-generation antipsychotic was effective for reducing repetitive behavior in youth with ASD.[16] However, the use of risperidone for repetitive behaviors would not be appropriate unless that particular behavior significantly interfered with function.

In Mary's case, the pediatrician considered the repetitive behavior as a target symptom but then assessed the depression and anxiety to be more salient. The appropriate treatment to target the combination of depression and anxiety was the SSRI, fluoxetine, at 5 mg every morning. Common adverse effects include nausea, stomach upset, hyperactivity (behavioral activation), and insomnia. Fluoxetine has a long half-life, so the dose was maintained for 4 weeks without change. For younger children, dosing may occur at even lower levels with a liquid preparation. Most children and adolescents will have an adequate response to 5 to 10 mg daily, although higher doses up to 40 mg may be needed for some patients.

CASE 3: Teddy

Teddy is a 7-year-old boy with ASD. He attends a special education program in a public school with mostly good results owing to the high level of supervision and tailored educational curriculum. He has a history of overactivity and reckless behavior such as climbing on furniture and jumping off. His parents report that he requires close supervision to limit his impulsive behavior. They keep the front door locked to prevent him from eloping out of the house. He cannot sit through dinner, instead taking a few bites and then again moving around the house. Despite the highly structured program at school, teachers report that since the start of this school year, he is often up out of his chair and wandering around the classroom. He cannot sit through small group time and needs one-on-one guidance to stay on task. He is redirectable but within a few minutes will get up and wander around the room again. He is not in any emotional distress, although sometimes is frustrated when redirected. At school, he has difficulty completing academic tasks and often refuses to participate. The family's pediatrician knew the history. When she heard about the current situation, she targeted hyperactivity.

Hyperactivity

Hyperactivity is a cardinal feature of attention deficit hyperactivity disorder (ADHD). As in children with ADHD, increased psychomotor activity may reflect sensory seeking activity in children with ASD. ADHD is a common childhood psychiatric condition and children with ASD appear to be at elevated risk for ADHD.[17] Agents used for hyperactivity in ASD include stimulants, alpha-adrenergic agents, and atomoxetine.

For Teddy, the pediatrician considered that his presentation was consistent with ADHD, and started methylphenidate extended release 10 mg every morning. Common adverse effects include decreased appetite, mood lability, or sleep disturbance. In children with ASD, there may be an increase in repetitive behavior.[18] Improvement is often apparent within the first week or two of treatment. The alpha-2 agonist, guanfacine, is another option. The extended-release preparation of guanfacine is FDA approved for the treatment of ADHD and has been studied in children with ASD and hyperactivity.[19] In that study, doses up to 3 mg/d were well tolerated. Adverse events included change in appetite, mood lability, fatigue, and midsleep waking.

Anxiety or mood symptoms

Individuals with ASD are vulnerable to depression or anxiety disorders. Findings from several studies have shown that the prevalence of anxiety disorders in youth and adults with ASD is higher than the general population.[20] Disentangling anxiety symptoms from features of ASD may be difficult. Clear communication of emotional states may be challenging for youth with ASD with impaired communication so parent ratings may be essential.[21] Social avoidance in ASD may be difficult to differentiate from social anxiety. Limited studies have been done studying treatment of mood disorders in ASD but most approaches involve use of psychotherapy and/or serotonergic antidepressant medicines.

Insomnia

Sleep dysregulation may be a challenging problem for children with ASD and their caregivers.[22] Sleep difficulties such as problems falling asleep or maintaining sleep are common reasons for neuropsychiatric consultation. Sleep architecture may be altered at baseline for those with ASD, which may add to the difficulty in assessment and treatment.[23] Sleep hygiene efforts or melatonin may be useful strategies to improve sleep onset. Sedating antidepressants, such as trazodone or mirtazapine, antihistamines, such as hydroxyzine or diphenhydramine, and the alpha-adrenergic clonidine are used in practice. However, the evidence to support the efficacy of these medications is extremely limited. Anecdotal information suggests that pharmacologic strategies often need to change when efficacy wanes regardless of the treatment used.

CLASSES OF MEDICINES COMMONLY USED

The evidence base for pharmacologic treatment of persons with ASD is improving but remains limited. This is especially true for the use of more than one medication. Clinicians routinely conduct medication management in the absence of empirically supported medication strategies. To date, only 2 medications, risperidone and aripiprazole, are FDA-approved for youth with ASD. These antipsychotic medications are approved for the treatment of irritability, not for core features of ASD. Several randomized, placebo-controlled trials have been done in recent years sponsored by industry or with federal funding and are detailed in **Tables 1–3**. Although most trials have been aimed at symptom targets described earlier, others have tested medications for core features of autism. For clinicians, practical and deliberate treatment

Table 1
Studies of antiseizure medicines targeting behavior difficulties in autism spectrum disorder

Medication	Study Report	Study Design	Outcome Measures	Results	Comments
Divalproex sodium	Hollander et al,[24] 2010	12 wk, RCT, placebo crossover, N = 27 (age 5–15 y)	CGI-I, ABC-I	Reduction in irritability in 62% treated vs 9% placebo	Irritability worsened in some cases
Valproate	Hellings et al,[25] 2005	8 wk, RCT, placebo crossover, N = 30 (age 6–20 y)	CGI-I, ABC	No effect on aggression or irritability	Mild weight gain and fatigue
Levetiracetam	Wasserman et al,[26] 2006	10 wk, RCT, placebo crossover, N = 20 (age 5–17 y)	CGI-I, ABC-I, CY-BOCS	No benefit for irritability or repetitive behaviors	Aggression and agitation worsened
Lamotrigine	Belsito et al,[27] 2001	18 wk RCT parallel, placebo, N = 28 (age 3–11 y)	ABC, Vineland	No improvement	Insomnia worse
Topiramate	Rezaei et al,[28] 2010	8 wk, RCT, added to risperidone, N = 40 (ages 4–12 y)	ABC	Reduction in stereotyped behavior and hyperactivity	Mild sedation and decreased appetite

Abbreviations: ABC, aberrant behavior checklist; ABC-I, aberrant behavior checklist—irritability subscale; CGI-I, clinical global impression-improvement; CY-BOCS, Children's Yale Brown Obsessive Compulsive Scale; RCT, randomized controlled trial.

Table 2
Randomized controlled trials of antipsychotics in autism spectrum disorder

Medication	Study Report	Study Design	Outcome Measures	Results	Comments
Risperidone	RUPP 2002[14]	8 wk, RCT, parallel placebo. N = 101 (age 5–17 y)	ABC, CGI-I	Reduced irritability on ABC and 75% improvement on CGI-I	Weight gain
Risperidone	Aman et al,[33] 2009; Scahill et al,[34,35] 2012	24 wk, RCT, RISP only vs RISP plus parent training. N = 124 (age 4–13 y)	ABC-I, Vineland, Adaptive Scales	RISP + PT superior to RISP only on ABC Irritability and Vineland	Parent training provide added benefits on daily living skills
Aripiprazole	Owen et al,[36] 2009	8 wk, RCT parallel, placebo. N = 98 (age 6–17 y)	ABC-I, CGI-I	Reduced ABC-Irritability, 52% improvement on CGI-I	Fatigue, weight gain, and tremors
Aripiprazole	Marcus et al,[37] 2009	8 wk, RCT parallel, fixed dose, placebo. N = 218 (age 6–17 y)	ABC, CGI-I,	Reduced ABC-Irritability, 50% improvement on CGI-I	Sedation common
Olanzapine	Hollander et al,[38] 2006	8 wk, RCT, placebo, N = 11 (age 6–14 y)	CGI-I, CY-BOCS	Improvement in CGI-I	Weight gain
Lurasidone	Loebel et al,[39] 2016	6 wk, RCT parallel, fixed dose, placebo. N = 150 (age 6–17 y)	ABC, CGI-I, CY-BOCS	No difference from placebo on ABC Irritability	Nausea and vomiting notable

Abbreviations: ABC, aberrant behavior checklist; ABC-I, aberrant behavior checklist—irritability subscale; CGI-I, clinical global impression-improvement; CY-BOCS, Children's Yale Brown Obsessive Compulsive Scale; PT, parent training; RCT, randomized controlled trial; RISP, risperidone; RUPP, research units on pediatric psychopharmacology.

Table 3
Studies of medicines used for attention deficit hyperactivity disorder in autism spectrum disorder

Medication	Study Report	Study Design	Outcome Measures	Results	Comments
Methylphenidate Immediate release	RUPP 2005[18]	4 wk, RCT, crossover, N = 66 (age 3–7 y)	CGI-I, ABC-hyperactivity	Improved hyperactivity	Adverse effects were dose related
Methylphenidate extended release plus methylphenidate immediate release	Pearson et al,[55] 2013	4 wk, RCT, crossover, N = 24 (age 7–13 y), high dose vs low dose	CGI-I	Improved ADHD symptoms at each dose level, more at higher doses	Stereotypies not exacerbated
Atomoxetine	Handen et al 2015[54,56]	10 wk, RCT, parallel, placebo, N = 128 (age 6–16 y)	SNAP-IV, CGI-I	47% vs 19% response rate	Less well tolerated than expected
Guanfacine, extended release	Scahill et al,[19] 2015 Politte et al,[57] 2018	8 wk, RCT, parallel, placebo, N = 62 (age 5–12 y)	ABC, CGI-I	Improved hyperactivity, on CGI-I 50% + response vs 9% placebo	Most common AE: sedation

Abbreviations: ABC, aberrant behavior checklist; ABC-I, aberrant behavior checklist—irritability subscale; CGI-I, clinical global impression-improvement; RCT, randomized controlled trial; RUPP, research units on pediatric psychopharmacology; SNAP-IV, Swanson, Nolan, and Pelham Scale, version 4.

choices have to be made. Prescribing cautiously, with low dosages and slow upward adjustment, is often the most appropriate strategy. In addition to the documented adverse events possible with any given medication, youth with ASD may have paradoxic reactions to medicines that require careful monitoring. Finally, with the exception of risperidone and aripiprazole, medication use, even medications with empirical support in ASD in children, are not FDA approved and are *off label*.

Antiseizure Medicines

ASMs include a wide range of what were previously referred to as antiepileptic or anticonvulsant drugs. Use of ASMs in ASD seems worth considering given the although speculative but theorized shared intrinsic hyperexcitability. ASMs have also been proven to be effective for managing manic episodes or as adjunctive treatment of major depressive episode in patients without ASD. ASMs may be useful for treating mood symptoms in ASD.

Mechanisms of ASMs vary. Some directly affect sodium or calcium ion channels. Other ASMs activate inhibitory gamma aminobutyric acid-ergic receptors. Although not empirically tested thus far, enhancing inhibitory networks may be a useful strategy for reducing spontaneous outbursts and impulsivity. Finally, many widely used ASMs have multiple or unknown mechanisms. To date, no clinical trials have directly targeted core features of ASD. Studies of ASMs in ASD are listed in **Table 1**.

Antipsychotics

Antipsychotics have been used to address aggressive outbursts in individuals with ASD for 50 years. In early studies, autism was defined as an uncommon and uniformly severe condition. Study samples may have included participants with autism, other developmental disabilities, or what was called childhood schizophrenia.[29,30] The long history of using these medicines served as the impetus to develop some of the most sophisticated clinical trials for ASD that have ever been done. The Research Units on Pediatric Psychopharmacology have provided large scale, multisite, placebo-controlled randomized clinical trial data on usage of 2 medicines, risperidone and aripiprazole, to address aggression and irritability in autism.[31,32] Both of those medicines have FDA indications for irritability associated with autism in pediatric age groups. Other antipsychotics have been attempted in persons with ASD, although not with the level of sophistication of the research units on pediatric psychopharmacology (RUPP) studies. Studies of antipsychotics in ASD are listed in **Table 2**.

Antidepressants

Clinicians in the autism field viewed the entry of the SSRIs in the 1990s with great interest. Although these serotonergic antidepressants are effective treatments of OCD, repetitive behaviors in youth with ASD may not reflect ego dystonic obsessions and compulsions fueled by anxiety. As noted above, repetitive behavior in ASD may include stereotypies, or preoccupation with circumscribed interests that a person with ASD may actually enjoy.

Several antidepressants are approved in pediatrics for the treatment of major depression and some anxiety disorders. Based on these approvals, clinicians often treat autistic children and adults with depression or anxiety disorders with SSRIs. The diagnosis of depression or anxiety disorders may be more difficult in ASD due to decreased capacity for verbal expression of self-perceived mood states. For children or adults with ASD who have decreased verbal capacity, clinicians rely on family members and reports of change in the autistic person's mood and functioning. This same challenge exists when evaluating change with treatment.

Several antidepressants, mostly SSRIs, have been studied in youth without ASD targeting depression, anxiety disorders, or OCD. Although several compounds have shown superiority to placebo across these conditions, the magnitude of effect is often modest.[40] A randomized placebo-controlled crossover trial with liquid fluoxetine was conducted with 39 participants aged 5 to 17 years. At a relatively low dose (mean final dose: 9.9 ± 4.35 mg/d), fluoxetine was superior to placebo for repetitive behaviors as measured by the CY-BOCS.[41] The crossover design, however, makes drawing conclusions about efficacy difficult. A placebo-controlled study with 149 participants during 12 weeks found that citalopram was not effective in reducing repetitive behaviors.[15] Sertraline has also been studied in pediatrics, although the pivotal trials for labeling purposes focused on obsessive compulsive disorder. Although the findings were positive, sertraline for depression or anxiety in pediatrics may still considered technically off-label.[42,43] An open label study of escitalopram in 28 children showed improvements in irritability on one rating scale but dose-related adverse effects were prominent. The adverse effects included irritability and hyperactivity.[44]

Antianxiety Medicines

Antidepressants are also first-line treatments of anxiety. Other medicines used in the treatment of anxiety include buspirone and benzodiazepines. Two randomized placebo-controlled trials with buspirone in children with ASD had mixed results.[45,46] Benzodiazepines, such as lorazepam, are commonly used as needed rather than as a standing dose. Adverse effects such as paradoxic hyperactivity in ASD often preclude routine usage. In practice, benzodiazepines are used for catatonia, which can occur in youth or adults with ASD.[47,48]

Stimulants and Adrenergic Agents

Stimulants have a long-standing history of effectiveness in the treatment of ADHD in children without ASD.[49] Because hyperactivity and impulsiveness are common in children with ASD, stimulants are commonly used in this population. The Research Units on Pediatric Psychopharmacology group conducted a multiple dose, placebo-controlled study of immediate release methylphenidate in children with ASD with high levels of hyperactivity and impulsiveness.[18] In that 4-change, crossover study, children were assigned to low, medium, or high-dose methylphenidate or placebo in random order for 4 weeks (1 week in each condition). Methylphenidate was superior to placebo. However, the effect size was lower in magnitude compared with the methylphenidate trial in children with ADHD but without ASD. In addition, adverse effects were common and dose related. The findings suggest that methylphenidate can be effective for the treatment of ADHD in children with ASD but the magnitude of improvement is lower and adverse effects may limit dose escalation. For practical purposes, clinicians should consider using lower doses of methylphenidate and carefully assess tolerability and response early in the treatment course.

Heightened autonomic nervous system activity may play a role in hyperactivity and insomnia in youth with ASD. Available evidence indicates that alpha-2 agonists, guanfacine and clonidine, are effective for ADHD. These agents are also used in the management of initial insomnia. Based on the reduction of sympathetic activity, guanfacine has also been used to manage posttraumatic stress disorder in children and adults.[50,51] Guanfacine has also been shown to be effective for the treatment of ADHD symptoms in children with tic disorders.[52] In a placebo-controlled trial with an average dose of 3 mg/d in 62 children with ASD, extended release guanfacine showed improvements in hyperactivity.[19] Treatment emergent side effects included fatigue, decreased appetite, and midsleep awakening. Effects on blood pressure were negligible and there were no electrocardiogram changes in either group.[19]

Atomoxetine is a specific norepinephrine reuptake inhibitor that is approved for the treatment of ADHD. Advantages include fewer apparent risks of cardiac arrythmias as compared with tricyclic antidepressants. Results tend to be mixed with a high placebo response rate.[53] Several randomized trials provide information on the use of atomoxetine in children with ASD, including one large trial that included parent training although found that response rates were higher with active atomoxetine regardless of parent training.[54]

Details of selected clinical trials of ADHD medicines in ASD are in **Table 3**.

Additional Medicines

A variety of other compounds have been studied in autism. A recent comprehensive meta-analysis of 45 randomized controlled trials in ASD noted a high risk of study bias in approximately a quarter of the studies reviewed. Sources of bias include whether investigators were blind to the random allocation sequence, whether blindness of treatment assignment was maintained, and whether the analysis followed intention-to-treat analysis.[58]

A large body of evidence from preclinical studies identified the role of the peptide, oxytocin, in pair bonding and social affiliation. These findings sparked interest in oxytocin as a candidate for enhancing social interest and behavior in autism. Several small studies followed, although most had equivocal results. A National Institute of Health funded study evaluated intranasal oxytocin versus placebo in 290 participants with ASD (age 3–17 years).[59] The primary outcome measure of the 24-week study was a modified version of the Aberrant Behavior Checklist—Social Withdrawal scale. The drug was well tolerated but there was no difference between oxytocin and placebo on the primary or secondary outcomes.

Naltrexone has been examined in clinical trials going back many years. As an opioid receptor antagonist, there has been interest in the possibility that naltrexone could reduce the reinforcing effect of self-injurious behavior in particular. Most studies had small samples and mixed results.[60] One study that included 41 subjects showed some improvement in hyperactivity but only modest effects on self-injurious behaviors were noted.[61]

Amantadine is an N-methyl-D-aspartate (NMDA) receptor antagonist. It also increases dopaminergic activity and has been used in the treatment of Parkinson disease. It has also been used for epilepsy and has some efficacy for recovery from traumatic brain injury.[62,63] King and colleagues conducted a placebo-controlled trial of amantadine (5 mg/kg/d) in 39 children with ASD targeting hyperactivity and irritability.[64] The study showed no significant group differences. In a randomized controlled trial of amantadine in 40 children, it was added to risperidone and compared to risperidone with placebo. The combined treatment group showed greater improvement on the ABC-Irritability scale than the risperidone only group.[65] Memantine is another NMDA receptor antagonist that is approved for the treatment of dementia. A Cochran review of available studies in ASD indicated small effect sizes for language and memory suggesting limited benefit.[66]

Cannabinoids are often discussed in clinical settings for various target symptoms in ASD. The popular press often expounds on purported medical benefits of cannabidiol as well as other cannabinoid products. Some survey results from the lay public suggest that mood and sleep may improve with cannabinoids.[67] To date, however, high-quality clinical trials in ASD have not been conducted. A pharmaceutical grade cannabidiol agent is approved for the treatment of seizures in Lennox-Gastaut syndrome, Tuberous Sclerosis Complex, and Dravet syndrome. Efficacy may also be present for psychiatric symptoms that are present in other conditions such as Sturge Weber Syndrome, which overlaps with ASD and epilepsy in many cases.[68]

REFERRAL TO SPECIALISTS

It is plausible for a primary care pediatrician to initiate a psychopharmacologic treatment plan and assess initial results. Pediatricians are often familiar with stimulants and antidepressants, and in recent years, some have gained acumen with many antipsychotics as well. If initial treatment responses with one medication are unsatisfactory, then increasing dosages is appropriate so long as tolerability is not compromised. An attempt with a second medicine either in the same class or in a different class that may address the same target symptom is also a reasonable approach to treatment. However, referral to a child psychiatrist or developmental pediatrician may be appropriate if initial treatment efforts prove to be ineffective. A specialist may offer opinions about treatment or even establish treatment with a new agent and then refer back to the primary care provider for treatment maintenance.

SUMMARY

ASD is a heterogeneous condition so a unifying approach to psychopharmacology treatment may be very difficult to elucidate. Symptom targets are still an essential way to design a treatment strategy and may be best used as a complement to nonpharmacologic strategies. Even though risperidone and aripiprazole have FDA indications for irritability associated with ASD, other medicines may also be effective. Associated conditions such as epilepsy or mood and anxiety disorders may suggest that other treatments could be used. As treatment targets become better specified and perhaps connected to genetic anomalies that may underlie pathophysiology, medication regimens will become more sophisticated. In the meantime, an increasing evidence base may allow psychopharmacology treatment decisions to be more rationally made with pragmatic goals in mind.

CLINICS CARE POINTS

- Symptom identification is key to developing a treatment approach.
- Medication decisions depend upon intensity and precursors of disruptive behavior.
- Many classes of medications may be effective, but the evidence base is most robust for risperidone and aripiprazole.

DISCLOSURES

Dr J.A. Salpekar has been a consultant for Cerevel Therapeutics and receives royalties from Springer and from Elsevier. Dr J.A. Salpekar's institution receives research funding from Jazz Pharmaceuticals. Dr L. Scahill has served as a consultant to Johnson and Johnson, Impel NeuroPharma & Cogstate Ltd. He has received licensing fees from Roche, Yamo Pharmaceuticals & Abbvie and book royalties from Oxford, Guilford, and American Psychological Association.

REFERENCES

1. APA. Diagnostic and statistical manual of mental disorders. 5th edition. American Psychiatric Association; 2013.

2. Howes OD, Rogdaki M, Findon JL, et al. Autism spectrum disorder: Consensus guidelines on assessment, treatment and research from the British Association for Psychopharmacology. J Psychopharmacol 2018;32(1):3–29.

3. Vasa RA, Mostofsky SH, Ewen JB. The Disrupted Connectivity Hypothesis of Autism Spectrum Disorders: Time for the Next Phase in Research. Biol Psychiatry Cogn Neurosci Neuroimaging 2016;1(3):245–52.

4. Owen MJ. Intellectual disability and major psychiatric disorders: a continuum of neurodevelopmental causality. Comment Editorial. Br J Psychiatry 2012;200(4): 268–9.

5. Baran B, Nguyen QTH, Mylonas D, et al. Increased resting-state thalamocortical functional connectivity in children and young adults with autism spectrum disorder. Autism Res 2023;16(2):271–9.

6. Salpekar J. Neuropsychiatric effects of epilepsy in developmental disorders. Curr Opin Psychiatr 2018;31(2):109–15.

7. Besag FM. Epilepsy in patients with autism: links, risks and treatment challenges. Neuropsychiatric Dis Treat 2018;14:1–10.

8. Galineau L, Arlicot N, Dupont AC, et al. Glutamatergic synapse in autism: a complex story for a complex disorder. Mol Psychiatr 2023;28(2):801–9.

9. Richard AE, Scheffer IE, Wilson SJ. Features of the broader autism phenotype in people with epilepsy support shared mechanisms between epilepsy and autism spectrum disorder. Neurosci Biobehav Rev 2017;75:203–33.

10. Hellings JA, Nickel EJ, Weckbaugh M, et al. The overt aggression scale for rating aggression in outpatient youth with autistic disorder: preliminary findings. J Neuropsychiatry Clin Neurosci. Winter 2005;17(1):29–35.

11. Aman MG, Burrow WH, Wolford PL. The Aberrant Behavior Checklist-Community: factor validity and effect of subject variables for adults in group homes. Am J Ment Retard 1995;100(3):283–92.

12. Frazier TW, Khaliq I, Scullin K, et al. Development and Psychometric Evaluation of the Open-Source Challenging Behavior Scale (OS-CBS). J Autism Dev Disord 2023;3(12):4655–70.

13. Scahill L, Jeon S, Boorin SJ, et al. Weight Gain and Metabolic Consequences of Risperidone in Young Children With Autism Spectrum Disorder. J Am Acad Child Adolesc Psychiatry 2016;55(5):415–23.

14. Network RUoPPA. Risperidone in Children with Autism and Serious Behavioral Problems. N Engl J Med 2002;347:314–21.

15. King BH, Hollander E, Sikich L, et al. Lack of efficacy of citalopram in children with autism spectrum disorders and high levels of repetitive behavior: citalopram ineffective in children with autism. Arch Gen Psychiatr 2009;66(6):583–90.

16. Scahill L, Sukhodolsky DG, Anderberg E, et al. Sensitivity of the modified Children's Yale-Brown Obsessive Compulsive Scale to detect change: Results from two multi-site trials. Autism 2016;20(2):145–52.

17. Handen BL, Taylor J, Tumuluru R. Psychopharmacological treatment of ADHD symptoms in children with autism spectrum disorder. Int J Adolesc Med Health 2011;23(3):167–73.

18. Research Units on Pediatric Psychopharmacology Autism N. Randomized, controlled, crossover trial of methylphenidate in pervasive developmental disorders with hyperactivity. Arch Gen Psychiatr 2005;62(11):1266–74.

19. Scahill L, McCracken JT, King BH, et al. Extended-Release Guanfacine for Hyperactivity in Children With Autism Spectrum Disorder. Am J Psychiatr 2015;172(12): 1197–206.

20. Towbin KE, Pradella A, Gorrindo T, et al. Autism spectrum traits in children with mood and anxiety disorders. J Child Adolesc Psychopharmacol 2005;15(3): 452–64.
21. Scahill L, Lecavalier L, Schultz RT, et al. Development of the Parent-Rated Anxiety Scale for Youth With Autism Spectrum Disorder. J Am Acad Child Adolesc Psychiatry 2019;58(9):887–896 e2.
22. Accardo JA, Malow BA. Sleep, epilepsy, and autism. Epilepsy Behav 2015;47: 202–6.
23. Limoges E, Mottron L, Bolduc C, et al. Atypical sleep architecture and the autism phenotype. Brain 2005;128(Pt 5):1049–61.
24. Hollander E, Chaplin W, Soorya L, et al. Divalproex sodium vs placebo for the treatment of irritability in children and adolescents with autism spectrum disorders. Neuropsychopharmacology 2010;35(4):990–8.
25. Hellings JA, Weckbaugh M, Nickel EJ, et al. A double-blind, placebo-controlled study of valproate for aggression in youth with pervasive developmental disorders. J Child Adolesc Psychopharmacol 2005;15(4):682–92.
26. Wasserman S, Iyengar R, Chaplin WF, et al. Levetiracetam versus placebo in childhood and adolescent autism: a double-blind placebo-controlled study. Int Clin Psychopharmacol 2006;21(6):363–7.
27. Belsito KM, Law PA, Kirk KS, et al. Lamotrigine therapy for autistic disorder: a randomized, double-blind, placebo-controlled trial. J Autism Dev Disord 2001;31(2): 175–81.
28. Rezaei V, Mohammadi MR, Ghanizadeh A, et al. Double-blind, placebo-controlled trial of risperidone plus topiramate in children with autistic disorder. Prog Neuro-Psychopharmacol Biol Psychiatry 2010;34(7):1269–72.
29. Kumra S, Jacobsen LK, Lenane M, et al. "Multidimensionally impaired disorder": is it a variant of very early-onset schizophrenia? J Am Acad Child Adolesc Psychiatry 1998;37(1):91–9.
30. Pontillo M, Averna R, Tata MC, et al. Neurodevelopmental Trajectories and Clinical Profiles in a Sample of Children and Adolescents With Early- and Very-Early-Onset Schizophrenia. Front Psychiatr 2021;12:662093.
31. Arnold LE, Aman MG, Martin A, et al. Assessment in multisite randomized clinical trials of patients with autistic disorder: the Autism RUPP Network. Research Units on Pediatric Psychopharmacology. J Autism Dev Disord 2000;30(2):99–111.
32. McDougle CJ, Scahill L, McCracken JT, et al. Research Units on Pediatric Psychopharmacology (RUPP) Autism Network. Background and rationale for an initial controlled study of risperidone. Child Adolesc Psychiatr Clin N Am 2000; 9(1):201–24.
33. Aman MG, McDougle CJ, Scahill L, et al. Medication and parent training in children with pervasive developmental disorders and serious behavior problems: results from a randomized clinical trial. J Am Acad Child Adolesc Psychiatry 2009; 48(12):1143–54.
34. Scahill L, McDougle CJ, Aman MG, et al. Effects of risperidone and parent training on adaptive functioning in children with pervasive developmental disorders and serious behavioral problems. J Am Acad Child Adolesc Psychiatry 2012;51(2):136–46.
35. Arnold LE, Aman MG, Li X, et al. Research Units of Pediatric Psychopharmacology (RUPP) autism network randomized clinical trial of parent training and medication: one-year follow-up. J Am Acad Child Adolesc Psychiatry 2012;51(11): 1173–84.

36. Owen R, Sikich L, Marcus RN, et al. Aripiprazole in the treatment of irritability in children and adolescents with autistic disorder. Pediatrics 2009;124(6):1533–40.

37. Marcus RN, Owen R, Kamen L, et al. A placebo-controlled, fixed-dose study of aripiprazole in children and adolescents with irritability associated with autistic disorder. J Am Acad Child Adolesc Psychiatry 2009;48(11):1110–9.

38. Hollander E, Wasserman S, Swanson EN, et al. A double-blind placebo-controlled pilot study of olanzapine in childhood/adolescent pervasive developmental disorder. J Child Adolesc Psychopharmacol 2006;16(5):541–8.

39. Loebel A, Brams M, Goldman RS, et al. Lurasidone for the Treatment of Irritability Associated with Autistic Disorder. J Autism Dev Disord 2016;46(4):1153–63.

40. Kolevzon A, Mathewson KA, Hollander E. Selective serotonin reuptak inhibitors in autism: a review of efficacy and tolerability. J Clin Psychiatry 2006;67(3):407–14.

41. Hollander E, Phillips A, Chaplin W, et al. A placebo controlled crossover trial of liquid fluoxetine on repetitive behaviors in childhood and adolescent autism. Neuropsychopharmacology 2005;30(3):582–9.

42. Wagner KD, Ambrosini P, Rynn M, et al. Efficacy of sertraline in the treatment of children and adolescents with major depressive disorder: two randomized controlled trials. JAMA 2003;290(8):1033–41.

43. Brawman-Mintzer O, Knapp RG, Rynn M, et al. Sertraline treatment for generalized anxiety disorder: a randomized, double-blind, placebo-controlled study. J Clin Psychiatry 2006;67(6):874–81.

44. Owley T, Walton L, Salt J, et al. An open-label trial of escitalopram in pervasive developmental disorders. J Am Acad Child Adolesc Psychiatry 2005;44(4):343–8.

45. Ghanizadeh A, Ayoobzadehshirazi A. A randomized double-blind placebo-controlled clinical trial of adjuvant buspirone for irritability in autism. Pediatr Neurol 2015;52(1):77–81.

46. Chugani DC, Chugani HT, Wiznitzer M, et al. Efficacy of Low-Dose Buspirone for Restricted and Repetitive Behavior in Young Children with Autism Spectrum Disorder: A Randomized Trial. J Pediatr 2016;170:45–53 e1, 4.

47. Hauptman AJ, Cohen D, Dhossche D, et al. Catatonia in neurodevelopmental disorders: assessing catatonic deterioration from baseline. Lancet Psychiatr 2023;10(3):228–34.

48. Vaquerizo-Serrano J, Salazar De Pablo G, Singh J, et al. Catatonia in autism spectrum disorders: A systematic review and meta-analysis. Eur Psychiatr 2021;65(1):e4.

49. Wolraich ML, Chan E, Froehlich T, et al. ADHD Diagnosis and Treatment Guidelines: A Historical Perspective. Pediatrics 2019;144(4).

50. Belkin MR, Schwartz TL. Alpha-2 receptor agonists for the treatment of posttraumatic stress disorder. Drugs Context 2015;4:212286.

51. Connor DF, Grasso DJ, Slivinsky MD, et al. An open-label study of guanfacine extended release for traumatic stress related symptoms in children and adolescents. J Child Adolesc Psychopharmacol 2013;23(4):244–51.

52. Scahill L, Chappell PB, King RA, et al. Pharmacologic treatment of tic disorders. Child Adolesc Psychiatr Clin N Am 2000;9(1):99–117.

53. Scahill L. Treating Hyperactivity in Children with Pervasive Developmental Disorders. In: Hollander EHR, Ferretti C, editors. Textbook of autism spectrum disorders. 2 edition. American Psychiatric Association Publishing; 2022. p. 512–4, chap 28.

54. Handen BL, Aman MG, Arnold LE, et al. Atomoxetine, Parent Training, and Their Combination in Children With Autism Spectrum Disorder and Attention-Deficit/Hyperactivity Disorder. J Am Acad Child Adolesc Psychiatry 2015;54(11):905–15.
55. Pearson DA, Santos CW, Aman MG, et al. Effects of extended release methylphenidate treatment on ratings of attention-deficit/hyperactivity disorder (ADHD) and associated behavior in children with autism spectrum disorders and ADHD symptoms. Research Support, N.I.H., Extramural Research Support, Non-U.S. Gov't. J Child Adolesc Psychopharmacol 2013;23(5):337–51.
56. Aman MG, Smith T, Arnold LE, et al. A review of atomoxetine effects in young people with developmental disabilities. Res Dev Disabil 2014;35(6):1412–24.
57. Politte LC, Scahill L, Figueroa J, et al. A randomized, placebo-controlled trial of extended-release guanfacine in children with autism spectrum disorder and ADHD symptoms: an analysis of secondary outcome measures. Neuropsychopharmacology 2018;43(8):1772–8.
58. Salazar de Pablo G, Pastor Jorda C, Vaquerizo-Serrano J, et al. Systematic Review and Meta-analysis: Efficacy of Pharmacological Interventions for Irritability and Emotional Dysregulation in Autism Spectrum Disorder and Predictors of Response. J Am Acad Child Adolesc Psychiatry 2023;62(2):151–68.
59. Sikich L, Kolevzon A, King BH, et al. Intranasal Oxytocin in Children and Adolescents with Autism Spectrum Disorder. N Engl J Med 2021;385(16):1462–73.
60. Elchaar GM, Maisch NM, Augusto LM, et al. Efficacy and safety of naltrexone use in pediatric patients with autistic disorder. Ann Pharmacother 2006;40(6):1086–95.
61. Herman BH, Asleson GS, Powell A, et al. Cardiovascular and other physical effects of acute administration of naltrexone in autistic children. J Child Adolesc Psychopharmacol. Fall 1993;3(3):157–68.
62. Hosenbocus S, Chahal R. Amantadine: a review of use in child and adolescent psychiatry. Journal of the Canadian Academy of Child and Adolescent Psychiatry 2013;22(1):55–60.
63. McLaughlin MJ, Caliendo E, Lowder R, et al. Prescribing Patterns of Amantadine During Pediatric Inpatient Rehabilitation After Traumatic Brain Injury: A Multicentered Retrospective Review From the Pediatric Brain Injury Consortium. J Head Trauma Rehabil 2022;37(4):240–8.
64. King BH, Wright DM, Snape M, et al. Case series: amantadine open-label treatment of impulsive and aggressive behavior in hospitalized children with developmental disabilities. J Am Acad Child Adolesc Psychiatry 2001;40(6):654–7.
65. Mohammadi MR, Yadegari N, Hassanzadeh E, et al. Double-blind, placebo-controlled trial of risperidone plus amantadine in children with autism: a 10-week randomized study. Clin Neuropharmacol 2013;36(6):179–84.
66. Brignell A, Marraffa C, Williams K, et al. Memantine for autism spectrum disorder. Cochrane Database Syst Rev 2022;8(8):CD013845.
67. Strickland JC, Jackson H, Schlienz NJ, et al. Cross-sectional and longitudinal evaluation of cannabidiol (CBD) product use and health among people with epilepsy. Epilepsy Behav 2021;122:108205.
68. Smegal LF, Vedmurthy P, Ryan M, et al. Cannabidiol Treatment for Neurological, Cognitive, and Psychiatric Symptoms in Sturge-Weber Syndrome. Pediatr Neurol 2023;139:24–34.

Profound Autism
An Imperative Diagnosis

Lee Elizabeth Wachtel, MD[a],*, Jill Escher, JD[a],
Alycia Halladay, PhD[a], Amy Lutz, PhD[a], Gloria M. Satriale, JD, EdD[a],
Arthur Westover, MD[b], Carmen Lopez-Arvizu, MD[c]

KEYWORDS

- Autism • Profound • Intellectual disability • Language disorder
- Challenging behaviors • Psychiatric disturbance • Treatment • Services

KEY POINTS

- Profound autism refers to autistic individuals with comorbid intellectual disability and minimal-to-no language who require lifelong 24-hour support.
- The Lancet Commission on autism offered this term in 2021 to capture the most severely afflicted autistic individuals who may not be readily identified by the American Psychiatric Association's Diagnostic and Statistical Manual, Fifth Edition (DSM-5) autism spectrum disorder (ASD) diagnosis.
- Individuals with profound autism and their families face many unique and dire challenges.
- Individuals with profound autism are underrepresented in ASD research and care models, despite their extensive needs.

INTRODUCTION

In 2021, the Lancet Commission of international clinicians and treatment providers, researchers, advocates, and parents convened to address the wide range of needs of autistic individuals and families worldwide. A sentinel contribution of the Lancet Commission was the newly coined entity of "profound autism." The authors emphasized the enormous heterogeneity of autism and the associated challenges with the fifth edition of the Diagnostic and Statistical Manual's (DSM-5) grouping of everyone under the single umbrella diagnosis of autism spectrum disorder (ASD). While the DSM-5 does allow for specifiers of intellectual disability (ID) and language impairment in an ASD diagnosis, as well as severity levels, these were underscored by the Lancet Commission as underutilized and insufficient. Most importantly, the global ASD diagnosis was

[a] Kennedy Krieger Institute, 707 North Broadway, Baltimore, MD 21205, USA; [b] University of Texas-Southwestern; [c] Kennedy Krieger Institute, 1741 Ashland Avenue, Baltimore, MD 21205, USA
* Corresponding author.
E-mail address: wachtel@kennedykrieger.org

Pediatr Clin N Am 71 (2024) 301–313
https://doi.org/10.1016/j.pcl.2023.12.005
0031-3955/24/© 2024 Elsevier Inc. All rights reserved.
pediatric.theclinics.com

felt to fall short in capturing and distinguishing those with the most severe forms of autism and associated ID, who are at risk of marginalization and insufficient treatment, service, and research opportunities despite their intense care needs.[1,2]

As such, the Lancet Commission proposed the profound autism rubric to identify those with autism and *all* of the following comorbidities.

1. ID with intelligence quotient (IQ) less than 50
2. Minimal or no language
3. Requires 24-hour supervision
4. Requires assistance with activities of daily living (ADLs)[1]

This new term was an important development toward more accurate and precise diagnosis. While the DSM is the most commonly used psychiatric classification system in the United States, it had become clear that the DSM-5's single autism diagnosis model was fraught with pitfalls: those who would qualify for a DSM-5 diagnosis of "ASD, Level III, with intellectual and language impairment" were not always characterized as such and were often tossed into the general ASD diagnostic pool, erroneously grouped with vastly different individuals who do not have intellectual or language impairment or intensive lifelong support needs. Many US autism advocates had also consistently decried any discussion of severity, capability, or care need differences amongst those with an ASD diagnosis, invoking claims of ableism and discrimination.[3,4] See **Box 1**.

The Lancet Commission is not alone in recognizing the need for diagnostic clarity in autism and recognition of all its forms. Waizhard-Bartov and colleagues[5] similarly emphasize DSM-5's limitations of ranking severity solely upon core autism symptoms, without regard for co-occurring ID, language impairment, or the wide range of additional medical, psychiatric, and behavioral comorbidities that are often present and can have significant deleterious effect on daily functioning and needs. They urge a multidisciplinary diagnostic approach that considers strengths and weaknesses and also evaluates support needs and resources to enhance overall clinical care. The Autism Phenome Project of the University of California Davis MIND Institute has similarly sought to identify "clinically meaningful" subtypes of autism separating the larger heterogeneous ASD population into homogenous groups based on biological, behavioral, medical, clinical, and developmental factors in order to *optimize patient care and enhance quality of life* for patients and families.[6] The US-based Autism Science Foundation has encouraged the autism community to accept the profound autism terms and their clinical utility for some rather than solely adhere to the cultural mantra that individuals with high-functioning autism represent and speak for the entire spectrum.[7] The shortcomings and heterogeneity in our current psychiatric classification systems have also led to the recent National Institutes of Mental Health initiative surrounding a novel classification known as the Hierarchical Taxonomy of Psychopathology, which

---

Box 1
Definition of profound autism

a. IQ < 50 (present in ~40% of ASD patients)

b. Little to no language

c. Requires 24-h supervision

d. Requires assistance with ADLs

Abbreviations: ADLs, activities of daily living; ASD, autism spectrum disorder; IQ, intelligence quotient.

seeks to classify disorders along dimensions and spectra and may ultimately offer a more accurate depiction of the range of ASD presentations.[8]

The diagnosis of autism has undeniably experienced much change. Autism was erroneously classified as a type of schizophrenia in the first 2 iterations of the DSM.[9,10] This classification was rectified in the 1980 DSM-III, in which a new diagnosis of "infantile autism" was offered and specifically distinguished from the core symptoms of schizophrenia. This change was a direct result of ongoing research establishing autism as a distinct biological condition with genetic determinants, as demonstrated in monozygotic versus dizygotic twin studies.[11,12] The DSM-III-Revision and DSM-III-Text Revision established the well-known triad of core deficits in (1) social interaction, (2) communication, and (3) restricted interests and activities, which was maintained through both iterations of the DSM-IV.[13] Symptom onset during childhood was mandated through the DSM-IV. The DSM-IV further established a pervasive developmental disorders "quintet" of autism, Asperger syndrome, pervasive developmental disorder—not otherwise specified, childhood disintegrative disorder, and Rett syndrome, arguably representing a wide range of individuals and clinical presentations (including the latter 2, which were subsequently recognized as separate neurodegenerative conditions).[14]

The DSM-5 brought about myriad relevant changes. The quintet was collapsed into a single unit, communication deficits were removed from the diagnostic criteria, and fewer and broader overall criteria were listed in a stated attempt to better express how ASD might manifest itself across sex, age, and culture. Childhood symptom onset was removed, and the possibility was offered of meeting criteria later in life when external demands exceeded internal capacity, by history or after a period of normal development. The spectrum became so wide that the stage was set for autism to take on a new character, often adopted as an identity, difference, or expression of culture and diversity and eschewed as a disorder by those who experienced it as a different way of life. This stood in contrast to autism as a biological condition with varying levels of impairments as well as multiple medical and psychiatric comorbidities necessitating care at varying degrees of intensity in order to offer optimal health and function.[2]

Temple Grandin,[15] a renowned autistic animal behaviorist and academic, commented in 2022 that "the spectrum is so broad it doesn't make much sense. Are we really going to put people with severe autism who cannot dress themselves in the same category as people with mild autism who work in Silicon Valley?"

This distinction is important given the growing body of worldwide literature surrounding long-term outcomes for autistic individuals, most poignantly those with concomitant ID and language impairment, that is, profound autism.

Indeed, studies have repeatedly shown suboptimal outcomes, higher needs, and decreased independence in autistic cohorts. A 2015 meta-analysis by van Heijst and Geurts of 485 autistic adults and 17,776 controls across 10 studies documented lower quality of life and physical health, as well as more dependence on parents in the ASD cohorts, and no evidence of core ASD symptom improvement compared to the time of initial diagnosis.[16] A 2016 meta-analysis of 828 ASD individuals across 12 samples reported that 47.7% had poor or very poor outcomes, defined respectively as "severely handicapped but some potential for social progress" and "no independent living at all." Importantly, 61.9% of those with DSM-IV ASD had poor or very poor outcomes as compared to only 26.4% with DSM-IV Asperger syndrome. A Greek study of 69 individuals diagnosed with ASD as children and re-evaluated in adulthood found that 47.1% had "very poor" or "poor" outcome as compared to 41.5% with "good" or "very good" outcome with severity of the initial ASD diagnosis and lower cognitive *function* as leading predictive factors in negative outcome.[17] A US study of 143 adults with ASD found that only 22% were employed, and only 7% were living independently, with *poorer outcomes directly associated lower IQ and verbal functioning* and higher autism severity, with *nonverbal mental age at 2 years old predictive of independence with ADLs at age 21.* Another American study followed 213 individuals diagnosed at age 2 and re-evaluated 17 years later; only 9% were found to have "overcome" autism, with significant ID at age 2 predictive 85% of the time of the same at age 19.[18] An Italian study of 22 ASD adults with comorbid ID and severe language disorder evaluated over a decade confirmed again that *outcome was predicted by severity of autism, cognitive, and language levels, as well as medical and psychiatric comorbidities.* The crucial element of treatment and residential services was also emphasized in best outcomes.[19] A 2020 Israeli study of 65 individuals followed from toddlerhood to adolescence split the subjects into lower and higher cognitive function based on an IQ of 85, documenting that while adaptive skills were similar at toddlerhood, higher IQ predicted adaptive skills in adolescence, and better communication skills and cognitive capacity in toddlerhood predicted better cognitive and adaptive skills in adolescence.[20] Finally, a 2020 UK study of 123 children reported that in adulthood, the greatest gains were made by children who had language progress by age 3 and average nonverbal skills at age 3, with the overriding conclusion that *"verbal and nonverbal IQ at age 2, and even more strongly at age 3, were strong indicators of independence at age 26."*[21]

These international data support the Lancet's emphasis on cognitive and language impairment as key components to a more severe or profound autism diagnosis and are a sobering reminder of the present suboptimal outcomes for an evergrowing patient population.

Indeed, autism is on the rise. In their 2023 report on 2020 surveillance, the Autism and Developmental Disabilities Monitoring (ADDM) Network of the Center for Disease Control (CDC) currently estimates an autism prevalence of 1 in 36 8-year-old children representing a 4-fold increase over the past 20 years. While the ADDM reports do not address profound autism per se, among the 4165 (66.7%) children with ASD with information on cognitive ability, 37.9% of them were classified as having an ID (an increase from 2 years prior), 23.5% had borderline ID (an increase from 2 years prior), and 38.6% had no ID (a decrease from 2 years prior). ADDM data also indicate that the population prevalence of ASD with comorbid ID and borderline ID has increased markedly since data were first collected in the 2008 surveillance year. For those with IQ 70 and below, the population prevalence was 0.429% in 2008; in 2020, it more than doubled to 1.046%. For those with borderline ID, or IQs 71 to 85, the population prevalence was 0.271% in 2008; in 2020, it more than doubled to 0.649% in 2020.[22,23] The CDC's 2023 study on profound autism also demonstrated that over 16 years of surveillance from 2000 to 2016, the prevalence of profound autism greatly increased, from 0.268% to 0.459% of 8-year-olds. Over the same period, the prevalence of nonprofound autism increased at even sharper rates from 0.394% to 1.426%.[24]

We seek to address multiple issues of particular salience to profound autism. Many of these concerns may come first to the pediatrician's attention, with parents desperate for guidance and solutions. These include (1) challenging behaviors; (2) comorbid psychiatric disturbance; (3) need for more extensive school, in-home, and residential services; and (4) insufficient research into profound autism.

Challenging Behaviors

Challenging behaviors are a daunting problem in autism, affecting 27% to 50% of individuals.[3,4] Those with profound autism are particularly at risk, given that heightened challenging behaviors are found among ASD individuals with more significant communication and cognitive delay, as well as those with medical and psychiatric comorbidities or genetic etiologies. Recent literature evaluating the characteristics of children meeting the precise Lancet criteria for profound autism across 15 US sites from 2000 to 2016 documented higher risk of self-injury as compared to those with non-profound autism. Maladaptive behaviors typically fall within the rubrics of self-injurious, aggressive, and disruptive acts, referring the challenging behaviors toward the self, others, and environment, respectively. There is enormous breadth in terms of these behaviors, which may include headbanging, hand-head or hand-body hitting, body slamming, scratching, biting, slapping, poking, kicking, punching, headbutting, property destruction, elopement, inappropriate excrement play, inappropriately sexualized behaviors, and dangerous pica. Many individuals display more than one kind of challenging behavior, and if left untreated, these behaviors have a propensity to worsen and intensify.[24–30]

There is also a tremendous range in terms of the sequelae of such behaviors, including localized abrasions, lacerations, bruises, swelling, broken limbs, cauliflower ears and other cosmetic tissue damage, traumatic cataract development, retinal detachment, skull fractures, cerebral hemorrhages, and even death.

Another unintended consequence of challenging behaviors is the frequent exclusion from community life as such conduct is generally not socially acceptable in public settings and may pose heightened safety risks outside of the immediate home. This affects an individual's ability to participate in educational, leisure, social, and family activities during childhood, and as they age, challenging behaviors negatively impact vocational and independent living options. Services available to facilitate integration into community life for this population can be declined on the basis of challenging behaviors being dangerous and disruptive or requiring a higher level of staffing to ensure safety.[31] Ironically, challenging behaviors may also lead to exclusion from necessary inpatient care due to facility safety policies and lack of management expertise, creating a unique health situation where one may be "too ill to be hospitalized."

Challenging behaviors in ASD are the most common reason for placement outside of the home as a child's problematic behavioral display often exceeds what caregivers can manage, especially as the child becomes an adult and the parents age as well. While many families receive some in-home supports from direct care staff, there is a national lack of sufficient in-home staff and supports that are familiar and comfortable to work with someone that can cause injury to a caregiver. There is related concern that individuals transitioning to adulthood may lose their funding for such supports due to age or insurance.[32,33] Behavioral emergency situations have significantly worsened since the coronavirus disease 2019 pandemic and have led to innumerable reports of individuals with autism and ID—most likely representative of profound autism—stranded in emergency departments unable to access services or discharge safely home.[34–37]

Multiple barriers exist in addressing challenging behaviors in profound autism, including the lack of access to expert clinicians and qualified care teams, as well as funds to pay for what are often very time-intensive, costly interventions. Treatment options are often limited to the pediatric population, may be part and parcel of educational accommodations and services through an individualized educational plan, and are often not covered by commercial insurances. Indeed, only recent legislature has mandated payment of applied behavioral analysis services, despite such being considered amongst the gold standard in the assessment and treatment of challenging behaviors in ASDs.[38]

Challenging behaviors may interfere with routine pediatric care, including well child-care and sick visits, procedures, testing, vaccination, and other preventative health measures. The pediatrician may be called upon to work in tandem with families and other providers in order to complete multiple necessary components of a child's care in the safest, most expeditious way. As individuals with profound autism and challenging behaviors age, the transition to adult health care is often fraught with difficulties. Individuals with neurodevelopmental disabilities have poorer health outcomes, with longer lengths of hospital stay, higher rates of readmission, poorer hospital experiences, and increased complications. Life expectancy for individuals with both autism and ID/developmental disabilities (DDs) is shorter than the average population.[16,39,40]

The American Academy of Pediatrics 2020 "Identification, Evaluation, and Management of Children with Autism Spectrum Disorder" discusses the critical role the pediatrician may play in establishing a "medical home" for the child and serving as a focused hub from which necessary medical and mental health services may be more readily coordinated and accessed.[41] The ADDM Network further underscores the frequent complex somatic needs of children with profound autism, likely inability to live independently or complete ADLs, issues which all may fall within the pediatrician's purview caring for such youth throughout childhood and transitioning into adulthood.[24]

Psychiatric Comorbidities

Psychiatric comorbidities in autism are common. A 2013 study demonstrated that 57.5% of autistic participants had at least 1 additional DSM diagnosis, and a 2019 study found that 91% of autistic children and 31% of autistic adults had at least 1 additional DSM diagnosis.[42,43] Multiple co-occurring diagnoses are often common, with a recent literature review documenting that 70% to 95% of youth with ASD had at least 1 DSM diagnosis, 41% to 60% had 2 or more DSM diagnoses, and fully 24% had 3 or more comorbid DSM diagnoses.[43,44] These comorbid diagnoses encompass the range of DSM pathology and are more fully addressed elsewhere in this edition. Briefly, anxiety is estimated to occur in 30% to 40% of autistic youth, ADHD in 14% to 70%, affective disorders in 5% to 10%, psychotic disorders in 4% to 11%, and catatonia in 12% to 20%.[44–48] The risk of development of schizophrenia in adolescents and young adults with ASD is around 10%.[49] Attention-deficit/hyperactivity disorder (ADHD) and anxiety are the most common psychiatric comorbidities of ASD.[48] All psychiatric comorbidities of ASD can contribute to overall impairment, for example, a 2021 study evaluating ASD and ADHD demonstrated that children with both diagnoses had higher scores on Vineland Adaptive and Social Responsiveness rating scales, indicating greater overall dysfunction and potential lower quality of life.[50]

ID is a complicating and additive comorbidity factor in ASD. The prevalence of ID in children and adolescents with autism in a meta-analysis of population-based studies was 23%,[51] and it is currently estimated that around 40% of individuals with ASD have ID.[22] Psychopathology of all forms is further known to occur at higher rates in individuals with ID as compared to those with normal cognitive functioning. Over a half century ago, the Isle of Wight studies demonstrated a 3-fold to 4-fold increased risk of psychiatry illness in youth with ID.[52] Multiple international studies have subsequently demonstrated the same heightened risk of psychopathology in those with ID, underscoring the need for vigilance in prompt diagnosis and treatment.[53,54]

Challenging behavior is also well recognized as an additional risk factor for psychiatric illness in ASD, and the best treatment paradigms for acute behavioral crises urge diagnosis and treatment of underlying psychopathology.[55–57]

By virtue of their autism and ID, individuals with profound autism are thus at significantly heightened risk for the development of additional psychiatric diagnoses and complications. This translates into a direct need for well-trained mental health providers who are available to promptly assess, diagnose, and treat a growing number of individuals with profound autism across the lifespan for a wide range of psychiatric concerns. Sadly, mental health services for individuals with autism are often limited and unequally available; a 2019 study of 8184 US mental health facilities found that only 43% accepted youth with ASD.[58]

Service Needs

Individuals with neurodevelopmental disabilities age out of federally mandated education, support, and services following high school graduation.[59] This abrupt cessation of services is commonly referred to as "falling off the cliff" into an adult-targeting human services system that is woefully inadequate to support the deluge of individuals with ASD entering that system. According to Gerhardt and Lanier,[60] the increasing number of children with autism exiting the educational system requiring life-sustaining adult services is creating "a looming crisis of unprecedented magnitude for adults with ASD, their families, and the ill-prepared and underfunded adult service system charged with meeting their needs". Families report fear and anxiety surrounding the process of securing adult services which often results in significant unmet needs leaving families struggling to fill the gaps.[61]

Currently, the dearth of services available to support individuals on the autism spectrum is a national concern. As a result, individuals with ASD, particularly individuals with profound ASD whose needs are so much greater, are often left to languish in the emergency departments of hospitals for months since there are no other services available to support their needs.[62] News stories and social media are replete with accounts of the growing hardship of families as they face, often unsuccessfully, the challenge of trying to meet the needs of their adult children themselves.[63] The lack of services is exacerbated by nationwide staffing shortages of direct care workers, a situation which is particularly dire for those with profound autism; agencies can pick and choose those they serve, and often decline those with the highest needs.[64]

In 2018, Anderson and Butt[65] performed a qualitative study of the perspectives of 36 families of individuals with ASD ages 19 to 31 regarding the availability and quality of publicly funded adult services. The study revealed common themes impacting access to and the caliber of services including an overall lack of funding, program suitability, and limited options, particularly appropriate to support individuals with more complex needs, a staffing crisis rooted in a lack of training, performance accountability, high turnover, and low pay, as well as a bureaucracy of confusing, complicated, and convoluted service systems that widely vary among states.

Predictably, individuals with ASD entering adulthood continue to experience more barriers and worse outcomes than those without ASD.[66] According to the National Longitudinal Transition Study (NLTS-2; National Center for Special Education Research 2018), nearly 40% of individuals with ASD receive no services in the first 2 years after high school, 66% were not employed within 2 years of graduation, and 42% remained unemployed after 4 years.[9] Only 19% were living independently.[10] Individuals with ASD are less likely to have ever worked or live independently than those with other learning, emotional, or DDs.[65,67]

A right to effective habilitation is well established in the literature. Habilitation services address skills considered key to meaningful engagement and financial stability in adulthood.[68] Without these support and services, quality of life cannot be achieved for individuals with autism and their families. Under-addressed funding and systems issues that impact the everyday life of individuals with autism and their families, especially those with profound autism, must be brought into the fore if post-secondary outcomes are expected to change.

Unequal Representation in Research

It is an undeniable, time-proven tenet of medicine that progress occurs through carefully orchestrated, objective research with results that are ultimately able to be replicated. This applies across the autism spectrum just as it would across the full spectrum of any other medical condition. Unfortunately, profound autism is not currently equally represented in autism research. While those with profound autism make up a significant portion (~30–50%) of those with autism, they are not equally represented in research. One study found that only 58% of autism studies included those with comorbid ID; such inclusion has also been found to be decreasing over time.[69,70] Inclusion of these individuals in research requires extra time and consideration, and recruitment goals for subjects with profound autism may lag behind for various reasons. They may be under-included, or researchers may be unclear as to the exact nature of their cognitive and language abilities. The reasons for the exclusion of these individuals are not malicious. In some cases, the goal is to stratify individuals in a highly heterogeneous group and to reduce the heterogeneity of the outcomes or the response. ASD heterogeneity has been noted as a key impediment in clinical trials involving drug development, a key area where progress is limited to the detriment of the entire ASD spectrum.[71] Oftentimes, grant reviewers recognize that autism is a broad concept and encourage scientists to narrow down the group in which their results will apply to ensure that within-group variability is controlled.[69,70]

In other cases, the reasons for exclusion are methodological or logistical. Research measures and instruments that rely on language as an outcome are not applicable to those who are minimally verbal. Certain tasks may require cognitive abilities that some people do not possess, and additional testing to ensure that IQ is obtained places an extra burden on family members. Certain tasks required for research such as reading, writing, processing directions, sitting still, or attention may not be feasible. Families may need alternative and augmentative communication devices to ensure participation, which may require additional Institutional Review Board approval or protocol modification. This leads to an under-inclusion and sometimes exclusion in research studies which, given the heterogeneity of autism, renders confident generalization of these results impossible to those with ASD who were unable to participate.[72]

In order to address this problem, researchers need to over-recruit individuals with ASD + ID, train research staff to work with families, and consider additional or alternative methods to collect information from families. Outcome measures need to be validated in those who have ID or who are minimally verbal, and alternatives to existing measures should be considered given that they may have floor effects for those with profound

---

Box 2
Challenges of profound autism

a. Challenging behaviors

b. Psychiatric comorbidities

c. Insufficient services

d. Insufficient resources

e. Semantic and political discord

Box 3
Take-home points for the pediatrician

a. Not all autism is the same.

b. Profound autism is real.

c. Patients and families affected by profound autism face different challenges from patients and families affected by non-profound autism.

d. Equity in care and research in profound autism currently eludes us.

e. The pediatrician can play an important role as the provider of a "medical home" for these youth.

---

autism.[69] This may require studies which focus on particular subgroups of individuals to determine the feasibility of protocols developed to accommodate the needs of those with ASD + ID or those who are minimally verbal, that is, those with profound autism.

Much work remains to be done to fully include those with profound autism in research. As Farmer and Thurm so aptly state, the current situation is sadly one where *"a vulnerable population is prevented from participating in and deriving full benefit from research."*[72] The ADDM Network has also emphasized the underrepresentation of individuals with profound autism in both research and intervention studies, despite the fact that they often have the greatest needs.[24] See **Box 2**.

SUMMARY

Profound autism is a novel term that refers to a subset of individuals with ASD who have ID with an IQ less than 50 and minimal-to-no language and require 24-hour supervision and assistance with ADLs. This term was offered in 2021 by the Lancet Commission in an effort to better capture the unique characteristics and needs of autistic individuals whose clinical presentation is not fully captured by the typical use of the DSM-5. Profound autism is associated with many significant issues across multiple arenas, including challenging behaviors, psychiatric comorbidities and associated limited access to mental health care, intensive service needs across the lifespan, and underrepresentation in scientific research. Recent data from the CDC indicate that the overall prevalence of autism in the United States is 1 in 36 children, with nearly 40% having concomitant ID. Quite simply, profound autism is on the rise and represents a health crisis of global concern demanding our immediate and upmost attention.

The general pediatrician will invariably work with autistic children across the spectrum and will likely encounter youth with profound autism. Awareness of profound autism as a real entity describing autistic children with concomitant ID and language impairment who require 24-hour care is the first step in developing a solid pediatric home for these youth, collaborating with families and other disciplines to access needed services and advocating for full inclusion in research to optimize long-term clinical outcomes in this unique subset of autistic children and adolescents. See **Box 3**.

CLINICS CARE POINTS

- Profound autism affects a not-insignificant number of autistic youth.

- Needs for those with profound autism are different and multiple.

- Ongoing awareness, research and advocacy are critical.

DISCLOSURE

The authors have no relevant disclosures.

REFERENCES

1. Lord C, Charman T, Havdahl A, et al. The Lancet Commission on the future of care and clinical research in autism. Lancet 2022;399(10321):271–334.
2. Association AP. Diagnostic and statistical manual of mental disorders. 5th Edition. Washington, DC: American Psychiatric Association; 2014. DSM 5.
3. Soke GN, Rosenberg SA, Hamman RF, et al. Brief Report: Prevalence of Self-injurious Behaviors among Children with Autism Spectrum Disorder-A Population-Based Study. J Autism Dev Disord 2016;46(11):3607–14.
4. Crocker AG, Mercier C, Lachapelle Y, et al. Prevalence and types of aggressive behaviour among adults with intellectual disabilities. J Intellect Disabil Res 2006; 50(Pt 9):652–61.
5. Waizbard-Bartov E, Fein D, Lord C, et al. Autism severity and its relationship to disability. Autism Res 2023. https://doi.org/10.1002/aur.2898.
6. Nordahl CW, Andrews DS, Dwyer P, et al. The autism phenome project: toward identifying clinically meaningful subgroups of autism. Front Neurosci 2021;15:786220.
7. Singer A. It's time to embrace 'profound autism'. Spectrum News 2022.
8. Ruggero CJ, Kotov R, Hopwood CJ, et al. Integrating the hierarchical taxonomy of psychopathology (HiTOP) into clinical practice. J Consult Clin Psychol 2019; 87(12):1069–84.
9. American Psychiatric Association. Diagnostic and Statistical Manual of Mental Disorders.
10. American Psychiatric Association. Diagnostic and statistical manual. 2nd Edition. Washington, DC: American Psychiatric Association; 1968.
11. American Psychiatric Association. Diagnostic and statistical manual of mental disorders. 3rd edition. Washington DC: American Psychiatric Association; 1980.
12. Folstein S, Rutter M. Infantile autism: a genetic study of 21 twin pairs. JCPP (J Child Psychol Psychiatry) 1977;18:297–321.
13. American Psychiatric Association. Diagnostic and statistical manual of mental disorders. 3rd edition. Washington, DC: American Psychiatric Association; 1987.
14. American Psychiatric Association. Diagnostic and statistical manual of mental disorders. 4th edition. Washington, D.C.: American Psychiatric Association; 1994.
15. Grandin T. www.templegrandin.com. Secondary www.templegrandin.com.
16. van Heijst BF, Geurts HM. Quality of life in autism across the lifespan: a meta-analysis. Autism 2015;19(2):158–67 [published Online First: Epub Date]].
17. Sevaslidou I, Chatzidimitriou C, Abatzoglou G. The long-term outcomes of a cohort of adolescents and adults from Greece with autism spectrum disorder. Ann Gen Psychiatr 2019;18:26.
18. Anderson DK, Liang JW, Lord C. Predicting young adult outcome among more and less cognitively able individuals with autism spectrum disorders. JCPP (J Child Psychol Psychiatry) 2014;55(5):485–94.
19. Fusar-Poli L, Brondino N, Orsi P, et al. Long-term outcome of a cohort of adults with autism and intellectual disability: A pilot prospective study. Res Dev Disabil 2017;60:223–31.
20. Ben-Itzchak E, Zachor DA. Toddlers to teenagers: long-term follow-up study of outcomes in autism spectrum disorder. Autism 2020;24(1):41–50.

21. Pickles A, McCauley JB, Pepa LA, et al. The adult outcome of children referred for autism: typology and prediction from childhood. JCPP (J Child Psychol Psychiatry) 2020;61(7):760–7.
22. Maenner MJ, Warren Z, Williams AR, et al. Prevalence and characteristics of autism spectrum disorder among children aged 8 years - autism and developmental disabilities monitoring network, 11 sites, United States, 2020. MMWR Surveill Summ 2023;72(2):1–14.
23. Investigators. Aaddmnsyp. Prevalance of autism spectrum disorders - autism and developmental disabilities monitoring network. Morb Mortal Wkly Rep - Surveillance Summ 2012;61(3):1–9.
24. Hughes MM, Shaw KA, DiRienzo M, et al. The prevalence and characteristics of children with profound autism, 15 Sites, United States, 2000-2016. Public Health Rep 2023;138(6):971–80.
25. Paclawskyj TR, Kurtz PF, O'Connor JT. Functional assessment of problem behaviors in adults with mental retardation. Behav Modif 2004;28(5):649–67.
26. Hagopian L, Caruso-Andersen M. Integrating behavioral and pharmacological interventions for severe problem behavior displayed by children with neurogenetic and developmental disorders. In: Shapiro B, Accardo P, editors. Neurobehavioral disorders: science and practice: brookes. 2010. p. 217–39.
27. Harris J. Developmental neuropsychiatry. Oxford UK: Oxford University Press; 1998. p. 251–7.
28. Schroeder S, Oster-Granite M, Berkson G, et al. Self-injurious behavior: gene-brain-behavior relationships. Ment Retard Dev Disabil Res Rev 2001;17:3–12.
29. Smith K, Matson J. Behavior problems: differences among intellectually disabled adults with co-morbid autism spectrum disorders and epilepsy. Res Dev Disabil 2010;31(5):1062–9.
30. McIntyre LL, Blacher J, Baker BL. Behaviour/mental health problems in young adults with intellectual disability: the impact on families. J Intellect Disabil Res 2002;46(Pt 3):239–49.
31. American Academy of C, American Academy of Child and Adolescent Psychiatry AACAP Committee on Community-Based Systems of Care and AACAP Committee on Quality Issues. Adolescent psychiatry committee on community-based systems of c, clinical@aacap.org acoqiea, american academy of c, adolescent psychiatry committee on community-based systems of c, issues acoq. clinical update: child and adolescent behavioral health care in community systems of care. J Am Acad Child Adolesc Psychiatry 2022. https://doi.org/10.1016/j.jaac.2022.06.001.
32. Shea LL, Koffer Miller KH, Verstreate K, et al. States' use of Medicaid to meet the needs of autistic individuals. Health Serv Res 2021;56(6):1207–14.
33. Carey ME, Tao S, Koffer Miller KH, et al. Association between medicaid waivers and medicaid disenrollment among autistic adolescents during the transition to adulthood. JAMA Netw Open 2023;6(3):e232768.
34. Beverly J, Giannouchos T, Callaghan T. Examining frequent emergency department use among children and adolescents with autism spectrum disorder. Autism 2021;25(5):1382–94.
35. Gomez-Ramiro M, Fico G, Anmella G, et al. Changing trends in psychiatric emergency service admissions during the COVID-19 outbreak: Report from a worldwide epicentre. J Affect Disord 2021;282:26–32.
36. ICD10Data.com. Secondary ICD10Data.com.
37. Pillai J, Dunn K, Efron D. Parent-reported factors associated with the emergency department presentation of children and adolescents with autism spectrum

disorder and/or intellectual disability with behaviours of concern: a qualitative study. Arch Dis Child 2022. https://doi.org/10.1136/archdischild-2022-325002.

38. Cerda N, Brinster M, Turner C, et al. Challenging case: leveraging community partnerships to address barriers to care for students with autism. J Dev Behav Pediatr 2023. https://doi.org/10.1097/DBP.0000000000001163.

39. Lauer E, McCallion P. Mortality of people with intellectual and developmental disabilities from select us state disability service systems and medical claims data. J Appl Res Intellect Disabil 2015;28(5):394–405.

40. Happe F, Charlton RA. Aging in autism spectrum disorders: a mini-review. Gerontology 2012;58(1):70–8.

41. Hyman SL, Levy SE, Myers SM, et al. Council on children with disabilities SOD, behavioral P. identification, evaluation, and management of children with autism spectrum disorder. Pediatrics 2020;145(1). https://doi.org/10.1542/peds.2019-3447.

42. van Steensel FJ, Bogels SM, de Bruin EI. Psychiatric comorbidity in children with autism spectrum disorders: a comparison with children with ADHD. J Child Fam Stud 2013;22(3):368–76.

43. Mosner MG, Kinard JL, Shah JS, et al. Rates of co-occurring psychiatric disorders in autism spectrum disorder using the mini international neuropsychiatric interview. J Autism Dev Disord 2019;49(9):3819–32.

44. Simonoff E, Pickles A, Charman T, et al. Psychiatric disorders in children with autism spectrum disorders: prevalence, comorbidity, and associated factors in a population-derived sample. J Am Acad Child Adolesc Psychiatry 2008;47(8): 921–9.

45. Varcin KJ, Herniman SE, Lin A, et al. Occurrence of psychosis and bipolar disorder in adults with autism: A systematic review and meta-analysis. Neurosci Biobehav Rev 2022;134:104543.

46. Wing L, Shah A. Catatonia in autistic spectrum disorders. Br J Psychiatry 2000; 176:357–62.

47. Billstedt E, Gilberg C, Gilberg C, et al. Autism after adolescence: population-based 13- to 22-year follow-up study of 120 individuals with autism diagnosed in childhood. J Autism Dev Disord 2005;35:351–60.

48. Kaat AJ, Gadow KD, Lecavalier L. Psychiatric symptom impairment in children with autism spectrum disorders. J Abnorm Child Psychol 2013;41(6):959–69.

49. Hsu TW, Chu CS, Tsai SJ, et al. Diagnostic progression to schizophrenia: a nationwide cohort study of 11 170 adolescents and young adults with autism spectrum disorder. Psychiatr Clin Neurosci 2022;76(12):644–51.

50. Liu Y, Wang L, Xie S, et al. Attention deficit/hyperactivity disorder symptoms impair adaptive and social function in children with autism spectrum disorder. Front Psychiatr 2021;12:654485.

51. Mutluer T, Aslan Genc H, Ozcan Morey A, et al. Population-based psychiatric comorbidity in children and adolescents with autism spectrum disorder: a meta-analysis. Front Psychiatr 2022;13:856208.

52. Rutter M, Graham P, Yule W. A neuropsychiatric study in childhood. Clin Dev Med 1970;35–6.

53. Platt JM, Keyes KM, McLaughlin KA, et al. Intellectual disability and mental disorders in a US population representative sample of adolescents. Psychol Med 2019;49(6):952–61.

54. White P, Chant D, Edwards N, et al. Prevalence of intellectual disability and comorbid mental illness in an Australian community. Aust N Z J Psychiatr 2005; 39:395–400.

55. Guinchat V, Cravero C, Diaz L, et al. Acute behavioral crises in psychiatric inpatients with autism spectrum disorder (ASD): recognition of concomitant medical or non-ASD psychiatric conditions predicts enhanced improvement. Res Dev Disabil 2015;38:242–55.

56. Myrbakk E, von Tetzchner S. Psychiatric disorders and behavior problems in people with intellectual disability. Res Dev Disabil 2008;29(4):316–32.

57. Moss S, Emerson E, Kiernan C, et al. Psychiatric symptoms in adults with learning disability and challenging behavior. Br J Psychiatry 2000;177:452–6.

58. Cantor J, McBain RK, Kofner A, et al. Fewer than half of us mental health treatment facilities provide services for children with autism spectrum disorder. Health Aff 2020;39(6):968–74.

59. Individuals with disabilities education act, 20 USC. p. 1400–19.

60. Gerhardt P, Lainer I. Addressing the needs of adolescents and adults with autism: a crisis on the horizon. J Contemp Psychother 2011;41(1):37–45.

61. Cheak-Zamora NC, Teti M, First J. 'Transitions are scary for our kids, and they're scary for us': family member and youth perspectives on the challenges of transitioning to adulthood with autism. J Appl Res Intellect Disabil 2015;28(6):548–60.

62. Schwieterman B. In: Omsbudman OoDD, editor. Stuck in the hospital. Washington State.; 2018.

63. Jenkins A. He's 13-years old, autistic and stuck in the hospital for the holidays. He's not the only one. Northwest News Network; 2021.

64. Scales K. It is time to resolve the direct care workforce crisis in long-term care. Gerontol 2021;61(4):497.

65. Anderson C, Butt C. Young adults on the autism spectrum: the struggle for appropriate services. J Autism Dev Disord 2018;48(11):3912–25.

66. Yamamoto SH, Alverson CY. From high school to postsecondary education, training, and employment: Predicting outcomes for young adults with autism spectrum disorder. Autism Dev Lang Impair 2022;7. https://doi.org/10.1177/23969415221095019. 23969415221095019.

67. Roux AM, Shattuck PT, Cooper BP, et al. Postsecondary employment experiences among young adults with an autism spectrum disorder. J Am Acad Child Adolesc Psychiatry 2013;52(9):931–9.

68. Shattuck PT, Garfield T, Roux AM, et al. Services for adults with autism spectrum disorder: a systems perspective. Curr Psychiatr Rep 2020;22(3):13.

69. Stedman A, Taylor B, Erard M, et al. Are children severely affected by autism spectrum disorder underrepresented in treatment studies? an analysis of the literature. J Autism Dev Disord 2019;49(4):1378–90.

70. Thurm A, Halladay A, Mandell D, et al. Making research possible: barriers and solutions for those with ASD and ID. J Autism Dev Disord 2021. https://doi.org/10.1007/s10803-021-05320-1.

71. McCracken JT, Anagnostou E, Arango C, et al. Drug development for autism spectrum disorder (ASD): progress, challenges, and future directions. Eur Neuropsychopharmacol 2021;48:3–31.

72. Farmer C, Thurm A. Inclusion of individuals with low IQ in drug development for autism spectrum disorder. Eur Neuropsychopharmacol 2021;48:37–9.

A Pediatrician's Practical Guide for Navigating Transition to Adulthood with Autistic Youth and Their Caregivers

Kristin Sohl, MD[a,b],*, Crystalena Oberweiser[c,1],
Elly Ranum, MD[a,2], Charles Oberweiser, CPA, PhD[d,1],
Wendy Cornell, MEd[b,e,3]

KEYWORDS

- Autism • Transition to adulthood • Pediatric guide

KEY POINTS

- Pediatricians are uniquely positioned to support autistic patients and their families during the transition from pediatric care to adult care.
- Pediatricians can use the longitudinal nature of pediatric care to monitor life and developmental milestones and provide anticipatory guidance to autistic people and their families.
- There are specific considerations at each stage of transition for clinicians to ask autistic patients and their families; carefully planning for transition from pediatric to adulthood can increase positive outcomes for autistic people.

INTRODUCTION AND BACKGROUND

For many adolescents, the transition to adulthood means changes in nearly every aspect of their lives: status in society, role with caregivers and friends, and even the environment where they spend their time.[1] With all of these changes, transition is a complex and ongoing process, beginning at birth, continuing through adolescence,

[a] Department of Pediatrics, University of Missouri School of Medicine, 400 North Keene Street, Columbia, MO 65211, USA; [b] ECHO Autism Communities, University of Missouri School of Medicine, 400 North Keene Street, Columbia, MO 65211, USA; [c] Human Differently, Nacogdoches, TX, USA; [d] Schlief School of Accountancy, Stephen F. Austin State University, 1936 North Street, Nacogdoches, TX, USA; [e] Department of Special Education, College of Education and Human Development, 611 Conley Avenue, Columbia, MO 65211, USA
[1] Present address: 828 Crooked Creek Drive, Nacogdoches, TX 75965.
[2] Present address: 3517 Briarmont Avenue, Apartment 206, Columbia, MO 65201.
[3] Present address: 804 Williams Court, Ashland, MO 65010.
* Corresponding author. 400 N. Keene Street, Columbia, MO 65211.
E-mail address: sohlk@health.missouri.edu

Pediatr Clin N Am 71 (2024) 315–326
https://doi.org/10.1016/j.pcl.2024.01.007
0031-3955/24/© 2024 Elsevier Inc. All rights reserved.

and evolving as a person enters into early adulthood. For the context of this article, pediatricians should consider age 12 years as the recommended time point for beginning transition planning with their patients. This process can be complex for any individual, making it important to consider the unique challenges individuals with autism face that require specialized considerations.

Arnett's research on transition shows that although the hallmarks of adulthood can be variable depending on culture or socioeconomic status, several aspects continually arise when parents, adolescents, and researchers are asked to define adulthood. Those aspects are relationships, life skills, financial literacy, higher education/vocational training, and health care literacy.[1]

The transition to adulthood can be especially challenging for autistic individuals, particularly without an intentional effort in planning. The lack of transition planning puts these individuals at risk for adverse effects that impact their ability to succeed and thrive as independent adults who can work, attend school, and participate in the community. Barriers to an autonomous life after transitioning to adulthood arise for many reasons, including impairments, forced dependence, additional skills one needs to acquire for health maintenance (considering co-occurring conditions), insufficient experience in activities, social isolation, and personal environmental factors.[2] Pediatric physicians and practitioners can leverage their unique longitudinal relationship with autistic patients by identifying potential areas in which transition to adulthood are progressing and areas that may require further intervention.

Pediatricians and pediatric clinicians are essential to helping guide the transition to adulthood process for youth on the autism spectrum and their families. Yet, clinicians feel ill-equipped to discuss many of the core topics related to transition to adulthood.[3] This practical guide (1) reviews the domains related to transition to adulthood, (2) reminds clinicians of practice standards outlined by major medical associations, and (3) offers decision support for implementing anticipatory guidance in a pediatric practice for transition to adulthood for autistic youth.

DOMAINS OF ADULTHOOD
Relationships

Social communication struggles are one of the hallmarks of autism spectrum disorder (ASD). As expected, poor social skills can make it difficult to interact and engage with others. These difficulties affect how an autistic person interacts with others in the way they express themselves, often creating the image that the individual is socially awkward or rude, as well as impacting how a person interprets social cues and understands and interprets the perspectives of others. These differences affect an individual's ability to form and maintain relationships with others. This includes both platonic friendships and, later, romantic relationships. Research suggests that individuals on the autism spectrum desire romantic relationships but may not have developed an understanding of how to initiate these relationships successfully.[4]

Asking autistic patients (and their caregivers/families) about their friendships and relationships is a good way to check in throughout the transition years. Because answering direct questions about friends can be difficult for all teens, asking patients to tell you one person they talk to at school or asking about activities/sports can be a good way to gauge if there needs to be further education around relationship building.

Life Skills

Life skills are sometimes referred to as daily living skills or independent living skills. These critical skills enable all individuals to function autonomously. The acquisition of life skills directly relates to adaptive functioning, executive functioning, and parental influence.

Adaptive functioning encompasses behaviors relevant to independent living, including social skills, communication skills, and daily living skills. Adaptive functioning is often delayed in autistic individuals. Recent research indicates that a high IQ is not protective against maladaptive behaviors.[5] Instead, research suggests that the gap for individuals with intact cognition seems to widen with age and is directly associated with poor outcomes in adulthood.[6,7] Average to above average IQ and intact language are not sufficient in predicting optimal outcomes for autistic individuals.[8]

Executive functioning challenges are directly associated with lower adaptive skills for autistic individuals with and without cognitive impairment[9,10] Specifically, individuals on the autism spectrum may have trouble with cognitive flexibility, organizational skills, problem-solving abilities, and attention, all strongly associated with adaptive functioning.[11] Executive dysfunction can hinder independence as it leads to problems managing time—a skill needed to maintain a schedule for work or school. Further, executive dysfunction can make skills like cleaning and maintaining one's space problematic.[12] Conversations that allow patients and their family to work on adaptive and executive functioning skills can help the person be more successful later in life. This can be as simple as checking in with autistic patients and their families/caregivers about morning and evening routines. Asking an autistic patient if they remember to take a shower on their own can be one way to gauge executive functioning.

Pediatricians are uniquely positioned to suggest various treatment options to target executive function deficits within school and clinic settings. For example, when executive function challenges impact academic achievement in school, parents can either request special accommodations if the child does not have an individualized education plan (IEP) or request services within an IEP through an occupational or speech therapist with goals that target executive dysfunction. In addition, pediatricians could also refer the individual to an outpatient clinic for occupational therapy. Cognitive behavioral therapy is another very effective treatment option for executive dysfunction, including problems with inhibition, emotion regulation, time management, and planning.

A sense of independence factors into a person's well-being and quality of life, making it appropriate to consider independent living and household circumstances when planning for the transition to adulthood for autistic patients. The National Autism Indicators Report: Transition into Young Adulthood reports that 68% of autistic individuals have never lived apart from their parents.[13] This statistical is not necessarily shocking as parents are often one of the largest sources of support for autistic people. Some parents may not acknowledge their child's true capabilities, as they sometimes cannot see past the disability. Typically, parents want what is best for their child and, with good intentions, may shelter their child and hinder independence. It is important for pediatricians to amplify the skills and capabilities of the autistic child while realistically assessing current and future support needs.

Being autonomous at a developmentally appropriate level allows for a sense of independence and self-confidence, complementing self-determination and supporting a successful transition to adulthood. Considering the parent perspective, preparing parents for this change is essential to help them transition to their new role as advisor. Many parents of children on the autism spectrum have spent a lifetime navigating services and advocating for their children. It can be challenging for parents to transition to a supporting role, as they have spent a considerable amount of time ensuring their child succeeds. Listening to parents' concerns and preparing them for this transition may be just as important as preparing youth on the autism spectrum for their transition to adulthood.

Financial

Social isolation may both contribute to, and be the result of, autistic individuals' lack of financial wellness. To the extent, a particular autistic individual is able to gain financial skills; socialization plays a role in both attainment of financial knowledge and in the choice of financial behaviors.[14] In interviews with autistic youth, Cheak-Zamora and colleagues find that "the majority of youth lacked confidence when it came to knowing how to manage their finances."[15] Although several authors have mentioned the lack of a national approach for financial education as a barrier to financial literacy for all youth, the situation is compounded for youth on the autism spectrum. Autistics transitioning to adulthood face both functional challenges from their autism and fewer opportunities to practice financial skills. In their literature synthesis, Anderson and colleagues note that parents are often uncertain about their role in transition.[16] Parents, particularly in western cultures, often see independence as a goal, but they may continue to perform daily living tasks, including managing finances for their child.

This is one aspect where the preparation for transition is just as much for the parent/caregiver as it is for the patient. Asking questions about chores, allowance, and savings not only checks in with the autistic person about financial skill development but also serves as a reminder to the parent/caregiver that their child is growing up and will need these important skills.

Developing financial skills is particularly critical for autistic youth who are able, as they navigate a dual challenge of additional support costs and lower expected earnings. Several studies show that young adults on the autism spectrum achieve low levels of postsecondary education and employment. The Howlin and colleagues' study of autistic adults without co-occurring ID found that 72% had no education beyond high school and 55% had never worked or were long-term unemployed.[17] Other studies found similarly low levels of employment for autistic adults.[13,18,19]

It is also essential to consider an autistic person's ability to engage in gainful employment, earn a livable wage, and independently manage their finances in thinking about discussions pertinent to financial matters with families. For example, individuals who have significant support needs due to co-occurring conditions, such as an intellectual disability, mental health conditions, or significant communication barriers, may not be able to engage in gainful and meaningful employment or manage their own finances. In cases such as this, it is important to begin discussions with families about sources of support before the individual turns 18 years. Some topics worthy of discussion include applying for Social Security and Medicaid benefits and applying for state-funded waiver programs, In addition, it may be appropriate to provide families with resources and guidance in establishing a special needs trust or an ABLE account to protect benefits that the individual may receive through Social Security and Medicaid.

For individuals with more significant support needs, this is also a good time to provide families with resources and information about guardianship, conservatorship, representative payee, and power of attorney options. Until the age of 18 years, parents are the "natural guardians" of their minor child, giving them the legal authority to make decisions about their child's health, safety, education, and support. The day a child turns 18 years, parents no longer have those rights. When an individual has significant support needs, discussions about the range of options for families should begin to better prepare families in consideration of the unique needs of the person with autism. For example, in cases where a person is not able to make legal decisions on his or her behalf, families may consider pursuing guardianship to retain the ability to make these decisions for the individual. In other cases, it may be appropriate for families to pursue less restrictive alternatives, such as a Power of Attorney, which grants shared authority to make financial and health-related decisions. In many cases, a family member or other person may be appointed to manage Social Security benefits for the individual with more significant support needs.

Education

Although there are programs such as vocational rehabilitation which work to help people with disabilities connect to postsecondary and vocational opportunities, it can still be difficult for autistic young people to finish those programs. Research indicates that approximately 26% of young adults on the autism spectrum received no services to help them become employed, continue their education, or live more independently.[13] Many individuals with autism have goals and aspirations to attend college and, in fact, do. These aspirations are not just attainable for autistic individuals with average to above average IQ but also are an option for individuals who have a co-occurring intellectual disability. Vocational Rehabilitation is one of the first agencies to direct families to learn about local programs that may be available and the services offered within those programs. Families should also be encouraged to call the college's disability center to learn about the supports and accommodations that can be provided. The College Autism Network is an excellent resource for degree-seeking autistic individuals. Think College is an excellent resource for students with intellectual disabilities seeking to go into postsecondary education opportunities.

According to Taylor and colleagues, "research demonstrates that job activities that encourage independence reduce autism symptoms and increase daily skills."[20] It is essential to encourage adolescents in the transition stage to participate in services that could help them practice job skills through volunteering in the community, becoming employed, and engaging in meaningful work experiences before high school graduation.

Although students who receive individualized education services are encouraged to attend and participate in their yearly IEP meetings, many do not. If an autistic person continues to postsecondary education or the workforce, the self-efficacy learned in through participation during their secondary education environment can pay dividends. This emphasizes the need to facilitate conversations with families and autistic patients with an intentional plan to help these patients and their parents/caregivers think ahead and prepare for this critical stage in life to capitalize on each opportunity to gradually release responsibility to the autistic individual.

An individual with more significant support needs may benefit from continued services in school up until age 22 years if it is demonstrated that the individual is not meeting IEP goals. It is important to discuss postsecondary options with families as the individual exits high school at 22 years of age. A range of options are available depending on the individual's needs, including transition to employment, day programs, and postsecondary education.

Health

A significant barrier to a transition to adulthood is moving from the pediatric care system to the separate adult care system in which a patient must cobble together a network of specialists to provide care for mental and physical health issues. The lack of holistic care is particularly challenging to autistics as autism often exists with a range of co-occurring physical and mental health conditions. For example, individuals who have a co-occurring intellectual disability, mental health condition, or significant communication needs may need a parent to assume guardianship or establish a

Table 1
Stages of transition planning by age

	Stages of Transition Planning	
Stage	Age	Suggested Discussion Topics
Preadolescence	Ages 8–11 y	• Discuss upcoming changes related to puberty (ie, height, weight, hair growth, mood/behavior changes) • Reassurance to parents/caregivers about changes they may see.
Preteen	Ages 12–13 y	• Discuss current mood/behavior and physical changes • Discuss medical diagnoses and/or medication indications to build engagement and decision-making skills • Begin short portions of the visit 1:1 with child
Early teen	Ages 14–15 y	• Discuss child's ideas for their future (ie, jobs, education, living) • Discuss steps to take toward their future (ie, skills required, money needed, limitations) • Discuss plans for a small step toward future goal (ie, learning a new chore, exploring degree requirements, job shadowing, learning more from teacher) • Briefly assess and discuss independent living skills (ie, driver's permit, money management, chores, hygiene) • Discuss relationships (ie, friends, romantic interests, family) • Review school transition (ie, IEP meeting for transition planning, graduation age)
Late teen	Ages 16–18 y	• Discuss community resources for transition support • Discuss pediatric health care transition policy (ie, age of last pediatric visit, options for adult health care clinicians) • Introduce legal considerations around adult decision-making • Discuss next steps toward future goals. • Discuss legal considerations around adult decision-making option
Early young adult	Ages 19–22 y	• Review daily living activities (ie, physical, social, vocational) • Discuss living arrangements (ie, independent, group, family, other) • First appointment with adult health care clinician

power of attorney so they can continue to communicate with medical professionals on behalf of their child.

The parents/caregivers of autistic people have often spent considerable time managing all the aspects of their child's medical care. Just as taking on the responsibility for health care needs can be scary for autistic patients, learning to step back and allow for independence can be just as scary for parents/caregivers.[13] With patients who are able to communicate on their own behalf, it is essential to include patients in conversations about medical care to encourage self-determination and self-advocacy skills, which are essential in establishing independent decision-making for individuals who are able.

Table 2
Anticipatory guidance for common transition topics

Mood/behavior changes	Mood changes become more common as a child transitions from being a child to a teenager. The body is making chemicals that help it grow more prominent and change. These chemicals can also make moods different. It is important to know that everyone experiences these mood changes. Help parents/caregivers recognize that sometimes a child does not have a lot of understanding about why they are suddenly acting differently. There may be more crying. There may be more laughing. There may be more arguing or refusing. Although some of these changes can be distressing to adults, it is common. The best thing to do is gently support the child with big emotions and be patient.
Physical body changes	Body changes for children on the autism spectrum can be upsetting. Some kids express that they do not like hair in new places. Some do not like changes happening to their body. Preparing kids for upcoming body changes or emotions can be very helpful.
Hygiene	Body odor and increased body oil are two common changes children need to learn to manage to stay healthy. Preparing children early for the role of deodorant, showers/baths, and keeping hair and skin clean are important. Helping prepare the child to take on more and more independence with these tasks is also important. Clinicians can support kids and families through these stages by offering tools and resources for these tasks, such as the Healthy Bodies Guide for Boys or Healthy Bodies Guide for Girls.
Understanding health and health care	As children move into the preteen phase of transition to adulthood, it is a good time to help them have more of a role in their health care. Clinicians and caregivers can shift their focus to the child and engage them more fully in decision-making. Help them learn the names of medications and health conditions. Clinicians can increase their interactions with the child to help them learn how to be engaged in health care decision-making. One way to do this is to introduce the transition process to adulthood by clearly talking with the child more and more at each visit. This process can initially feel funny to the child, but they generally enjoy becoming more involved in their doctors' visits.
Supporting change in parent/caregiver's role	It is critical for pediatric clinicians to recognize their role in helping a parent/caregiver move from an active manager to a consultant in the life of their developing teen. It is helpful to be clear with parents/caregivers about the changing expectations of your visits as the child grows. Helping parents/caregivers see the transition journey can be invaluable and establish essential steps for a successful transition to adulthood. For parents/caregivers, it will be important to ensure they have information about the spectrum of supported decision-making options. Just like their teens, they will also have many decisions to consider. Preparing and learning about those decisions is critical so they are not making decisions with limited information or time to feel confident about them.

(continued on next page)

Table 2 (continued)	
Supporting self-determination	It is critical to establish that a child has a voice in their body and health care voice in their body, and health care is a vital step. When the child recognizes that their doctor will ask them about their opinions and discuss treatment options with them and their parents, they learn that they have a role in the conversations around them.
Employment	Support youth and their parents/caregivers to identify various employment opportunities. Variety is important so they may experience different tasks and environments. Sometimes getting experience with something they enjoy, like cooking, cleaning, or helping with animals, are great places to start. Vocational rehabilitation programs are available in every state. Be sure to connect your patient with this vital resource or similar programs in your area. They have expertise in navigating employment and post-high school education options for people who may benefit from additional support.

The American Academy of Pediatrics (AAP) has recognized health care transition for all young adults as a critically important tenant of maintaining health during adolescence and early adulthood. In a clinical report co-authored by representatives from the AAP, the American Academy of Family Practice, and the American College of Physicians, clinical practice guidelines were developed to help health care clinicians support all adolescents as they transition from pediatric to adult health care.[21] This includes youth in family medicine and medicine-pediatric clinics who will still complete a transition to an adult model of care even if their clinician remains the same. Although these guidelines are not specific to ASD, the principles and concepts apply. The initial clinical report updated in 2018 focuses on the importance of a clinic and patient-specific model of transition.

Some of the key recommendations include the following.

1. Start early: Health care transition planning should begin at the age of 12 years. For children with any special health care needs, it is recommended that this process begin even earlier to provide additional time to discuss self-care, independent living, and guardianship concerns if necessary.
2. Involve the patient and family: Health care transition is a collaborative process involving the health care team and the patient and family. Youth should be given maximum independence throughout the transition process to ultimately help them adapt to an adult health care model.
3. Coordinate care: Essential to the transition process is coordination with adult primary providers and subspecialists. An adult provider should be identified, and an appointment made before the patient's final contact with the pediatric provider.
4. Provide education: Throughout the transition process, patients should receive in-office education on the adult care model.
5. Individualized transition process: The transition timeline and components should be tailored to meet the needs of each patient, considering their unique health conditions, developmental level, and cultural background.
6. Chronic condition management: For children with chronic medical conditions, the transition may require additional consideration. Regardless of whether guardianship is likely to be required, youth should always be involved in transition planning to the greatest extent possible. Patients should receive the same education and transition

Table 3
Suggested questions for discussion by domains of adulthood

	Relationships	Life Skills	Financial	Education	Health
8–11 y	Who is someone you talk to at school? Who do you eat lunch with? What does it mean to be a good friend?	What are the numbers you would call if there was an emergency? What do you like to eat? Do you help take care of younger siblings or a pet?	Do you know how many pennies are in a nickel or dime? If you go to the store with an adult, do you know how to tell how much something costs?	What do you like about school?	Tell me about how you sleep at night. Do you take any medicine every day?
12–14 y	Are you in any clubs at school? (Do you want to be?) Do you talk to people online?	What is one food that you can cook? How often do you shower/brush teeth/etc? Have you thought about getting your driver's permit?	Do you earn money for doing chores at home? Do you save your money for a special purchase?	What do you want to do after you finish school?	Have you been to the hospital since our last visit? If you take medicine, what do you take medicine for?
15–17 y	Do you have/want a boyfriend or girlfriend? How do you know if someone likes you? Are you sexually active? How can you stay safe? Who do you talk to if someone touches your body in a way that you don't want?	Do you know how to do laundry? Are you learning to drive?	Do you have a job or place you volunteer? Do you have a bank account or a way to manage a small amount of money?	Do you know what your IEP goals are for this semester? Do you know who to talk to if you have concerns about your learning?	Do you know the name of your doctor? Do you know the name of your pharmacy?
18–21+ y	How do you ask someone out on a date? What do you do if they say no? (If they say they are busy?)	Are you thinking about getting your own place to live? Do you want to live by yourself or with roommates?	Who can help you make decisions about big purchases like a car?	How do you spend your day? What do you like to do for fun?	Do you know how to call the doctor's office to make an appointment? Where would you call if you need a refill on a medicine?

planning as their peers; however, special attention should be paid to ensure adult providers are knowledgeable and comfortable with the management of the patient's condition and that subspecialty transition also occurs in an organized manner.[21]

The AAP recommends that all clinical settings where minors are treated have a written transition policy that is given to all providers, patients, and families. The process for creating such a system is outlined in the "Six Core Elements of Health Care Transition," which are built into the Got Transition program.[21] Got Transition is a federally funded resource center that provides information, tools, and resources to both health professionals and patients and their families to support successful health care transition. These are not clinical recommendations, but rather a framework for developing a transition policy that is appropriate for each clinic's unique needs. Got Transition recommends that all clinics develop a transition plan and discuss it with each patient when beginning the transition process.[22]

A comprehensive, individualized transition packet should be developed with collaboration from patients that includes a medical summary, outlines their health care needs and goals, and includes their transition readiness assessment. The American College of Physicians has developed several condition-specific toolkits, including one for adolescents with intellectual or developmental disabilities. These toolkits include transition and self-care readiness forms to track each patient's progress through the transition process as well as a health care summary form that can be filled out and used as their transition packet to be given to their adult provider.[21]

DISCUSSION

Transition to adulthood is a critical time for patients and their families. When considering the aspects of progressing through childhood and into adult life, pediatric clinicians play an integral role in providing essential anticipatory guidance for their patients and the patient's caregivers. Just like other essential periods of development like moving from infancy to toddler years and prepuberty to puberty, pediatricians and other pediatric clinicians play a vital role in the successful transit through to adulthood. It is critical that pediatricians learn and embrace their role in preparing teens, and especially teens on the autism spectrum, to navigate relationships, life skills, finances, education, and health decisions.

SUMMARY

Primary care pediatric clinicians have an important role in supporting youth and their caregivers through the transition to adulthood. Particularly for autistic patients, transition planning is crucial to improved patient outcomes.

Transition out of primary pediatric care can be divided into stages. Outcomes are often better for autistic people who are allowed to gradually take on responsibility for their care in the supportive environment of pediatric care. It is important for primary care physician/practitioner (PCPs) to educate themselves, their patients, and their patient's parents/caregivers about these changes long before they occur to help for a smoother entry into adolescence.

CLINICS CARE POINTS

The following are resources for clinicians to guide their practice for autistic youth and establish a smooth transition between child and adulthood.

- It may be helpful to consider the stages of transition planning by age in a broad sense to ensure that anticipatory guidance is communicated in a longitudinal, continuous, and culturally sensitive approach (**Table 1**).
- Similarly, consideration of anticipatory guidance topics by topic is another way to consider the stages of transition planning and serve as a practical guide for pediatric clinicians' consideration (**Table 2**).
- Pediatricians can help patients and their families transition to adulthood by taking a few minutes during appointments to ask questions about the domains of adulthood. Suggested questions by age and domain are included for consideration (**Table 3**).
- Asking these questions early will allow the clinician to know if there are any pressing issues that need to be addressed. If so, patient and family education can begin in earnest.

DISCLOSURE

K. Sohl is a practicing physician who serves children, youth and adults on the autism spectrum. C. Oberweiser is an autistic adult who also provides life coaching to neurodiverse youth and adults through Human Differently. W. Cornell is the parent of a young adult with autism spectrum disorder. E. Ranum and C. Oberweiser do not have relevant financial or nonfinancial disclosures as relates to this article.

REFERENCES

1. Arnett JJ. Conceptions of the transition to adulthood: Perspectives from adolescence through midlife. J Adult Dev 2001;8:133–43.
2. Zhang-Jiang S, Gorter JW. The use of the Rotterdam Transition Profile: 10 years in review. J Transit Med 2019;1(1). https://doi.org/10.1515/jtm-2018-0002.
3. Cheak-Zamora N, Farmer JG, Crossman MK, et al. Provider perspectives on the extension for community healthcare outcomes autism: Transition to adulthood program. J Dev Behav Pediatr 2021;42(2):91–100.
4. Stokes MA, Kaur A. High-functioning autism and sexuality: a parental perspective. Autism Int J Res Pract 2005;9(3):266–89.
5. Baker E, Stavropoulos KKM, Baker BL, et al. Daily living skills in adolescents with autism spectrum disorder: Implications for intervention and independence. Res Autism Spectr Disord 2021;83:101761.
6. Kanne SM, Gerber AJ, Quirmbach LM, et al. The role of adaptive behavior in autism spectrum disorders: implications for functional outcome. J Autism Dev Disord 2011;41(8):1007–18.
7. Tillmann J, San José Cáceres A, Chatham C, et al. Investigating the factors underlying adaptive functioning in autism in the EU-AIMS longitudinal european autism project. Autism Res 2019. https://doi.org/10.1002/aur.2081.
8. Alvares GA, Bebbington K, Cleary D, et al. The misnomer of "high functioning autism": Intelligence is an imprecise predictor of functional abilities at diagnosis. Autism Int J Res Pract 2020;24(1):221–32.
9. Pugliese CE, Anthony L, Strang JF, et al. Increasing adaptive behavior skill deficits from childhood to adolescence in autism spectrum disorder: role of executive function. J Autism Dev Disord 2015;45(6):1579–87.
10. Pugliese CE, Anthony LG, Strang JF, et al. Longitudinal examination of adaptive behavior in autism spectrum disorders: influence of executive function. J Autism Dev Disord 2016;46(2):467–77.

11. Lynch CJ, Breeden AL, You X, et al. Executive dysfunction in autism spectrum disorder is associated with a failure to modulate frontoparietal-insular hub architecture. Biol Psychiatry Cogn Neurosci Neuroimaging 2017;2(6):537–45.
12. Hill EL. Executive dysfunction in autism. Trends Cogn Sci 2004;8(1):26–32.
13. National Autism Indicators Report: Transition into Young Adulthood. Autism Outcomes. Published April 8, 2022. Accessed May 31, 2023. https://drexel.edu/autismoutcomes/publications-and-reports/publications/National-Autism-Indicators-Report-Transition-to-Adulthood/.
14. financialeducationyouthdisabilitiesliteraturereview.pdf. Accessed May 31, 2023. https://www.dol.gov/sites/dolgov/files/odep/research/financialeducationyouthdisabilitiesliteraturereview.pdf.
15. Cheak-Zamora NC, Teti M, Peters C, et al. Financial capabilities among youth with autism spectrum disorder. J Child Fam Stud 2017;26(5):1310–7.
16. Anderson C, Butt C, Sarsony C. Young adults on the autism spectrum and early employment-related experiences: aspirations and obstacles. J Autism Dev Disord 2021;51(1):88–105.
17. Howlin P, Moss P, Savage S, et al. Social outcomes in mid- to later adulthood among individuals diagnosed with autism and average nonverbal IQ as children. J Am Acad Child Adolesc Psychiatry 2013;52(6):572–81.e1.
18. Schmidt L, Kirchner J, Strunz S, et al. Psychosocial functioning and life satisfaction in adults with autism spectrum disorder without intellectual impairment: psychosocial functioning in autism. J Clin Psychol 2015;71(12):1259–68.
19. Farley M, Cottle KJ, Bilder D, et al. Mid-life social outcomes for a population-based sample of adults with ASD. Autism Res 2018;11(1):142–52.
20. Taylor JL, Smith LE, Mailick MR. Engagement in vocational activities promotes behavioral development for adults with autism spectrum disorders. J Autism Dev Disord 2014;44(6):1447–60.
21. White PH, Cooley WC, et al, Transitions clinical report authoring group, American academy of pediatrics, american academy of family physicians, american college of physicians. Supporting the health care transition from adolescence to adulthood in the medical home. Pediatrics 2018;142(5):e20182587.
22. GotTransition.org. Got Transition® - Six Core Elements of Health Care TransitionTM. GotTransition.org. Accessed May 31, 2023. https://www.gottransition.org/six-core-elements/.

The Autism Constellation and Neurodiversity

Long-Term and Adult Outcomes in Autism Spectrum Disorder

Inge-Marie Eigsti, PhD[a,b,c,d,*]

KEYWORDS

- Developmental trajectory • Behavioral outcomes • Neural changes in autism
- Early intervention • Self-reported priorities in autistic adults

KEY POINTS

- Research on autistic adults suggests significant heterogeneity in outcomes. A significant proportion of individuals struggle with intellectual disability and limited communication skills.
- Of the 67% who have age-appropriate cognitive skills, around half are expected to attain a college education, and 25% are likely to hold a full-time job.
- Outcomes have been improving over time, in part, because of earlier diagnosis and earlier intervention. Indeed, an estimated 10% to 20% are expected to lose all symptoms of autism by adolescence.

Autism spectrum disorder (ASD)[1] is a neurodevelopmental condition characterized by difficulties in social communication and the presence of repetitive behaviors, unusually strong and sometimes unusual interests, and sensory hypersensitivity and hyposensitivity. Epidemiologic estimates[2] suggest a global autism prevalence of 1 in 100 with precise estimates ranging from 1.09 in 10,000 to 436.0 in 10,000. The wide variation in estimates reflects community-specific differences in access to services, awareness, and sociodemographic factors; for example, one recent survey of a racially and ethnically diverse caregiver cohort ($n = 744$) reported that Latínx and multiracial caregivers were significantly more likely than African-American/Black, White, and Asian parents to report that their autistic child had support needs that were unmet.[3] Some 33% of autistic individuals have co-occurring intellectual disability

[a] Connecticut Autism and Language Lab (CALL), University of Connecticut; [b] Cognitive Neuroscience of Communication T32 Training Program; [c] Institute for the Brain and Cognitive Sciences; [d] Department of Psychological Sciences, University of Connecticut, 406 Babbidge Road, Unit 1020, Storrs, CT 06269, USA
* Department of Psychological Sciences, University of Connecticut, 406 Babbidge Road, Unit 1020, Storrs, CT 06269.
E-mail address: inge-marie.eigsti@uconn.edu

Pediatr Clin N Am 71 (2024) 327–341
https://doi.org/10.1016/j.pcl.2024.01.003
0031-3955/24/© 2024 Elsevier Inc. All rights reserved.

(ID)[2]; thus, approximately two-thirds of autistic individuals have cognitive abilities that are broadly commensurate with chronologic age.

ADULT OUTCOMES IN AUTISM

The transition into adulthood for autistic individuals is a difficult one, even in comparison to outcomes for other developmental disabilities.[4–7] The educational system provides many forms of support; after exiting school at age 18 or 21 years, autistic adults struggle significantly with underemployment or unemployment,[8] nonindependent living arrangements,[9] unmet service needs,[9] psychiatric comorbidities,[10] and a lack of meaningful social relationships and loneliness.[4] One study reported that more than 50% of autistic adolescents were not engaged in either employment or educational activities during the 2-year period following high school graduation.[4] Some American parents have described this difficult experience as "falling off the cliff,"[11] reflecting the sudden suspension of services on which they previously relied.

Most autism research focuses on childhood and adolescence; only limited research has quantified the experiences and outcomes of autistic adults. Reviewed in later discussion, this research includes studies that code and quantify *broad* outcomes that typically measure multiple outcome variables, such as occupation, friendships, independent living, and physical health, and activities, and collapse these into a global outcome score. Other research examines *trajectories of change*, typically by focusing on a small number of focal outcome variables.

BROAD OUTCOMES IN COHORTS OF ADULTS

Studies have used a global outcomes rating, including employment, living situation, and friendships developed by Howlin,[12] and were modified by Gillespie-Lynch.[13] Results of these studies suggest that most autistic adults were "very dependent"; few lived alone, had close friends or permanent employment; stereotyped behaviors and interests persisted into adulthood. More than half of individuals with ASD who had left high school in the past 2 years reported *no participation in employment or education*.[5] Social isolation was described as a particularly prevalent and painful concern, with one-half to two-thirds of adults with autism reporting no real friendships.[12,14,15] In a 2008 study, few individuals (4%) are described as having a "very good" outcome; some 17% had *good* outcomes, and the remainder had *fair* to *very poor* outcomes.[9] Social isolation, stress, depression, and anxiety were frequent concerns *even with high intelligent quotient (IQ)*; see[16] for a review. There is evidence that these difficulties tend to *increase* with age in ASD.[17,18] Some negative outcomes are mitigated by higher family income, better adaptive skills in activities of daily living, fewer behavioral issues and co-occurring psychiatric conditions, milder autism symptoms, and lack of ID.[4,5,8,10,19,20] Even so, adult outcomes of individuals diagnosed in the 1970s and 1980s (forming the bulk of the scant evidence base) are often poor.[21] Although evidence is too limited to draw firm conclusions, research hints at improvement in global outcomes over time, as shown in **Table 1**. For example, the most recent reports suggest positive outcomes in approximately half of participants.[31]

LONGITUDINAL CHANGES

Research conducted in the early 2000s examined developmental change for individuals with a childhood diagnosis of autism. Piven and colleagues described adult

Table 1
Longitudinal and adult outcomes as a function of publication year

Reference	Sample	Outcomes	Predictors of Better Outcomes
Global outcomes			
Howlin et al,[13] 2004	68 autistic adults with IQ > 50, from age 7 to 29 y	Outcomes rated as: 12% = Very Good, 10% = Good, 19% = Fair, 46% = Poor, 12% = Very Poor	Not reported
Billstedt et al,[7] 2005	120 autistic children followed to ages 17–40 y	Outcome rated as: 78% = Poor	Higher child IQ, phrase speech at age 6 y
Billstedt et al,[15] 2007	105 autistic adults with rigorous childhood diagnosis	Social impairments most consistent over time	Speech < age 5 y, higher IQ, male gender, no medical conditions, and no seizures in early childhood, predicted social, communication, and self-direction skills
Eaves & Ho,[10] 2008	48 autistic adults, age 24 y	Outcomes rated as follows: 50% = Good to Fair, 46% = Poor. Comorbid conditions, obesity and medication use were common	IQ and CARS score at the age of 11 y
Shattuck et al,[5] 2012	680 autistic youth ages 13–16	35% had attended college and 55% had paid employment; however, more than 50% had no employment or education in the 2 y after high school graduation	Higher income and higher functional ability were associated with postsecondary employment and education
Mhatre et al,[22] 2016	80 autistic children aged older than 10 y	80% = fluent verbal skills; 43% = spoken abilities with significant challenges; 25% = meaningful friendships; 46% = age-appropriate adaptive abilities	Lower symptomatology, parent participation, and higher maternal education

(continued on next page)

Table 1
(continued)

Reference	Sample	Outcomes	Predictors of Better Outcomes
Longitudinal outcomes			
Piven et al,[23] 1996	38 autistic adolescents and adults with age-appropriate IQ, from age 5 to ages 13–28 y	Improvements in social, communicative, and repetitive behaviors; 13% of these individuals no longer met criteria for ASD, though had significant impairment. Health, psychiatric and behavioral problems were common	IQ of 70 or higher
Turner et al,[24] 2006	26 autistic children from age 2 to 9 y	12% lost the diagnosis, 88% remained autistic; 67% had significant cognitive improvements (average increase: 23 IQ points)	Age of diagnosis, cognitive and language scores at 2 y, and hours of speech-language therapy at ages 2–3 y
Fountain et al,[25] 2012	6975 autistic children, from age 2 to 14 y	10% of the sample displayed a very steep trajectory, with significant delays at Time 1 but age-appropriate levels of functioning at Time 2	Parental education, ethnicity/race, and lesser severity of ASD symptoms at diagnosis, predicted faster improvements
Fein et al,[26] 2013	Compared 34 LAD, 44 autistic individuals with rigorously evaluated ASD histories, and 34 nonautistic individuals	The LAD group had no symptoms of ASD and was in the nonautistic range for social and communication skills. LAD/ nonautistic groups did not differ in social communication, language, or face recognition	Milder early social symptoms and earlier engagement in intervention predicted LAD outcome

Anderson et al,[27] 2014	85 autistic children from age 2–19 y	Of those with age-appropriate cognitive abilities, 9% no longer met criteria for ASD. 62% had verbal IQ (VIQ) scores under 70%, and 38% had VIQ scores of 71+	Early behavioral intervention, and a sharp reduction in repetitive and stereotyped behaviors between ages 2–3 y
Gillberg et al,[11] 2016	50 adult man with Asperger syndrome, IQ > 70, older than 20 y	54% of full sample had co-occurring ADHD, depression or both. 22% had no ASD symptoms at follow-up; of these, 6% had no co-occurring psychiatric conditions	Absence of co-occurring psychiatric conditions associated with better outcomes
Mukaddes, Mutluer, Ayik & Umut (2017).[28] Pediatrics International, 59, 416–421.	26 autistic children who lost the diagnosis followed for 2–8 y	92% lifetime, 81% current co-occurring psychiatric conditions (ADHD, specific phobia, obsessive–compulsive disorder)	Not reported
Torenvliet et al,[29,30] 2023	128 autistic with IQ > 70 and 112 nonautistic adults at 3 timepoints	No group differences in verbal memory, visual working memory, prospective memory, theory of mind, fluency, response speed, inhibition, planning, or switching	Not reported

Note. All ages are shown in years.

outcomes in $n = 38$ autistic individuals with high IQ, reporting that communication and social abilities were more likely to improve compared with repetitive and stereotyped behaviors.[22] Psychiatric, behavioral, and health difficulties were common; however, 13% of these individuals no longer met criteria for ASD (although still had unspecified "significant impairments"). Research by Turner, Stone, and colleagues[23,32] followed 48 children diagnosed at the age of 2 years to follow-up at ages 4 and 9 years. They found that 38% no longer met criteria at the age of 4 years and that earlier age at diagnosis was a predictor of this outcome, suggesting earlier treatment is more effective. In a different sample of 25 children followed until the age of 9 years, 88% retained the ASD diagnosis, and IQ scores were more than 70 for 72% (and in the average range or higher for 56%); this was a significant improvement from the age of 2 years. An estimated 32% of participants had conversational language skills, 56% had multiple words but were not able to engage in conversational exchanges, and 12% had very limited productive speech; none of the participants who were verbal at the age of 2 years fell into the limited speech group at the age of 9 years. A study of 80 children followed during 10 years, conducted in India,[31] indicated that 80% had fluent verbal skills, 43% had spoken abilities with significant challenges, 25% had meaningful friendships, and 46% displayed age-appropriate adaptive abilities. Fountain and colleagues followed a very large cohort of children ($n = 6975$) from ages 2 to 14 years and identified 6 distinct statistical trajectories.[24] One group, comprising 10% of the sample, displayed a very steep trajectory, with significant delays at time one and age-appropriate levels of functioning by the age of 14 years. These individuals were more likely to have been White and non-Latinx, and to have parents with more education. Altogether, results of more recent studies suggest that *most autistic children make meaningful gains in functioning*. The variability in outcomes reflects the timing of treatment onset (with better outcomes when treatment is initiated at younger ages), as well as individual differences in communication skills, milder autism symptoms, higher cognitive abilities, stronger adaptive skills, and parental involvement in intervention.[25]

One of the strongest predictors of better outcomes is engagement in early intervention (EI). Most such interventions are grounded on the principles of applied behavioral analysis; current approaches (eg, Early Intensive Behavioral Intervention, EIBI),[33] and the Early Start Denver Model (ESDM)[34] are designed to address developmentally appropriate and socially relevant treatment goals, and are oriented toward a child's own interests and choices. These approaches aim to motivate a child to participate and engage with the interventionist via play, home routines, naturalistic teaching, and structured learning environments; most are highly flexible and responsive to a child's current behavior and affect. Related Naturalistic Developmental Behavioral Interventions[35] incorporate a mixture of both therapist-led and child-initiated approaches; these include programs such as Incidental Teaching,[36] Social Communication/Emotional Regulation/Transactional Supports,[37] Enhanced Milieu Teaching,[38] Joint Attention, Symbolic Play, Engagement and Regulation[39] and Early Achievements[40]; see Waddington, van der Meer and Sigafoos (2016) for more detailed description.[41] Children in both ESDM and EIBI programs make significant gains in general cognitive ability after 1 year, with average gains in Developmental Quotient of 7.8 points (ESDM) or 14.8 points (EIBI), with no significant difference between the 2 approaches.[25] A systematic review of EIBI intervention studies compared with "care as usual" found significant gains in spoken language with a mean effect size of $g = 0.26$ and a confidence interval of 0.11 to 0.42[42]; effects were largest when parents and clinicians collaborated in the intervention. Although there more double-blind randomized treatment trials are needed, the evidence clearly demonstrates that gains are greater when individuals participate in EIBI.

The results of outcomes research describing individuals diagnosed in earlier decades may not generalize fully to individuals who are diagnosed now. We know that effective early detection tools have led to steady decreases in the current age at diagnosis. For example, the MCHAT-R[43,44] is a 23-item parent report checklist that can be completed in 5 to 10 minutes, ideally during pediatric well-child visits. When paired with a follow-up phone call for cases that fail the written screening, the MCHAT has excellent reliability ($\alpha = .85$), with a positive predictive value (sensitivity) of .80 and a negative predictive value (specificity) of .99. Effective early screening leads to earlier diagnosis and thus to earlier engagement in behavioral intervention. Indeed, epidemiologic study suggests that, currently, significantly more autistic children are being identified early (defined as before the age of 4 years) than in the past, with significant changes observed during the period of 2002 to 2016.[45] Children were *4 times more likely* to be identified by age 48 months in 2016, compared with 2002, with the largest increases observed for cases without concurrent ID. Of course, the median age of diagnosis varies widely from state to state in the United States, for example, from 36 months in California to 63 months in Minnesota,[46] due to differential access to services.[47]

MORE RECENT OUTCOMES RESEARCH

Given significant changes in the timing of diagnosis and the provision of EI and other services, updated information about long-term and adult outcomes in ASD is of high interest. A recent meta-analysis reported that 20% had "good" outcomes, with typical or near-typical social lives and satisfactory school/work functioning, 31% had a fair outcome, and 48% had a poor outcome.[48] Outcomes were defined as follows: "very good" indicated a high level of independence; "good" indicated that some degree of support in daily living was required; "fair" indicated some degree of independence, where support and supervision was needed but not placement outside the home; "poor" indicated that residential placement and a high level of support was needed; and "very poor" indicated a need for high-level institutional care. These findings represent an improvement compared with older studies. An extended longitudinal study followed autistic individuals aged from 2 to 13 years to 29 to 64 years.[49] Measures of language and cognitive abilities suggested stability or some improvement in 75% but ongoing difficulty in language for 23%. Regarding aging in autism, a recent study found no evidence for heightened risk of cognitive decline or dementia in autistic adults without ID.[50] Several groups have been following individuals who were diagnosed with ASD before the age of 5 years, using gold-standard measures, into adulthood, with strongly positive outcomes. Anderson and colleagues[51] saw 85 autistic children diagnosed with ASD at the age of 2 years when those children were aged 19 years. Of these, 62% had verbal IQ (VIQ) scores less than 70%, and 38% had VIQ scores of 71 or higher, and 9% no longer met criteria for ASD. These latter individuals were more likely to have had early behavioral intervention, and to have shown a reduction in repetitive and stereotyped behaviors between 2 and 3 years.

LOSS OF THE AUTISM DIAGNOSIS

Although autism is generally assumed to be lifelong, there is evidence that 3% to 25% of children who meet clear diagnostic criteria for ASD will enter the typical range of cognitive, adaptive, and social skills by adolescence, displaying *no* symptoms of autism.[29] Mukaddes and colleagues[27] described a sample of 39 children who met clear diagnostic criteria at the age of 2 years but who no longer met criteria, according to expert clinical judgment, at the age of 6 years. Gillberg and colleagues reported that individuals who moved *off* the spectrum were largely free of other psychiatric disorders[10] although there were increased rates of psychiatric comorbidity. One study has followed individuals who were rigorously diagnosed early in the development, who had no detectable symptoms of ASD by the time of adolescence[52]; a series of articles describing these individuals has examined multiple domains of functioning and reported that individuals who had lost the ASD diagnosis (loss of the autism diagnosis [LAD]) were generally indistinguishable from their nonautistic peers. Studied domains include social skills,[26] personality and traits of the "Broader Autism Phenotype,"[53] academic skills,[54] standardized assessments of language,[55] and experimental assessments of subtle pragmatic language skills.[56–58] Executive Global Executive Composite scores as reported by parents using the BRIEF[59] were in the clinical range for significantly more autistic participants (50%) compared with LAD (4%) and nonautistic (0%) peers.[60] On direct assessment using the D-KEFS,[61] all executive functioning scores for LAD individuals were in the average range (although they had lower scores than nonautistic peers on measures of impulsivity, set-shifting, problem-solving, working memory, and planning). Although present in childhood, restricted and repetitive behaviors in LAD individuals had resolved at the time of study.[62] Our recent study indicates that LAD individuals maintain their non-ASD status in adulthood,[63] according to brief impressions during the first few minutes of an interaction, and according to gold-standard expert clinician diagnoses. LAD young adults display heterogenous language outcomes (see also[64]); although most have structural (morphosyntactic) abilities that are in the average range or higher, they display significantly more language impairments than nonautistic peers.[65]

A study of psychiatric profiles indicated equivalent *lifetime* prevalence of psychiatric diagnoses in LAD and autistic groups[66]; although concurrent diagnoses persisted in the autism group, they waned in the LAD group, leaving the latter with elevated rates only of attention-deficit/hyperactivity disorder (ADHD; inattentive or combined types) and specific phobias. Consistent with findings of meaningful syndromic overlap between ADHD and autism at both behavioral and genetic levels,[67] there is evidence that autism can "evolve" into ADHD, with age-appropriate social and communication skills alongside impairments and delays in executive function and adaptive skills.[68] Recent study by our group finds that, as young adults, LAD individuals have elevated rates of depression and anxiety relative to their neurotypical peers,[69] suggesting a relatively greater vulnerability to other psychiatric conditions in those with a history of autism; ongoing study is examining the role of treatment but the predictors of this vulnerability are unknown to date. A careful ascertainment of internalizing disorders is warranted, given their higher prevalence in autistic young adults; estimates suggest that 23% to 37% of autistic young adults experience depression.[70]

NEURAL FUNCTIONING IN LOSS OF THE AUTISM DIAGNOSIS

Although behaviorally indistinguishable from typically developing peers, functional neuroimaging results suggest that "normalized" behavior in LAD individuals reflects the action of compensatory neural systems.[71] Results of a functional MRI study performed during a sentence comprehension task indicated similar activations in frontal and temporal regions (left middle frontal, left supramarginal, and right superior temporal gyri) and posterior cingulate in LAD and autistic participants, where both differed from neurotypical peers. In addition, the LAD group had heightened activation in left precentral/postcentral gyri, right precentral gyrus, left inferior parietal lobule, right supramarginal gyrus, left superior temporal/parahippocampal gyrus, left middle occipital gyrus, and cerebellum. These results suggested that in the context of highly typical language abilities, brain functioning differed.

PREDICTORS OF POSITIVE LONG-TERM OUTCOMES

Acquiring useful language by age 5 years is often listed as a predictor of positive outcomes in ASD; for example, in a study of 119 children, producing first words (other than "mama" or "dada") by the age of 24 months was a particularly strong predictor of better outcomes early in life.[64] Important predictors of clinically or functionally meaningful adolescent and adult outcomes, such as higher IQ scores and age-appropriate and unimpaired social and language abilities, include age-appropriate or higher cognitive abilities; relatively stronger verbal and motor imitation skills; better pretend play; milder earlier symptoms; and stronger motor skills; see Helt and colleagues for a review.[29] Note that earlier age of diagnosis, earlier engagement in intervention, and quicker response to intervention, are each associated with more age-appropriate outcomes and greater reductions in deficits and impairments. The presence of seizures, intellectual disabilities, and genetic syndromes are predictors of greater developmental delays and more ASD symptomatology in the long term. Interestingly, gender is not an important predictor of long-term outcomes.

NEURODIVERSITY PERSPECTIVE

What does a change in diagnostic status mean for an individual's functioning and well-being[a]? Advocates of the neurodiversity perspective have argued that autistic individuals need support and acceptance, rather than treatment and change, and that autism should be treated as a continuum of abilities rather than a categorical condition (as it is under the medical model). This argument is compelling given the enormous heterogeneity in abilities and long-term outcomes that characterizes autism as a clinical condition. Social impairments can range from an apparent disinterest in others (including family members) to a desire to socialize but with poor social judgment. Language abilities can range from a complete lack of spoken language with very limited comprehension, to language that is fluent and structurally within the normal range but with poor pragmatic abilities. Cognitive functioning can encompass severe disability to the superior range. Repetitive behaviors and stereotyped interests encompass both debilitating self-injurious behaviors and idiosyncratic but functional strong interests.

Although the neurodiversity approach to autism as a continuum of abilities rather than a clinical diagnosis is appealing for these and other reasons, we argue that the categorical medical model presents important practical advantages.[64] Relevant constructs are the notions of impairment and distress, which are central to diagnostic and statistical manual of mental disorders (DSM) definitions of disorders; thus, in a DSM diagnosis of an anxiety disorder but not in "everyday anxiety" individuals struggle to function and feel pervasive, disabling distress due to their symptoms. Following this logic, if LAD individuals display no symptoms, experience no functional impairments, and experience little or no distress, they no longer fall into the diagnostic category of autism. Autistic self-advocates and others have argued that calling the loss of an ASD diagnosis a "positive outcome" implies that meeting criteria for the diagnosis is *ipso facto* a negative outcome.[72] We agree that society needs to accommodate both the

---

[a] Note that studies of LAD individuals focus on an individual's clinical strengths and challenge; the goal is to understand individual profiles of strengths and weaknesses, not to reduce access to services.

strengths and weaknesses of autism and other neurodiverse conditions; the primary goal of diagnosis and intervention should *not* be the loss of the ASD diagnosis but rather maximizing an individual's autonomy, relationships, and daily living skills (including the ability to participate in employment or activities outside the home), in a manner that is consistent with an individual's preferences and interests.[73] We believe that the LAD outcome reflects one such positive outcome. We also note that services that support autistic individuals are sometimes helpful to all. For example, a qualitative interview study of autistic adults and their experiences in the health-care system[74] reported concerns about logistical barriers to accessing services (eg, insurance, fees, and transportation); concerns about the clinical environment (eg, wait times, sensory qualities, and anxiety-provoking procedures); and concerns about health-care provider knowledge about autism, communication and rapport, individualized care, and approaching the relationship as a partner. Improving clinical care in these dimensions would better serve not only autistic individuals but also everyone.

SUMMARY

Because of the enormous heterogeneity in long-term and adult outcomes, it would be clinically irresponsible to promise a particular prognosis to a child diagnosed with autism early in development. That said, the results reviewed here indicate that because of success in earlier screening and diagnosis, and provision of early behavioral interventions, autistic children can currently anticipate more positive outcomes than their counterparts in past decades, including the possibility of losing the diagnosis altogether. Clinicians can encourage parents to engage children in treatment and intervention, with the realistic expectation that many children will achieve significant independence later in life; as our group's study indicates, a significant minority will function at the level of their nonautistic peers in adulthood, and can realistically hope to engage in meaningful social relationships, daily activities, and to be healthy and happy. Individuals who receive earlier behavioral interventions are likely as adults to display age-appropriate skills, fewer social communication challenges, and fewer repetitive behaviors or interests that present difficulties to those individuals. One important caveat is the likelihood of anxiety and depression symptoms in young adulthood for autistic individuals. Clinicians can recommend with confidence that individuals and families consider early behavioral interventions as a critical component of developmentally appropriate care.[75,76,77]

CLINICS CARE POINTS

- Producing first words (other than "mama" or "dada") by the age of 24 months is a strong predictor of better *childhood* outcomes in autism.

- The best predictors of *adult* outcomes are early diagnosis, early engagement in intervention, milder early symptoms, and quicker response to intervention. Other important predictors of positive adult outcomes are higher IQ scores, using verbal communication in childhood, motor skills, motor imitation skills, pretend play, and milder earlier symptoms. The effect size of EI on later outcomes is of large magnitude, although more randomized controlled trials are needed.

- Parents and caregivers seek guidance on maximizing communication abilities, social relationships with peers, adaptive skills, managing challenging behaviors and, in the long term, a child's prospects for employment, education, independence, and having a family. In

- addition, families prioritize access to EI and other critical supports; the financial means to cover these supports is a significant stressor for many families.
- Adult outcomes are improving over time, due to earlier diagnosis and engagement in intervention. Reflecting input from community stakeholders, clinical priorities of adults include improving access to informed and individualized health care, management of highly prevalent co-occurring psychiatric conditions including depression, anxiety, and ADHD, and promoting broader social acceptance of autistic behaviors.

DISCLOSURE

The author has no commercial or financial conflicts of interest to disclose. This research was funded by NIMH, United States-1R01MH112687-01A1 to I.M. Eigsti and D.A. Fein (MPIs).

REFERENCES

1. American Psychiatric Association. Diagnostic and statistical manual of mental disorders. 5th edition. Washington, DC: American Psychiatric Association; 2013.
2. Zeidan J, Fombonne E, Scorah J, et al. Global prevalence of autism: A systematic review update. Autism Res 2022;15(5):778–90.
3. Rivera-Figueroa K, Milan S, Quinn D, Dumont-Mathieu T, Eigsti IM. Oral Presentation. Racial and ethnic group differences in service utilization in children with autism spectrum disorder: The role of parental stigma. presented at: International Society for Autism Research (INSAR); 2023, May 3-6; Stockholm, Sweden.
4. Shattuck PT, Narendorf SC, Cooper B, et al. Postsecondary education and employment among youth with an autism spectrum disorder. Pediatrics 2012; 129(6):1042–9.
5. Shattuck PT, Roux AM, Hudson LE, et al. Services for adults with an autism spectrum disorder. Can J Psychiatr 2012;57(5):284–91.
6. Billstedt E, Gillberg IC, Gillberg C. Autism after adolescence: population-based 13- to 22-year follow-up study of 120 individuals with autism diagnosed in childhood. J Autism Dev Disord 2005;35(3):351 60.
7. Henninger NA, Taylor JL. Outcomes in adults with autism spectrum disorders: a historical perspective. Autism 2013;17(1):103–16.
8. Schall CM, Wehman P, Brooke V, et al. Employment interventions for individuals with ASD: The relative efficacy of supported employment with or without prior Project SEARCH Training. J Autism Dev Disord 2015;45(12):3990–4001.
9. Eaves LC, Ho HH. Young adult outcome of autism spectrum disorders. J Autism Dev Disord 2008;38(4):739–47.
10. Gillberg IC, Helles A, Billstedt E, et al. Boys with Asperger syndrome grow up: Psychiatric and neurodevelopmental disorders 20 years after initial diagnosis. J Autism Dev Disord 2016;46(1):74–82.
11. Children with autism 'fall off the cliff' after graduation. Available at: abcnews.go.com/Health/kids-autism-fall-off-cliff-turn-21/story?id=19068035.
12. Howlin P, Goode S, Hutton J, et al. Adult outcome for children with autism. J Child Psychol Psychiatry 2004;45(2):212–29.
13. Gillespie-Lynch K, Sepeta L, Wang Y, et al. Early childhood predictors of the social competence of adults with autism. J Autism Dev Disord 2012;42(2):161–74.
14. Billstedt E, Gillberg IC, Gillberg C. Autism in adults: symptom patterns and early childhood predictors. Use of the DISCO in a community sample followed from childhood. J Child Psychol Psychiatry 2007;48(11):1102–10.

15. Orsmond GI, Krauss MW, Seltzer MM. Peer relationships and social and recreational activities among adolescents and adults with autism. J Autism Dev Disord 2004;34(3):245–56.

16. Howlin P. Outcome in adult life for more able individuals with autism or Asperger syndrome. Autism 2000;4:63–83.

17. Anderson DK, Maye MP, Lord C. Changes in maladaptive behaviors from mid-childhood to young adulthood in autism spectrum disorder. Research Support, N.I.H., Extramural. Am J Intellect Dev Disabil 2011;116(5):381–97.

18. Howlin P, Moss P, Savage S, et al. Social outcomes in mid- to later adulthood among individuals diagnosed with autism and average nonverbal IQ as children. J Am Acad Child Adolesc Psychiatry 2013;52(6):572–581 e1.

19. Holwerda A, van der Klink JJ, Groothoff JW, et al. Predictors for work participation in individuals with an Autism spectrum disorder: a systematic review. J Occup Rehabil 2012;22(3):333–52.

20. Wei X, Christiano ER, Yu JW, et al. Reading and math achievement profiles and longitudinal growth trajectories of children with an autism spectrum disorder. Autism 2015;19(2):200–10.

21. Howlin P, Moss P. Adults with autism spectrum disorders. Can J Psychiatry 2012; 57(5):275–83.

22. Mhatre D, Bapat D, Udani V. Long-Term Outcomes in Children Diagnosed with Autism Spectrum Disorders in India. J Autism Dev Disord 2016;46(3):760–72.

23. Piven J, Harper J, Palmer P, et al. Course of behavioral change in autism: a retrospective study of high-IQ adolescents and adults. Journal of the American Academy of Child and Adolescent Psychiatry 1996;35(4):523–9.

24. Turner LM, Stone WL, Pozdol SL, et al. Follow-up of children with autism spectrum disorders from age 2 to age 9. Autism 2006;10(3):243–65.

25. Fountain C, Winter AS, Bearman PS. Six developmental trajectories characterize children with autism. Pediatrics 2012;129(5):e1112–20.

26. Fein D, Barton M, Eigsti IM, et al. Optimal outcome in individuals with a history of autism. JCPP (J Child Psychol Psychiatry) 2013;54(2):195–205.

27. Anderson DK, Liang JW, Lord C. Predicting young adult outcome among more and less cognitively able individuals with autism spectrum disorders. Research Support, N.I.H., Extramural. JCPP (J Child Psychol Psychiatry) 2014;55(5): 485–94.

28. Mukaddes NM, Mutluer T, Ayik B, et al. What happens to children who move off the autism spectrum? Clinical follow-up study. Pediatr Int 2017;59(4):416–21.

29. Torenvliet C, Groenman AP, Radhoe TA, et al. One size does not fit all: An individualized approach to understand heterogeneous cognitive performance in autistic adults. Autism Res 2023;16(4):734–44.

30. Turner LM, Stone WL. Variability in outcome for children with an ASD diagnosis at age 2. J Child Psychol Psychiatry 2007;48(8):793–802.

31. Bent C, Glencross S, Mckinnon K, et al. Predictors of Developmental and Adaptive Behaviour Outcomes in Response to Early Intensive Behavioural Intervention and the Early Start Denver Model. J Autism Dev Disord 2023. https://doi.org/10.1007/s10803-023-05993-w.

32. Leaf R, McEachin JA. Work in Progress: behavior Management Strategies and a Curriculum for Intensive behavioral Treatment ofAutism. New York: DRL; 1999.

33. Rogers SJ, Dawson G. Early Start Denver Model for Young children with autism. New York: Guilford; 2009.

34. Schreibman L, Dawson G, Stahmer AC, et al. Naturalistic Developmental Behavioral Interventions: Empirically Validated Treatments for Autism Spectrum Disorder. J Autism Dev Disord 2015;45(8):2411–28.

35. Hart B, Risley TR. Incidental teaching of language in the preschool. J Appl Behav Anal 1975;8(4):411.

36. Prizant B, Wetherby A, Rubin E, et al. The SCERTS Model: a comprehensive educational approach for children with autism spectrum disorders. Baltimore, MD: Paul Brookes; 2006.

37. Yoder PJ, Warren SF. Intentional communication elicitslanguage-facilitating maternal responses in dyads with children whohave developmental disabilities. Am J Ment Retard 2001;106(4):327–35.

38. Kasari C, Freeman S, Paparella T. Joint attention and symbolic play in young children with autism: a randomized controlled intervention study. J Child Psychol Psychiatry 2006;47(6):611–20.

39. Landa RJ, Holman KC, O'Neill AH, et al. Intervention targeting development of socially synchronous engagement in toddlers with autism spectrum disorder: a randomized controlled trial. J Child Psychol Psychiatry 2011;52(1):13–21.

40. Waddington H, van der Meer L, Sigafoos J. Effectiveness of the Early Start Denver Model: A systematic review. Review Journal of Autism and Developmental Disorders 2016;3:93–106.

41. Hampton LH, Kaiser AP. Intervention effects on spoken-language outcomes for children with autism: a systematic review and meta-analysis. J Intellect Disabil Res 2016;60(5):444–63.

42. Dumont-Mathieu T, Fein D. Screening for autism in young children: The Modified Checklist for Autism in Toddlers (M-CHAT) and other measures. Ment Retard Dev Disabil Res Rev 2005;11(3):253–62.

43. Robins DL, Casagrande K, Barton M, et al. Validation of the modified checklist for Autism in toddlers, revised with follow-up (M-CHAT-R/F). Pediatrics 2014;133(1):37–45.

44. Shaw KA, Mcarthur D, Hughes MM, et al. Progress and Disparities in Early Identification of Autism Spectrum Disorder: Autism and Developmental Disabilities Monitoring Network, 2002-2016. Journal of the American Academy of Child & Adolescent Psychiatry 2022;61(7):905–14.

45. Sohl K, Levinstein L, James A, et al. ECHO (Extension for Community Healthcare Outcomes) Autism STAT: A Diagnostic Accuracy Study of Community-Based Primary Care Diagnosis of Autism Spectrum Disorder. J Dev Behav Pediatr 2023; 44(3):e177–84.

46. Pham HH, Sandberg N, Trinkl J, et al. Racial and Ethnic Differences in Rates and Age of Diagnosis of Autism Spectrum Disorder. JAMA Netw Open 2022;5(10): e2239604.

47. Steinhausen H-C, Mohr Jensen C, Lauritsen MB. A systematic review and meta-analysis of the long-term overall outcome of autism spectrum disorders in adolescence and adulthood. Acta Psychiatr Scand 2016;133(6):445–52.

48. Howlin P, Magiati I. Autism spectrum disorder: outcomes in adulthood. Curr Opin Psychiatr 2017;30(2):69–76.

49. Torenvliet C, Groenman AP, Radhoe TA, et al. A longitudinal study on cognitive aging in autism. Psychiatry Res 2023;321:115063.

50. Helt M, Kelley E, Kinsbourne M, et al. Can children with autism recover? If so, how? Neuropsychology Reviews 2008;18(4):339–66.

51. Mukaddes NM, Tutkunkardas MD, Sari O, et al. Characteristics of children who lost the diagnosis of autism: a sample from istanbul, Turkey. Journal Article. Autism Research and Treatment 2014;2014:472120.

52. Orinstein AJ, Suh J, Porter K, et al. Social function and communication in optimal outcome children and adolescents with an autism history on structured test measures. J Autism Dev Disord 2015;45(8):2443–63.

53. Suh J, Orinstein AJ, Barton M, et al. Ratings of broader autism phenotype and personality traits in optimal outcomes from autism spectrum disorder. J Autism Dev Disord 2016;46(11):3505–18.

54. Troyb E, Orinstein AJ, Tyson K, et al. Academic abilities in children and adolescents with a history of autism spectrum disorders who have achieved optimal outcomes. Autism 2014;18(3):233–43.

55. Tyson K, Kelley E, Fein D, et al. Language and verbal memory in individuals with a history of autism spectrum disorders who have achieved optimal outcomes. J Autism Dev Disord 2014;44(3):648–63.

56. Canfield AR, Eigsti IM, de Marchena A, et al. Story goodness in adolescents with autism spectrum disorders and in optimal outcomes from ASD. Journal of Speech, Language and Hearing Research 2016;59:533–45.

57. Fitch A, Fein DA, Eigsti IM. Detail and gestalt focus in individuals with optimal outcomes from autism spectrum disorders. Research Support, N.I.H., Extramural. J Autism Dev Disord 2015;45(6):1887–96.

58. Irvine CA, Eigsti IM, Fein DA. Uh, Um, and autism: Filler disfluencies as pragmatic markers in adolescents with optimal outcomes from autism spectrum disorder. Journal article. J Autism Dev Disord 2016;46(3):1061–70.

59. Gioia GA, Isquith PK, Guy SC, et al. Behavior rating inventory of executive function. Child Neuropsychol 2000;6(3):235–8.

60. Troyb E, Rosenthal M, Eigsti IM, et al. Executive functioning in individuals with a history of ASDs who have achieved optimal outcomes. Child Neuropsychol 2014; 20(4):378–97.

61. Delis D, Kaplan E, Kramer J. Delis Kaplan Executive Function system. Psychological Corporation; 2001.

62. Troyb E, Knoch K, Herlihy L, et al. Restricted and Repetitive Behaviors as Predictors of Outcome in Autism Spectrum Disorders. J Autism Dev Disord 2016;46(4): 1282–96. https://doi.org/10.1007/s10803-015-2668-2.

63. Canale R, Larson C, Thomas RP, et al. Frank autism in adolescents and adults who have lost the autism diagnosis: Impressions during the first five minutes of an interaction. presented at: International Society for Autism Research (INSAR); 2023, May 3-6; Stockholm, Sweden.

64. Larson C, Rivera-Figueroa K, Thomas HR, et al. Structural language impairment in Autism Spectrum Disorder versus Loss of Autism Diagnosis: Behavioral and neural characteristics. Neuroimage: Clinical. 2022;34:103043.

65. Larson C, Mohan A, Taverna E, et al. The role of structural language in social-emotional, educational, and vocational outcomes in autism spectrum disorder and loss of autism diagnosis. presented at: Meeting on Language in Autism; 2023, March 9-11; Durham, NC.

66. Orinstein AJ, Tyson KE, Suh J, et al. Psychiatric symptoms in youth with a history of autism and optimal outcome. J Autism Dev Disord 2015;45(11):3703–14.

67. Mattheisen M, Grove J, Als TD, et al. Identification of shared and differentiating genetic architecture for autism spectrum disorder, attention-deficit hyperactivity disorder and case subgroups. Nat Genet 2022;54(10):1470–8.

68. Fein D, Dixon P, Paul J, et al. Brief report: pervasive developmental disorder can evolve into ADHD: case illustrations. Case Reports. J Autism Dev Disord 2005; 35(4):525–34.
69. Thomas HR, Crutcher J, Canale R, Fein DA, Eigsti IM. Psychiatric disorders in individuals who have lost the autism diagnosis. presented at: International Society for Autism Research (INSAR); 2024, May 15-18; Melbourne, Australia.
70. Hollocks MJ, Lerh JW, Magiati I, et al. Anxiety and depression in adults with autism spectrum disorder: a systematic review and meta-analysis. Psychol Med 2019;49(4):559–72.
71. Eigsti IM, Stevens M, Schultz R, et al. Language comprehension and brain function in individuals with optimal outcomes from autism. Neuroimage: Clinical. 2016; 10:182–91.
72. Mayo J, Chlebowski C, Fein DA, et al. Age of first words predicts cognitive ability and adaptive skills in children with ASD. J Autism Dev Disord 2013;43(2):253–64.
73. Eigsti IM, Fein DA. Insights from losing the autism diagnosis: Autism spectrum disorder as a biological entity. Front Psychiatry 2022;13:972612.
74. Pellicano E, Houting J. Annual Research Review: Shifting from 'normal science' to neurodiversity in autism science. JCPP (J Child Psychol Psychiatry) 2022;63(4): 381–96.
75. McCauley JB, Pickles A, Huerta M, et al. Defining positive outcomes in more and less cognitively able autistic adults. Autism Res 2020;13(9):1548–60.
76. Mazurek MO, Sadikova E, Cheak-Zamora N, et al. Health Care Needs, Experiences, and Perspectives of Autistic Adults. Autism Adulthood 2023;5(1):51–62.
77. Brandsen S, Dawson G, Gilberg M, et al. Making informed decisions: Understanding and navigating Applied Behavior Analysis (ABA). 2023.

Mortality and Autism

Suicide and Elopement

Suzanne Rybczynski, MD, MSHCM[a,b,c],*

KEYWORDS

- Autism • Autism spectrum disorder • Elopement • Wandering • Suicide
- Suicidal thoughts and behaviors

KEY POINTS

- Autistic individuals are at increased risk for premature mortality.
- Two preventable causes of premature mortality are due to elopement and suicide.
- Caregivers should be educated regarding the risks of elopement, prevention strategies, and make plans in the event of a missing child.
- Suicide is a leading cause of death in autistic individuals.
- Suicide risk for autistic children and youth is often not identified and therefore underdiagnosed.

INTRODUCTION

Past research demonstrated an increased risk of premature and excess mortality for autistic individuals.[1–3] One review noted that the risk of death in autism spectrum disorder (ASD) is 2 to 3 times higher than in peers matched for age and sex.[4] Deaths are commonly attributed to comorbid neurologic conditions, especially epilepsy, and accidents such as choking or drowning.[5–7] In a longitudinal study of Danish children, Schendel and colleagues reported a low absolute mortality rate for those with autism (0.3% of all deaths). However, the overall risk of mortality was 1.7 to 2.0-fold greater for those with autism compared to those without ASD. Most of those decedents (83.8%) had comorbid mental health or neurologic conditions.[8] Hirvikoski and colleagues noted a significant delineation of causes of death based on the functional level of autistic decedents. In individuals with co-occurring intellectual disability (ID) and ASD, premature mortality was most often due to neurologic illness or congenital malformations. In autistic individuals without ID, excess mortality was significantly more likely to be due to suicide.[9]

[a] East Tennessee Children's Hospital, 2018 Clinch Avenue, Knoxville, TN 37916, USA; [b] Kennedy Krieger Institute, Baltimore, MD, USA; [c] Department of Pediatrics, Johns Hopkins School of Medicine, Baltimore, MD, USA
* East Tennessee Children's Hospital, 2018 Clinch Avenue, Knoxville, TN 37916.
E-mail address: SRybczynski@etch.com

Pediatr Clin N Am 71 (2024) 343–351
https://doi.org/10.1016/j.pcl.2023.12.006
0031-3955/24/© 2023 Elsevier Inc. All rights reserved.

Prevention of premature mortality in autistic youth can be achieved through awareness of risks. While the association of epilepsy and autism is well known,[10–12] sudden unexplained death in patients with both epilepsy and autism is an area that could benefit from additional research.[13–15] Prevention of morbidity and mortality in ASD due unintentional and intentional self-harm, likewise, could be impacted by increased awareness of medical and educational professionals, patients, and their caregivers. The author will first address unintentional self-harm in ASD due to wandering and elopement behaviors (WAEB) followed by an analysis of the intentional self-harm of suicide and suicidal behaviors in ASD.

WANDERING AND ELOPEMENT BEHAVIOR

Mortality for autistic individuals from unintentional injuries is $3 \times$ that of the general population.[16] This is especially high in children younger than 15. Almost 80% of all mortality in autistic children is due to drowning, suffocation, or asphyxiation.[17] Drowning often occurs when an autistic child wanders off from the safety of caregivers. WAEB can be defined as events where a person, who requires supervision to be safe, leaves a safe area or the supervising person, and is exposed to possible harm or injury. These potential dangers include environmental hazards, such as water, traffic, terrain, and weather, or encounters with predatory strangers.[18] WAEB can be seen in typically developing children, individuals with autism and other neurodevelopmental disabilities, individuals with traumatic or acquired brain injury,[19] or those with dementia.[20]

While stressful and anxiety provoking, it is common toddler behavior to wander away from caregivers as they explore the environment and establish independence. Common reasons for toddlers to wander include escape from overwhelming situations, lack of awareness of their environment, searching for something specific, or inadvertent separation from adult supervision. After age 4 or 5, WAEB typically decrease.[21] However, the risk for significant morbidity or mortality for autistic children does not always decrease with age. In a study of children with special health care needs, elopement was inversely correlated to age but positively associated with an ASD diagnosis.[22]

The National Autism Association collected data on autistic individuals who eloped or wandered long enough to require police or media intervention over a 6-year period. Of the 808 reported missing persons with autism spectrum disorder (ASD), 17% died, 13% required medical attention, and 38% were at risk of physical harm. The most common cause of death was drowning (71%) followed by traffic injuries (18%). Children aged 5 to 9 had the highest number of deaths while fatalities occurred in almost 60% of children under age 5.[23]

While the full impact of WAEB is not yet known, caregivers of autistic children can provide added insight into risks and burdens for families. In a study of caregivers, almost half of all children with ASD attempted to elope at least once after age 4. More than a quarter of these elopements lasted long enough to raise concern. The most common locations to elope from included home (74%), stores (40%), and schools. The peak age for elopement was 5.4 years.[24]

Another study described the most common triggers for WAEB. It is notable that not all triggering circumstances are adverse. Most common negative motivators included attempt to escape from a stressful or anxiety-provoking situation (43%) and escape from uncomfortable sensory stimuli (34%). Caregivers also reported that WAEB also occurred while their child was enjoying running or exploring the environment (41%) or pursuing a special interest (27%).[25]

Research has demonstrated that more severely impacted autistic children were more likely to have WAEB. Children who were unable to communicate their name or address, have a language disorder, or had intellectual disability along with ASD were significantly more likely to elope. Other co-morbid conditions which increased the risk of WAEB included aggressive, self-injurious, or disruptive behaviors. Of note, the only co-morbid psychiatric diagnosis that significantly increased risk for elopement was Attention-Deficit Hyperactivity Disorder. Mood and anxiety disorders did not independently increase risk of WAEB.[26] Additionally, research has shown that sociodemographic factors of families do not significantly impact the risk of elopement.[22,24,25]

PREVENTION OF WANDERING AND ELOPEMENT BEHAVIORS

The prevention of tragic outcomes from WAEB requires collaboration between caregivers, medical team members, schools, and law enforcement. One study, tellingly, noted that only a third of parents received any counseling about WAEB from a professional contact, including pediatricians, developmental pediatricians, neurologists, psychologists, or teachers. The most common source of information was via autism advocacy groups.[27] An excellent resource for prevention is the National Autism Association's "Big Red Safety Box" which provides families with proactive strategies to prevent injury from WAEB. A safety "toolbox" provides concrete measures for prevention along with plans for what to do in the event a child does wander.[17] One study of prevention strategies indicated that the most implemented prevention measures included locks on the top of doors, followed by applied behavioral analysis therapy to target triggering circumstances, and a home alarm system.[28]

Engagement with schools can troubleshoot situations that are likely to trigger WAEB. Parents should request an adjustment to an individual education plan to address WAEB and set up a plan if a child leaves a classroom or school grounds.[25] It is important that each child undergo a functional-based assessment which can idenify relationships and situations that increase or alleviate the risk for WAEB.[27–29] Lastly, while the use of electronic tracking devices can prove useful in decreasing parental stress regarding WAEB, they are not a sole solution for prevention of events. Children may not tolerate wearing the devices. Also, cost and lack of awareness of the technology can be barriers to implementation.[30]

SUICIDE AND AUTISM

According to the World Health Organization, in 2019, the global rate of suicide was 9 deaths per 100,000 people.[31] Rates of suicide in the United States have increased 30% from 2000 to 2020. The peak rate was noted in 2018 at 14.2 deaths per 100,000. A decline was noted for the subsequent 2 years (2019–2020) but rates returned near peak level in 2021 at 14.0 per 100,000 people.[32] Additionally, the American Foundation for Suicide Prevention reports that there were an estimated 1.2 million suicide attempts in 2020 in the United States.[33]

Autistic individuals are not immune from suicidal ideation and attempts. A Danish nationwide retrospective cohort study spanning from 1995 to 2016 followed all individuals 10 years of age or older diagnosed with ASD and those without ASD. The rate of suicide attempts in individuals with ASD was 266.8 per 100,000 person years compared to 63.4 per 100,000 person years in those without ASD. Autistic women were more than 4 times as likely to attempt suicide when compared to autistic men. A total of 72.5% of individuals with ASD who attempted suicide had a psychiatric co-morbidity, most commonly attention-deficit/hyperactivity disorder followed by anxiety disorders. Autistic people in this cohort were 3.75 times as likely to die by suicide compared to the general population. This is a work in progress. More than 90% of decedents with ASD had a psychiatric co-morbidity, most commonly affective or anxiety disorders.[34] A study from Finland analyzed risk for premature mortality in ASD in general and due to self-harm, including suicide. Autistic individuals without intellectual disability (ID) were more at risk for death from suicide compared to those with ID. Of note, this study did not stratify level of ID associated with ASD diagnosis. Researchers did find an increased risk for death for ASD overall but did not find an increased risk for death from suicide in autistic individuals without psychiatric comorbidities.[35] A study of suicide deaths in the state of Utah (USA) from 1998 to 2017 noted a significant increase in suicide rates in the ASD population compared to the general population. This study revealed increased risk for death in autistic women.[36]

Much of the research on suicide in the autistic population is based on adult data. A recent study of deaths by suicide in England noted that 10.7% of all decedents were autistic or had elevated autistic traits. This was 11 × higher than the prevalence of autism in the United Kingdom (1.1%). Interviews with family members of the deceased revealed possible autism in 41% of those who died, indicating risk for suicide in adults with undiagnosed ASD.[37] In a study of autistic adults, Cassidy and colleagues noted that 72% had risk for suicide compared to the general population of adults (33%).[38] In another study by Cassidy of adults diagnosed with Asperger's Syndrome (high functioning ASD), 66% of participants reported suicidal ideation and 35% reported suicide plans or attempts. A total of 31% of this group reported depression as well.[39]

Current research has noted the challenge in estimating the true prevalence of suicidal thoughts and behaviors in autistic youth. This is due to factors including lack of clarity on the impact of non-suicidal self-injury and the exclusion of youth with both ASD and ID.[40] For example, Storch and colleagues found that suicidal thoughts and behaviors were present in approximately 11% of subjects based on patient and parent reporting.[41] Mayes and colleagues found that almost 32% of autistic children aged 12 to 18 sampled in a psychiatric outpatient clinic had suicide ideation and 10.5% had actual suicide attempts.[42] Horowitz and colleagues reported that 22% of verbally fluent youth with ASD who were hospitalized for psychiatric care frequently talked about suicide or death.[43] Rybczynski and colleagues found that patients presenting to a specialty center for autism and related disorders demonstrated a positive screening 12% rate for suicide risk in a universal screening setting.[44] Finally, a meta-analysis of suicidality in autistic youth by O'Halloran demonstrated an overall pooled prevalence of suicidal ideation of more than 25%, prevalence of suicide attempts of 8.3%, and fatality rate of 0.2%.[45]

FACTORS IMPACTING SUICIDE RISK

Most of the information regarding risk factors for suicide can be learned from studies of autistic adults. Small studies have described characteristics of autistic adults that seem to increase risk. For example, Richards and colleagues studied a small sample of adults for suicide attempts and autistic traits using the Autism Spectrum Quotient (AQ). They found high levels of autistic traits in participants who had attempted suicide, including those who did not self-report an ASD diagnosis.[46] Hooijer and Sizoo studied a small group of autistic adults and did not identify any temperament or character traits that predisposed subjects to suicidal ideation or attempts. They did find that depression was a significant issue in those who did have suicidality.[47] Given the increased risk of suicide in autistic individuals with psychiatric co-morbidities and autistic girls and women,[35] it is important to understand additional factors which impact this patient population.

In a study by Crane and colleagues of autistic youth aged 16 to 25 years, several themes emerged from interviews which help describe the special circumstances faced by this group. As autistic youth experience the world, they are often challenged to negotiate whether their struggles are due to ASD or mental health conditions.[48] This translates into further difficulty as their health care providers may not diagnose psychiatric co-morbidities due to focus on ASD. This is called diagnostic overshadowing. However, it is more likely that ASD is not recognized in patients with psychiatric disorders. It is important to recognize that autistic individuals, especially girls and women, are often forced to behave in a more neurotypical manner to fit in to society. This is known as camouflaging. An example of camouflaging is making eye contact despite its resultant internal emotional distress for the autistic individual. Camouflaging behavior can be exhausting and increases risk for mental health conditions along with risk for suicidality.[49] Crane also reported that these youth faced stigmatization along with a lack of access to appropriate mental health care. Autistic youth desperately desired mental health care providers who understood both their mental health needs along with ASD.[48] This was also noted in a study of clinicians treating autistic adolescents and adults. Clinicians were less likely to screen autistic individuals for suicide compared to neurotypical clients and less likely to use evidence-based safety planning intervention for autistic individuals.[50] McDonnell et al found that increasing age of the child, lower parental educational achievement, restrictive and repetitive behaviors, increased verbal IQ, co-morbid affective and conduct disorders, and being overweight increased the risk for suicide-related behaviors.[51]

PREVENTION OF SUICIDE IN AUTISTIC CHILDREN AND YOUTH

The first step to prevention of suicide in autistic youth and children is awareness and recognition of elevated risk for suicidal thoughts and behaviors in this group. Strengthened with this knowledge, clinicians can begin to understand and explore risks for their individual patients. Patients should be assessed holistically with consideration of risk for diagnostic overshadowing along with camouflaging. Risk factors described previously should be noted and explored, especially psychiatric co-morbidities.

Universal suicide risk screening can provide initial insight into the mindset of a patient at the start of an encounter. Screening has demonstrated to be efficiently and effectively implemented in neurodevelopmental disorders clinics, including clinics focused on autism.[44] If screening indicates increased risk, further safety assessment should be performed, including a safety planning intervention when indicated. As is true for adults, there are no suicide risk screenings, suicide safety assessments, or safety planning interventions validated for autistic children and adolescents.[52] While updating current tools for the ASD population are currently under study, clinicians should use the currently available tools, such as the Columbia Suicide Severity Rating Scale[53] or the Ask Suicide-Screening Questions Youth ASQ Toolkit,[54] to help determine disposition for those at risk. The American Academy of Pediatrics provides an excellent resource on how to implement suicide prevention in the Blueprint for Youth Suicide Prevention. One important guidance for pediatricians in the blueprint is to establish and reinforce connections to mental health resources prior to implementing any screening program. This will help expedite entry points to care for autistic youth in crisis.[55]

A child's pediatrician is often their most trusted partner in health care. Pediatricians should take advantage of school-aged well child visits to discuss mental health before any concerns may be raised. Recent studies have indicated that children think about suicide at a much earlier age than previously recognized.[56] Having established mental health–focused dialogues with parents will allow open conversations in times of crisis. This intentional and proactive approach can help destigmatize mental illness. Parents should be counseled to take signs of mental illness, especially suicidal thoughts and behaviors, seriously. In all children, not just those with ASD, signs of emotional distress can be confusing and subtle. Caregivers should take explicit statements of suicidal ideation seriously and seek help immediately for their child. An excellent online resource for parents is from the American Academy of Pediatrics and focuses on actions parents can do to prevent suicide. Perhaps the most important lifesaving tip for parents is to remove potentially lethal means of suicide from the home, especially firearms.[57] Additionally, parents should be made aware of the 988 Suicide & Crisis Lifeline. This service is available across the nation and is accessible by phone call or by text.[58]

SUMMARY

Both WAEB and suicidal thoughts and behaviors can lead to tragic consequences for autistic children and their caregivers. However, pediatricians can take an active role in prevention of these potentially devastating events through increased awareness of the problem and recognizing the specific risks faced by each individual autistic child and adolescent. Providing anticipatory guidance regarding risks to caregivers is essential.

CLINICS CARE POINTS

- WAEB are common in autistic children. Parents should be counseled about risk, identify triggers for the behavior, and strategize prevention in the home, school, and community.
- Parents should proactively establish a plan to find a missing child involving family, friends and neighbors, community groups, and law enforcement.
- Autistic individuals are at increased risk of excess and premature mortality with suicide a significant cause in all ages.
- Increased risk for suicide is seen in autistic girls and women along with those with psychiatric co-morbidities.
- Suicidal thoughts and behaviors in autistic youth are often under identified.
- Pediatricians should be aware of the impact of camouflaging on the mental health of autistic individuals and its potential to increase suicide risk.

REFERENCES

1. Catalá-López F, Hutton B, Page MJ, et al. Mortality in persons with autism spectrum disorder or attention-deficit/hyperactivity disorder: a systematic review and meta-analysis. JAMA Pediatr 2022;176(4):e216401.
2. Bilder D, Botts EL, Smith KR, et al. Excess mortality and causes of death in autism spectrum disorders: a follow up of the 1980s Utah/UCLA autism epidemiologic study. J Autism Dev Disord 2013;43(5):1196–204.
3. Gillberg C, Billstedt E, Sundh V, et al. Mortality in autism: a prospective longitudinal community-based study. J Autism Dev Disord 2010;40(3):352–7.
4. Woolfenden S, Sarkozy V, Ridley G, et al. A systematic review of two outcomes in autism spectrum disorder - epilepsy and mortality. Dev Med Child Neurol 2012; 54(4):306–12. Erratum in: Dev Med Child Neurol. 2012 Jul;54(7):672. PMID: 22348343.

5. Mouridsen SE, Brønnum-Hansen H, Rich B, et al. Mortality and causes of death in autism spectrum disorders: an update. Autism 2008;12(4):403–14.

6. Shavelle RM, Strauss DJ, Pickett J. Causes of death in autism. J Autism Dev Disord 2001;31:569–76.

7. Pickett JA, Paculdo DR, Shavelle RM, et al. Letter to the Editor. 1998-2022 Update on "Causes of death in autism". J Autism Dev Disord 2006;36:287–8.

8. Schendel DE, Overgaard M, Christensen J, et al. Association of psychiatric and neurologic comorbidity with mortality among persons with autism spectrum disorder in a danish population. JAMA Pediatr 2016;170(3):243–50.

9. Hirvikoski T, Mittendorfer-Rutz E, Boman M, et al. Premature mortality in autism spectrum disorder. Br J Psychiatry 2016;208(3):232–8.

10. Lukmanji S, Manji SA, Kadhim S, et al. The co-occurrence of epilepsy and autism: a systematic review. Epilepsy Behav 2019;98(Pt A):238–48.

11. Levisohn PM. The autism-epilepsy connection. Epilepsia 2007;48(Suppl 9):33–5.

12. Berg AT, Plioplys S. Epilepsy and autism: is there a special relationship? Epilepsy Behav 2012;23(3):193–8.

13. Kløvgaard M, Lynge TH, Tsiropoulos I, et al. Epilepsy-related mortality in children and young adults in denmark: a nationwide cohort study. Neurology 2022;98(3): e213–24.

14. Devinsky O, Spruill T, Thurman D, et al. Recognizing and preventing epilepsy-related mortality: a call for action. Neurology 2016;86(8):779–86.

15. Tomson T, Walczak T, Sillanpaa M, et al. Sudden unexpected death in epilepsy: a review of incidence and risk factors. Epilepsia 2005;46(Suppl 11):54–61.

16. Guan J, Li G. Injury mortality in individuals with autism. Am J Publ Health 2017; 107(5):791–3.

17. National Autism Association. About Autism and Wandering. Available at: https://nationalautismassociation.org/resources/wandering/. Accessed March 18, 2023.

18. Belanger HG, King-Kallimanis B, Nelson AL, et al. Characterizing wandering behaviors in persons with traumatic brain injury residing in veterans health administration nursing homes. Arch Phys Med Rehabil 2008;89(2):244–50.

19. Alzheimer's Association. Wandering. Available at: https://www.alz.org/help-support/caregiving/stages-behaviors/wandering.Accessed March 18, 2023.

20. Frost A. What to Do if Your Toddler Keeps Running Away. June 27, 2022. What to Expect website. Available at: https://www.whattoexpect.com/toddler/behavior/wandering-off.aspx Accessed March 18, 2023.

21. Barnard-Brak L, Richman DM, Moreno R. Predictors of elopement exhibited by school-aged children with special health care needs: towards the development of a screening instrument for elopement. J Prim Prev 2016;37:543–54.

22. McIlwain L. and Fournier W., Mortality & risk in ASD wandering/elopement 2011–2016, 2018, National Autism Association. Available at: https://nationalautismassociation.org/wp-content/uploads/2017/04/NAAMortalityRiskASDElopement.pdf. Accessed March 18, 2023.

23. Anderson C, Law JK, Daniels A, et al. Occurrence and family impact of elopement in children with autism spectrum disorders. Pediatrics 2012;130(5):870–7.

24. Andersen AM, Law JK, Marvin AR, et al. Elopement patterns and caregiver strategies. J Autism Dev Disord 2020;50(6):2053–63.

25. McLaughlin L, Keim SA, Adesman A. Wandering by children with autism spectrum disorder: key clinical factors and the role of schools and pediatricians. J Dev Behav Pediatr 2018;39(7):538–46.

26. Pereira-Smith S, Boan A, Carpenter LA, et al. Preventing elopement in children with autism spectrum disorder. Autism Res 2019;12(7):1139–46.

27. Phillips LA, Briggs AM, Fisher WW, et al. Assessing and treating elopement in a school setting. Teach Except Child 2018;50(6):333–42.
28. Scheithauer M, Call NA, Lomas Mevers J, et al. A feasibility randomized clinical trial of a structured function-based intervention for elopement in children with autism spectrum disorder. J Autism Dev Disord 2021;51(8):2866–75.
29. Boyle MA, Keenan G, Forck KL, et al. Treatment of elopement without blocking with a child with autism. Behav Modif 2019;43(1):132–45.
30. McLaughlin L, Rapoport E, Keim SA, et al. Wandering by children with autism spectrum disorders: impact of electronic tracking devices on elopement behavior and quality of life. J Dev Behav Pediatr 2020;41:513–21.
31. World Health Organization. Suicide worldwide in 2019. Available at: https://www. who.int/publications/i/item/9789240026643. Accessed October 15,2023.
32. Curtin SC, Garnett MF, Ahmad FB. Provisional numbers and rates of suicide by month and demographic characteristics: United States, 2021. Vital Statistics Rapid Release; no 24. September 2022. DOI: https://dx.doi. org/10.15620/cdc:120830.
33. American Foundation for Suicide Prevention. Suicide Statistics website. Available at: https://afsp.org/suicide-statistics/. Accessed March 18, 2023.
34. Kõlves K, Fitzgerald C, Nordentoft M, et al. Assessment of suicidal behaviors among individuals with autism spectrum disorder in Denmark. JAMA Netw Open 2021;4(1):e2033565.
35. Jokiranta-Olkoniemi E, Gyllenberg D, Sucksdorff D, et al. Risk for premature mortality and intentional self-harm in autism spectrum disorders. J Autism Dev Disord 2021;51(9):3098–108.
36. Kirby AV, Bakian AV, Zhang Y, et al. A 20-year study of suicide death in a state-wide autism population. Autism Res 2019;12(4):658–66.
37. Cassidy S, Au-Yeung S, Robertson A, et al. Autism and autistic traits in those who died by suicide in England [published online ahead of print, 2022 Feb 15]. Br J Psychiatry 2022;1–9. https://doi.org/10.1192/bjp.2022.21.
38. Cassidy S, Bradley L, Shaw R, et al. Risk markers for suicidality in autistic adults. Mol Autism 2018;9:42.
39. Cassidy S, Bradley P, Robinson J, et al. Suicidal ideation and suicide plans or attempts in adults with Asperger's syndrome attending a specialist diagnostic clinic: a clinical cohort study. Lancet Psychiatr 2014;1(2):142–7.
40. Oliphant RYK, Smith EM, Grahame V. What is the prevalence of self-harming and suicidal behaviour in under 18s with asd, with or without an intellectual disability? J Autism Dev Disord 2020;50(10):3510–24.
41. Storch EA, Sulkowski ML, Nadeau J, et al. The phenomenology and clinical correlates of suicidal thoughts and behaviors in youth with autism spectrum disorders. J Autism Dev Disord 2013;43:2450–9.
42. Dickerson Mayes S, Calhoun SL, Baweja R, et al. Suicide ideation and attempts in children with psychiatric disorders and typical development. Crisis 2015;36(1):55–60.
43. Horowitz LM, Thurm A, Farmer C, et al. Talking about death or suicide: prevalence and clinical correlates in youth with autism spectrum disorder in the psychiatric inpatient setting. J Autism Dev Disord 2018;48(11):3702–10.
44. Rybczynski S, Ryan TC, Wilcox HC, et al. Suicide risk screening in pediatric outpatient neurodevelopmental disabilities clinics. J Dev Behav Pediatr 2022;43(4):181–7.
45. O'Halloran L, Coey P, Wilson C. Suicidality in autistic youth: a systematic review and meta-analysis. Clin Psychol Rev 2022;93:102144.

46. Richards G, Kenny R, Griffiths S, et al. Autistic traits in adults who have attempted suicide. Mol Autism 2019;10:26.
47. Hooijer AAT, Sizoo BB. Temperament and character as risk factor for suicide ideation and attempts in adults with autism spectrum disorders. Autism Res 2020; 13(1):104–11.
48. Crane L, Adams F, Harper G, et al. 'Something needs to change': Mental health experiences of young autistic adults in England. Autism 2019;23(2):477–93.
49. South M, Costa AP, McMorris C. Death by suicide among people with autism: beyond zebrafish [published correction appears in jama netw open. 2021 feb 1;4(2):e210724. JAMA Netw Open 2021;4(1):e2034018.
50. Jager-Hyman S, Maddox BB, Crabbe SR, et al. Mental health clinicians' screening and intervention practices to reduce suicide risk in autistic adolescents and adults. J Autism Dev Disord 2020;50(10):3450–61.
51. McDonnell CG, DeLucia EA, Hayden EP, et al. An exploratory analysis of predictors of youth suicide-related behaviors in autism spectrum disorder: implications for prevention science. J Autism Dev Disord 2020;50(10):3531–44.
52. Howe SJ, Hewitt K, Baraskewich J, et al. Suicidality among children and youth with and without autism spectrum disorder: a systematic review of existing risk assessment tools. J Autism Dev Disord 2020;50(10):3462–76.
53. The Columbia Lighthouse Project. The Columbia Protocol for Healthcare and Other Community Settings website. Available at: https://cssrs.columbia.edu/the-columbia-scale-c-ssrs/healthcare/. Accessed October 15, 2023.
54. National Institute of Mental Health. Youth ASQ Toolkit website. Available at: https://www.nimh.nih.gov/research/research-conducted-at-nimh/asq-toolkit-materials/youth-asq-toolkit. Accessed October 15, 2023.
55. American Academy of Pediatrics. Suicide: Blueprint for Youth Suicide Prevention website. Available at: https://www.aap.org/en/patient-care/blueprint-for-youth-suicide-prevention/. Accessed October 15, 2023.
56. Lanzillo EC, Horowitz LM, Wharff EA, et al. The importance of screening preteens for suicide risk in the emergency department. Hosp Pediatr 2019;9(4):305–7.
57. "12 Things Parents Can Do to Help Prevent Suicide." American Academy of Pediatrics. Health children.org website. Available at: https://www.hcalthychildren.org/English/health-issues/conditions/emotional-problems/Pages/ten-things-parents-can-do-to-prevent-suicide.aspx. Accessed October 15, 2023.
58. 988 Suicide and Crisis Lifeline. 988 Lifeline Chat and Text website. Available at: https://988lifeline.org/chat/. Accessed October 15, 2023.

Moving?

Make sure your subscription moves with you!

To notify us of your new address, find your **Clinics Account Number** (located on your mailing label above your name), and contact customer service at:

Email: journalscustomerservice-usa@elsevier.com

800-654-2452 (subscribers in the U.S. & Canada)
314-447-8871 (subscribers outside of the U.S. & Canada)

Fax number: 314-447-8029

Elsevier Health Sciences Division
Subscription Customer Service
3251 Riverport Lane
Maryland Heights, MO 63043

*To ensure uninterrupted delivery of your subscription, please notify us at least 4 weeks in advance of move.